WORKBOOK TO ACCOMPANY DELMAR'S

CLINICAL MEDICAL ASSISTING

Fourth Edition

Gerry A. Brasin, AS, CMA (AAMA), CPC
Corporate Education Coordinator
Premier Education Group
Springfield, MA

Barbara M. Dahl, CMA (AAMA), CPC
Program Director
Whatcom Community College
Bellingham, WA

Comprehensive Examination by:
Tricia Berry, MATL, OTR/L
Assistant Dean of Clinical Placement
School of Health Sciences
Kaplan University
Johnston, IA

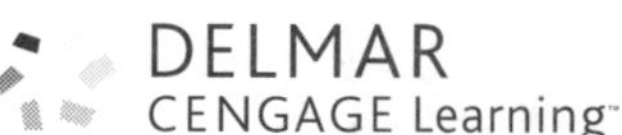

DELMAR CENGAGE Learning

Australia • Brazil • Japan • Mexico • Singapore • Spain • United Kingdom • United States

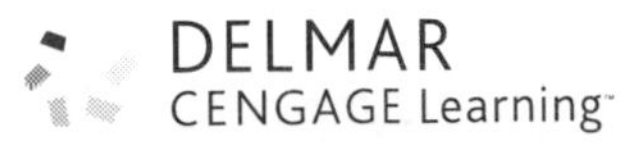

DELMAR
CENGAGE Learning™

Workbook to Accompany Delmar's Clinical Medical Assisting, Fourth Edition
Gerry A. Brasin, Barbara M. Dahl, and Tricia Berry

Vice President, Career and Professional Editorial: Dave Garza

Director of Learning Solutions: Matthew Kane

Senior Acquisitions Editor: Rhonda Dearborn

Managing Editor: Marah Bellegarde

Senior Product Manager: Sarah Prime

Editorial Assistant: Chiara Astriab

Vice President, Career and Professional Marketing: Jennifer McAvey

Executive Marketing Manager: Wendy E. Mapstone

Senior Marketing Manager: Nancy Bradshaw

Marketing Coordinator: Erica Ropitzky

Production Director: Carolyn Miller

Content Project Manager: Anne Sherman

Senior Art Director: Jack Pendleton

Production Technology Analyst: Tom Stover

Library of Congress Control Number: 2008930399

ISBN-13: 978-1-4354-1926-1

ISBN-10: 1-4354-1926-X

Delmar
5 Maxwell Drive
Clifton Park, NY 12065-2919
USA

Cengage Learning is a leading provider of customized learning solutions with office locations around the globe, including Singapore, the United Kingdom, Australia, Mexico, Brazil, and Japan. Locate your local office at: **international.cengage.com/region**

Cengage Learning products are represented in Canada by Nelson Education, Ltd.

To learn more about Delmar, visit **www.cengage.com/delmar**
Purchase any of our products at your local college store or at our preferred online store **www.ichapters.com**

For your lifelong learning solutions, visit **delmar.cengage.com**
Visit our corporate website at **www.cengage.com**

Notice to the Reader

Publisher does not warrant or guarantee any of the products described herein or perform any independent analysis in connection with any of the product information contained herein. Publisher does not assume, and expressly disclaims, any obligation to obtain and include information other than that provided to it by the manufacturer. The reader is expressly warned to consider and adopt all safety precautions that might be indicated by the activities described herein and to avoid all potential hazards. By following the instructions contained herein, the reader willingly assumes all risks in connection with such instructions. The publisher makes no representations or warranties of any kind, including but not limited to, the warranties of fitness for particular purpose or merchantability, nor are any such representations implied with respect to the material set forth herein, and the publisher takes no responsibility with respect to such material. The publisher shall not be liable for any special, consequential, or exemplary damages resulting, in whole or part, from the readers' use of, or reliance upon, this material.

Printed in the United States of America
2 3 4 5 6 7 12 11 10

CONTENTS

TO THE LEARNER

This workbook is part of a dynamic learning system that will help reinforce the essential competencies you need to enter the field of medical assisting and become a successful, multiskilled medical assistant. It has been completely revised to challenge you to apply the chapter knowledge from *Delmar's Clinical Medical Assisting*, Fourth Edition, to develop basic competencies, use critical thinking skills, and integrate your knowledge effectively.

WORKBOOK ORGANIZATION

The Chapter Assignment Sheets are divided into the following sections: Chapter Pre-Test, Vocabulary Builder, Learning Review, Certification Review, Learning Application, Chapter Post-Test, and Self-Assessment. The content of the workbook has been designed to give you a creative and interpretive forum to apply the knowledge you have learned, not simply to repeat information to answer questions. Realistic simulations appear throughout the workbook that reference the characters in the textbook. This gives the material a real-world feel that comes as close as possible to your future experiences in an ambulatory setting. Clinical principles, such as infection control or communication and patient education, are repeatedly reinforced through simulation exercises that require the ability to use your knowledge effectively and readily.

COMPETENCY ASSESSMENT CHECKLISTS

Competency Assessment Checklists are designed to set criteria or standards that should be observed while a specific procedure is being performed. The procedural steps are listed in the textbook, and the Competency Assessment Checklist scoring reflects the major milestones, or outcomes, of following the specific procedural steps. As you perform each procedure, the evaluation section of this checklist can be used to judge your performance. The instructor will use this checklist to evaluate your competency in performing this skill. Your instructor may combine some Competencies and adjust others to suit individual program schedules. These checklists are provided for guidance.

A master Competency Assessment Tracking Sheet is also provided for you prior to this section of the workbook to use as an overview of all competency assessment checklists. This tracking sheet can serve as a table of contents for all checklists, as well as a guide to easily view your performance on the assessment checklists.

The format of the Competency Assessment Checklists is designed to provide specific conditions, standards, milestone steps, and evaluation and documentation sections for essential skills necessary for an entry-level medical assistant. Forms are provided on the Student Online Companion for use with the competency assessment checklists as you complete the procedures in your textbook. To access the Student Online Companion, use the instructions on the tear-out Access Card in your book to create your account and log in.

COMPREHENSIVE EXAMINATION

Feel certain that each procedure and concept you master is an important step toward preparing your skills and knowledge for the workplace. A final comprehensive examination is presented at the conclusion of the workbook, covering all the essential topic areas that medical assisting graduates must master. This examination has 200 questions and provides excellent practice for national certification examinations.

FINAL THOUGHTS

The textbook, software CDs, workbook, and online companion have all been coordinated to meet the core objectives. Review the performance objectives at the beginning of each chapter in the textbook before you begin to study; they are a road map that will take you to your goals.

Remember that you are the learner, so you can take credit for your success. The instructor is an important guide on this journey, and the text, workbook, student software CD, and practicums are tools, but whether or not you use the tools wisely is ultimately up to you.

Evaluate yourself and your study habits. Take positive steps toward improving yourself, and avoid habits that could limit your success. Do family responsibilities and social opportunities interfere with your study? If so, sit down with your family and plan a schedule for study that they will support and to which you will adhere. Find a special place to study that is free from distraction.

Because regulations vary from state to state regarding which procedures can be performed by a medical assistant, it will be important to check specific regulations in your state. A medical assistant should never perform any procedure without being aware of legal responsibilities, correct procedure, and proper authorization.

As you pursue a wonderful career in medical assisting, make the most of your education and training.

Chapter Assignment Sheets

Name ______________________ Date ____________ Score ______

CHAPTER 1

The Medical Assisting Profession

CHAPTER PRE-TEST

Perform this test without looking at your book. If an answer is "false," rewrite the sentence to make it true.

1. Circle all that apply: Are medical assistants licensed, registered, or certified?
2. True or False? Anyone can take the AAMA medical assisting examination without going through a special program.

 ____

 ____

3. True or False? Medical assistants are allowed to work only in the clinical area of the office.

 ____

 ____

4. True or False? Medical assistants can become office managers.

 ____

 ____

5. Circle all that apply: Medical assistants work as administrative medical assistants in such positions as medical bookkeepers, medical insurance coders and billers, transcriptionists, office managers, and as clinical medical assistants in such positions as laboratory assistants, surgical assistants, phlebotomists, electrocardiography technicians, patient educators.
6. True or False? Choosing to attend an accredited medical assisting program is not as important as getting trained as quickly as possible so you can find employment.

 ____

 ____

7. True or False? Medical assistants do not have to be credentialed to work in their profession.

 ____

 ____

VOCABULARY BUILDER

Misspelled Words

Find the words below that are misspelled; underline them, and then correctly spell them in the space provided.

acredits	complience	integrate
ambulatory care setting	credential	licensure
associate's	disposition	liscensed
attributes	empathy	litigous
certify	facilitates	practicums
competancy	improvising	versatile

____________________ ____________________ ____________________

____________________ ____________________

Fill in the Blanks

From the vocabulary list below, select the term that best fits in the blank in each sentence. (Hint: not all terms will be used.)

accreditation	CMAS	practicum
ambulatory care facilities	competency	RMA
CCMA	compliance	scope of practice
certification examination	credential	versatile
certify	diploma	
CMA (AAMA)	litigious	

1. The medical assistant is a __________________________ health care professional.
2. The medical assistant performs many clinical and administrative duties in providers' offices and __________________________.
3. In today's __________________________ society, health care consumers are demanding educated, skilled health care professionals.
4. The AAMA and AMT provide national __________________________ examinations which certify the skills of medical assistants at entry level.
5. Medical assisting programs undergo __________________________ processes that prove they are covering the appropriate curriculum and are properly serving the education/learning needs of their students.
6. When you graduate from your medical assisting program, you will be given a __________________________ (sometimes called a certificate), which proves that you have taken all the courses necessary to graduate from the program.
7. Upon successfully passing the AAMA's certification examination, you will be credentialed as a ____________.
8. The American Medical Technologists offers examinations to become an __________________________ and/or __________________________.
9. The National Healthcareer Association offers an examination to become a __________________________.

Word Search

Find the words in the grid below. They may go in any direction.

B L E C O M E C E R T I F I E D Z B E C G O
M I P I H S N R E T X E E I N L I C E N S E
V T O L V E D Q Y C N E T E P M O C I C O S
N I T C I N I U E E L E A R N I N T G S Z I
B G C L E E T N Z M Z W Q M Z K T K H C P V
M I D H J R C L T R P Y V M T E K D L O R O
N O L T X X T N G E R A F Q S A R M R P O R
O U D V N K L I A G G A T E B R M D N E F P
I S W Z G N C L F I C R R H J R E O Q O E M
T P J R W M F X J I L A A G Y L R D L F S I
A R J K A M K B L P C P X T A F W D D P S L
T R L Y X R J I I Y P A M I E B P I E R I N
I D B R R X T H R R M Z T O K R T S T A O D
D T J V R A S O A Y T N P I C Q M P A C N Y
E R T Q T N T C K P E W N C O C C O V T A V
R F K E R A T T P D Z K P R W N Z S I I L Y
C Z W E L I R V E F N D G F K L M I T C I F
C Y T U C M W R X K Q P N A D N Z T L E S N
A N B U L T C T N H L K N R M R T I U D M V
I M M T T R W R N D H K V M R R Z O C J M R
A M B Y H A T T R I B U T E V Y D N Z Q K Z
G D E X T E R I T Y Y R A T E I R P O R P K

Accreditation
Ambulatory care setting
Attribute
Certification
Certified
CMA (AAMA)
Competency
Compliance
Credentialed

Cultivate
Dexterity
Diploma
Disposition
Empathy
Facilitate
Improvise
Integrate
Internship

License
Litigious
Practicum
Professionalism
Proprietary
RMA
Scope of practice

LEARNING REVIEW

True or False

Mark a true statement with a T *and a false statement with an* F. *If an answer is "false," rewrite the sentence to make it true.*

____ 1. Medical assistants are licensed by each state.

____

____

___ 2. All medical assisting programs are accredited by either CAAHEP or ABHES.

___ 3. Anyone can call himself or herself a medical assistant, but professional medical assistants have graduated from an accredited program and obtained a credential to prove their competency.

___ 4. If you graduate from a medical assisting program and get a diploma or certificate, then you are automatically credentialed.

___ 5. Medical assistants continue their education by attending seminars, workshops, and professional meetings.

___ 6. Individuals with RMAs and CMA (AAMA)s are required to obtain continuing education units (CEUs) to recertify.

___ 7. Medical assistants must be either CMA (AAMA)s or RMAs to join the AAMA or the AMT.

___ 8. The AAMA "owns" the CMA (AAMA) credential, and individuals may not call themselves CMA (AAMA)s unless they have passed the national AAMA certification examination.

___ 9. Possessing empathy is not considered important in the health care profession.

___ 10. It is extremely important that medical assistants demonstrate a positive attitude toward the patient.

___ 11. Emotionalism can sometimes cloud the medical assistant's judgment.

___ 12. When dealing with a patient, in certain circumstances it is acceptable for the medical assistant to demonstrate an unpleasant disposition.

___ 13. Certification is mandatory for medical assistants to become employed.

___ 14. The CMA (AAMA) exam is a computer-based examination offered on a continuous basis throughout the year.

___ 15. Two agencies that accredit medical assisting programs are ABHES and CAAHEP.

___ 16. Becoming certified or registered depends solely on the accrediting body of the institution where the student is enrolled in the program.

___ 17. All CMA (AAMA)s who are currently employed must have current status as CMA (AAMA)s to use the credential.

___ 18. The AAMA does not encourage continuing education for medical assistants.

___ 19. The NHA offers several allied health certifications, including CCMA, CMT, and MLA.

___ 20. The federal government and most states require a medical assistant to be registered or certified to practice the profession.

___ 21. Neither the CMA (AAMA) or the RMA is higher than the other.

___ 22. Another profession the AMT certifies is that of certified medical administrative specialist.

Matching

A medical assisting curriculum should provide a variety of clinical, administrative, and general skills courses. Write a C next to each clinical course, an A next to each administrative course, and a G next to each general course.

______ 1. Medical Records

______ 2. Medical Law and Ethics

______ 3. Urine and Blood Testing in the Laboratory

______ 4. Insurance, Billing, and Coding

______ 5. Pharmacology

______ 6. Medical Terminology

______ 7. Word Processing

______ 8. Anatomy and Physiology

______ 9. Appointments and Scheduling

______ 10. Electronic Medical Records

______ 11. Patient Education

______ 12. Infection Control

______ 13. Temperature, Pulse, Respirations, and Blood Pressure

______ 14. Drawing Blood Samples

Web Search

Search the Web and find the site for both the AAMA, the AMT, and the NHA. List the Web site, address, and phone number for each.

American Association of Medical Assistants

____

____

American Medical Technologists

____

____

National Healthcareer Association

____

____

The Nines

The following word bank consists of the nine attributes of a medical assistant. Choose the word that best describes the listed attribute and fill in the blank.

Ability to communicate	Desire to learn	Flexibility
Attitude	Empathy	Initiative
Dependability	Ethical behavior	Professional appearance

_______________ 1. Considering the patient's welfare and being kind

_______________ 2. Helping your patients feel more at ease by portraying a warm and friendly disposition and possessing a sense of humor

_______________ 3. Being punctual; limiting absences from work

_______________ 4. Being willing and able to work independently, being observant of work to be done, and taking the action to complete the tasks

_______________ 5. Being adaptable and developing alternative action plans

_______________ 6. Acquiring information and updating knowledge and skills

_______________ 7. Having an appearance that reflects good health habits

Write a sentence for each attribute describing how each contributes to better patient care and the development of good relationships with both coworkers and employers.

1. Ability to communicate

____

____

2. Empathy

____

____

3. Flexibility

____

____

4. Dependability

____

____

5. Attitude

____

____

6. Desire to learn

____

____

7. Ethical behavior

____

____

8. Initiative

9. Physical attributes

Short Answer

1. Name four reasons why the medical assisting profession has grown to require more formal, skilled education and credentialing for medical assistants.

2. The U.S. Department of Labor, Bureau of Statistics, lists medical assisting as the fastest-growing allied health profession. Name eight settings where medical assistants are usually employed.

3. What is the purpose of the CARE bill?

4. State the significance of being credentialed.

5. State the benefits of graduating from a program accredited by either CAAHEP or ABHES.

6. Define the profession of medical assisting.

7. List at least four benefits of the practicum experience.

8. What are some of the benefits that medical offices receive as a result of being a practicum site?

9. Define the acronym CAAHEP and state its purpose.

10. Membership in the AAMA is at three levels. Name them.

11. List at least six components that constitute the professional appearance of a health care provider.

12. List the three terms used to define the transition period between the classroom and actual employment.

13. Circle all that apply. The Occupational Analysis for the CMA (AAMA) and the AMT's Medical Assisting Task List are lists of competencies compiled by practicing medical assistants. These competencies can be used by medical assisting program directors to develop curricula that ensure:

    a. certification

    b. employment preparedness

    c. continuing education

    d. high-quality medical assisting education

CERTIFICATION REVIEW

These questions are designed to mimic the certification examination. Select the best response.

1. Medical assistants may take the AAMA examination to obtain which credential?

   a. CMAS

   b. RMA

   c. CMA (AAMA)

   d. CPC

   e. AMT

2. Select the following statement(s) that best describes the professional medical assistant.

   a. Has good written and oral communication skills

   b. Looks and acts professional at all times

   c. Is aware of the scope of practice and stays within the legal boundaries

   d. Assists the provider in all areas of the ambulatory care setting

   e. All of the above

3. Good medical assistants portray their professional attitude by:

   a. discussing their personal lives at work because it is therapeutic for them

   b. talking with their coworkers to help them with their problems

   c. reminding their providers that they work only 7.5 hours per day

   d. helping patients in a friendly and empathetic manner

   e. doing a basic workload

4. To become involved with their professional organization, medical assistants could:

   a. attend local chapter or state meetings

   b. attend a national conference or state convention

   c. join their national organization

   d. offer to serve on a local, state, or national committee

   e. do all of the above

5. A system of values that each individual has that determines perceptions of right and wrong is called:

   a. laws

   b. ethics

   c. attributes

   d. attitudes

6. Stepping into a patient's place, discovering what the patient is experiencing, then recognizing and identifying with those feelings is:

   a. sympathy

   b. association

   c. flexibility

   d. empathy

7. Which of the following contribute to a professional appearance?

   a. Good nutrition and exercise

   b. Healthy looking skin, teeth, and nails

   c. Daily showering and use of deoderant

   d. All of these answers

8. Courses in a professional medical assisting program include a complement of general knowledge classes such as anatomy and physiology and:

   a. assisting with minor surgery

   b. CPR

   c. medical terminology

   d. computer applications

9. The type of regulation for health care providers that is legislated by each state and is mandatory in order to practice is:

   a. licensure

   b. registration

   c. certification

   d. a and c

LEARNING APPLICATION

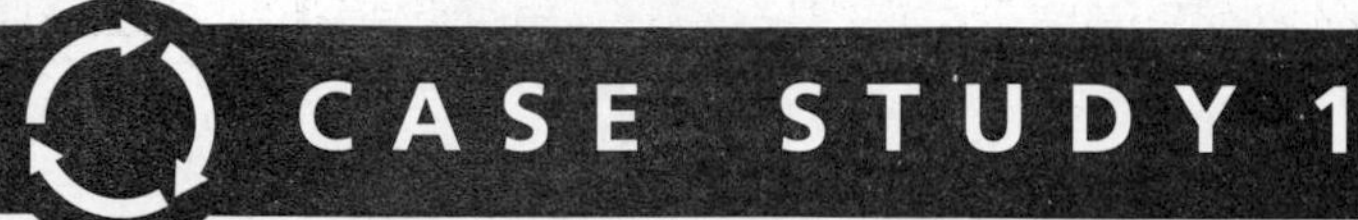

CASE STUDY 1

During your course of studies to become a medical assistant, you have an opportunity to volunteer to help out at a multiprovider urgent care center downtown in a large city to gain some firsthand experience in a professional setting.

CASE STUDY REVIEW QUESTIONS

1. Would this opportunity be interesting to you? Would you want to volunteer in this professional setting?

____

____

____

____

2. Even though you are a volunteer, why is it important to look and behave like a professional?

____

____

____

____

____

____

____

CASE STUDY 2

Michelle Lucas is preparing for her practicum. Michelle is an excellent student, detail oriented, responsible, and professional in her dress and attitude. Michelle is eager to experience her practicum with a large general practice or clinic with open hours built into the schedule for emergency patients, such as Inner City Health Care. Michelle is intrigued by the idea of working with a group of providers and a diverse patient population where she can really work on improving her screening skills. Michelle, however, is shy and quiet; she has difficulty meeting new people and relies on a core group of friends.

CASE STUDY REVIEW QUESTIONS

1. Is Michelle really suited to practicum at Inner City Health Care? What are the potential advantages or disadvantages of this practicum placement?

____

____

____

____

____

____

____

2. What would be some ways in which Michelle could overcome the difficulty she experiences when meeting new people?

____

____

3. Being able to work with diverse populations is just a small part of being a health care professional. What suggestions would you offer Michelle in reaching her goal of professional growth?

____

____

4. Consider your own short- and long-range goals. How important is it to challenge yourself, personally and professionally, with experiences that contribute to your growth and knowledge? How can you use your practicum placement to work toward fulfilling your goals?

____

____

CHAPTER POST-TEST

Perform this test without looking at your book. If an answer is "false," rewrite the sentence to make it true.

1. True or False? Medical assistants may be either licensed, registered, or certified.

2. True or False? The AAMA medical assisting certification examination is available to anyone, even people who have not been formally trained.

3. True or False? Medical assistants work in only the administrative part of the office.

4. True or False? The position of office manager is a career option for a medical assistant.

5. Circle all that apply: Medical assistants work as administrative medical assistants in such positions as medical bookkeepers, medical insurance coders and billers, transcriptionists, office managers, and as clinical medical assistants in such positions as laboratory assistants, surgical assistants, phlebotomists, electrocardiography technicians, patient educators.

6. True or False? Getting trained as quickly as possible is more important than attending an accredited medical assisting program.

7. True or False? Medical assistants may work in their profession even without being credentialed.

SELF-ASSESSMENT

1. As you begin your education as a medical assistant, you may not be sure whether you want to work in the administrative and clerical area or in the clinical and laboratory areas. What are some ways for you to explore the various options?

2. For each of the attributes listed in your textbook to describe a professional, identify individuals from your family, circle of friends, work, or community who possess one or more of those traits. Explain why you chose them.

____

____

____

3. Imagine your first day in your practicum. What will you wear? How will you prepare the night before? How will you look? Would you change your hairstyle? Makeup? Jewelry?

____

____

____

____

____

____

Name ________________________ Date ____________ Score ______

CHAPTER **2**

Health Care Settings and the Health Care Team

CHAPTER PRE-TEST

Perform this test without looking at your book. If an answer is "false," rewrite the sentence to make it true.

1. True or False? Providers who work in sole proprietorships work alone and employ no other providers.

____

____

2. True or False? When two or more providers join under legal agreement, a partnership is formed.

____

____

3. True or False? Urgent care centers are like emergency rooms and do not offer routine care services.

____

____

4. True or False? Medical assistants do not generally work in urgent care centers.

____

____

5. True or False? An HMO is one example of a managed care operation that hosts a network of providers within a defined geographic area.

____

____

6. True or False? Providers are licensed to practice nationally so they can move freely from state to state.

____

____

7. True or False? Doctors of chiropractic medicine work only on the musculoskeletal system.

____

____

8. True or False? Acupuncturists treat pain in a variety of disorders in the gastrointestinal, urogenital, gynecologic, circulatory, respiratory, neuromusculoskeletal, and many other systems.

____

____

VOCABULARY BUILDER

Misspelled Words

Find the words below that are misspelled; circle them and correctly spell them in the spaces provided. Then insert the correct vocabulary terms from the list that best fit the descriptions below.

accupuncture
ambulatory care settings
concerge
frindge benefits
health maintainance organizations (HMOs)
homeopathy
independent provider association (IPA)
intagrative medicine
managed care options
prefered provider organization (PPO)
screening
urgant care

_______________ _______________ _______________
_______________ _______________ _______________
____

1. _______________ Organizations designed to provide a full range of health care services under one roof or, more recently, through a network of participating providers within a defined geographic area
2. _______________ Advantages added to the terms of employment, such as health insurance and vacation time
3. _______________ An independent organization of providers, whose members agree to treat patients for an agreed-upon fee
4. _______________ Treatment using highly diluted doses of certain substances derived from plants, animals, or minerals that are manufactured by pharmaceutical companies under strict guidelines
5. _______________ Medical setting that provides services on an outpatient basis
6. _______________ A form of oriental medicine where sterile fine needles are inserted in specified sites of the body
7. _______________ Organizations in which providers network to offer discounts to employers and other purchasers of health care
8. _______________ Alternative forms of health care increasingly perceived as complements to traditional health care

9. ____________________ A for-profit center that provides services for primary care, routine illnesses, and injury, as well as minor surgery

10. ____________________ Another avenue of health care that provides exclusive services for fees ranging from $2,000 to $6,000.

11. ____________________ Assessment of patient needs to determine the priority of medical action

12. ____________________ A standard of patient care that seeks to provide quality care while containing costs

LEARNING REVIEW

Short Answer

1. How has managed care changed medical settings as the health care profession works to offer high-quality, cost-effective care to patients? What is the medical assistant's role in contributing to the efforts of the health care team in an era of managed care?

____

____

____

____

____

____

____

2. Since medical assistants are often patients' first contact with the facility and the provider, what attributes must medical assistants possess?

____

____

____

3. Name six administrative duties of the medical assistant as a member of the health care team.

____

____

____

4. Name five clinical duties of the medical assistant as a member of the health care team.

____

____

____

____

5. In the medical field, the abbreviation Dr. is used, and the title of doctor is addressed to the person qualified by education, training, and licensure to practice medicine. List the medical degree associated with each of the following credentials, and define each specialty.

M.D. ______________________________

____

D.P.M. ______________________________

D.C. ______________________________

____

N.D. ______________________________

____

D.O. ______________________________

____

O.D. ______________________________

____

D.D.S. ______________________________

6. Using a medical dictionary or encyclopedia to help you, define the following eight medical and surgical specialists. Refer to your textbook for a complete listing of medical and surgical specialties.

Radiologist ______________________________

____

Obstetrician/gynecologist ______________________________

____

Ophthalmologist ______________________________

Pediatrician ______________________________

____

Allergist and Immunologist ______________________________

____

Dermatologist ______________________________

Cardiologist ______________________________

7. Medical assistants are only one of many allied health and other health care professionals who form the health care team. Although medical assistants may not work directly with each professional, they are likely to come into contact with many of them through telephone, written, or electronic communication. List six of those types of professionals.

____

____

____

____

____

8. In an effort to receive alternative therapies, many health care providers and patients are pursuing integrative medicine as a complement to traditional health care. Name eight alternative forms of health care that may be currently perceived to supplement traditional health care.

____

____

____

9. List at least five services that a so-called boutique or concierge medical practice offers.

____

____

____

____

10. What is the role of the physician assistant? How does a physician assistant relate to a medical assistant?

____

____

____

____

____

11. What are the licensure requirements for a physician assistant?

____

____

____

____

____

Medical Settings Activity

For each of the three forms of medical practice management, list appropriate medical settings. Describe the patient's experience with care under each form of medical practice management. Note how patient experiences may differ and why this is possible.

1. Sole Proprietorships

   Medical settings: ____

   Patient experience: ____

   ____

   ____

2. Partnerships

   Medical settings: ____

   Patient experience: ____

   ____

   ____

   ____

   ____

3. Corporations

Medical settings: ____________________

Patient experience: ____________________

____

____

CERTIFICATION REVIEW

These questions are designed to mimic the certification examination. Select the best response.

1. The form of medical practice management that states that personal property cannot be attached in litigation is a:

   a. partnership

   b. sole proprietorship

   c. corporation

   d. group practice

2. The minimum amount of time it takes to become an M.D. without specialization is:

   a. 6 years

   b. 8 years

   c. 12 years

   d. 4 years

3. In the ambulatory care setting, the medical assistant may prefer what tasks?

   a. Educating patients

   b. Administration such as coding and billing

   c. Performing various laboratory tests

   d. All of the above

4. The American Society of Clinical Pathology is the professional organization that oversees credentialing and education in what allied health area?

   a. Nurses

   b. Medical laboratory

   c. Registered dietician

   d. Physical therapy

5. The specialty that is based on the belief that the cause of disease is violation of nature's laws is called:

   a. chiropractic

   b. osteopathy

   c. podiatry

   d. naturopathy

6. A branch of the healing arts that gives special attention to the physiologic and biochemical aspects of the body's structure, including manipulation of the spine, is:

   a. acupuncture

   b. chiropractic

   c. massage

   d. oriental medicine

7. HMOs are organizations designed to:

   a. provide a full range of health care service under one roof

   b. employ providers who network to offer discounts to employers and other purchasers of health care

   c. include environments such as a medical office and a primary care center

   d. serve as an emergency room

8. In order to practice medicine, a physician must:

   a. go to college

   b. pay a fee

   c. take online courses

   d. obtain a license to practice from a state or jurisdiction of the United States

9. Another name of the organization where providers network to offer discounts to employees and other purchasers of health insurance is:

   a. IPA

   b. HMO

   c. PPO

   d. group practice

10. Another term for assessing the patient's needs is:

    a. screening

    b. prescribing

    c. taking vital signs

    d. monitoring

LEARNING APPLICATION

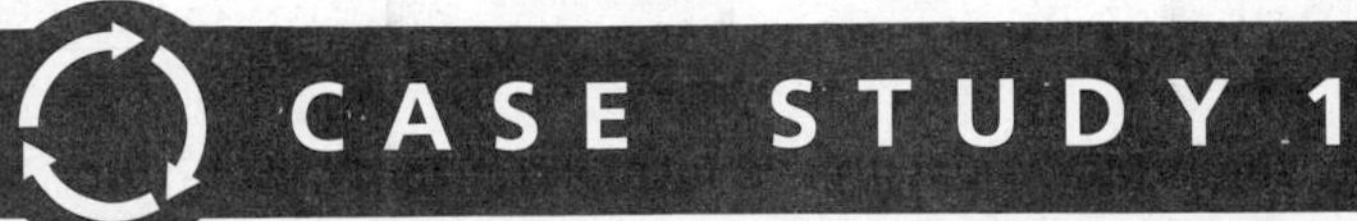

CASE STUDY 1

Abigail Johnson is an older woman in her 70s with mature-onset diabetes. She is having trouble managing her diet; she lives alone but craves social contact and seems to enjoy her visits to the family provider's office. She has an appointment today for dietary counseling.

CASE STUDY REVIEW QUESTIONS

1. How can Mrs. Johnson be encouraged to consider herself part of the health care team?

___

___

___

2. What is the role of the medical assistant?

___

___

___

CASE STUDY 2

Herb Fowler is an African American man in his early 50s. Herb is a heavy smoker, is significantly overweight, and has a chronic cough. He believes the cough is caused by bronchitis and stubbornly insists on being prescribed antibiotics. Today, Herb is at the medical office for a preventive medicine appointment.

CASE STUDY REVIEW QUESTIONS

1. How can Mr. Fowler be encouraged to consider himself part of the health care team?

___

___

___

2. What is the role of the medical assistant?

___

___

CASE STUDY 3

Juanita Hansen is a single mother in her mid-20s with one son, Henry. Juanita arrives at the urgent care clinic for the fourth time in a month. Henry has fallen down the stairs twice, suffered a burn on the hand, and is now refusing to eat. There are bruises on various parts of Henry's body, as well.

CASE STUDY REVIEW QUESTIONS

1. How can the mother be encouraged to consider herself part of the health care team?

____

____

2. What is the role of the medical assistant?

____

____

____

CASE STUDY 4

Lenore McDonell is a disabled woman in her early 30s who lives independently with the aid of a motorized wheelchair. Lenore functions well in her home environment but has grown fearful of venturing out, even to the provider's office for her routine follow-up examinations. She has canceled three appointments in a row. Today she is in for her yearly physical.

CASE STUDY REVIEW QUESTIONS

1. How can Mrs. McDonell be encouraged to consider herself part of the health care team?

____

____

____

2. What is the role of the medical assistant?

____

____

____

CHAPTER POST-TEST

Perform this test without looking at your book. If an answer is "false," rewrite the sentence to make it true.

1. True or False? Sole proprietors work alone and do not employ other providers.

2. True or False? Partnerships are made up of two or more providers who share the total business operation of the practice.

3. True or False? Urgent care centers are for emergencies only.

4. True or False? Urgent care centers require skills that medical assistants do not generally have.

5. True or False? A form of managed care is the HMO, whose providers form a network within a geographic area.

6. True or False? Providers are licensed to practice state by state.

7. True or False? Chiropractors work on only musculoskeletal conditions.

8. True or False? Acupuncture can be helpful when dealing with pain and a variety of disorders in the gastrointestinal, urogenital, gynecologic, circulatory, respiratory, neuromusculoskeletal, and many other systems.

SELF-ASSESSMENT

As you were deciding to become a medical assistant, what other career were you considering? List the three reasons you were considering that other career, and then list three reasons you chose medical assisting instead. Keep in mind not just the time, money, and education involved, but also the profession itself, the day-to-day duties, the type of work, the people involved, and so forth. Think about the similarities between the careers. Are there more similarities than differences? Are you going to be using some of the same skills? Is there a way these different careers will come together at any point in the future?

___

___

___

___

___

Name ______________________ Date ____________ Score ______

CHAPTER 3

History of Medicine

CHAPTER PRE-TEST

Perform this test without looking at your book. If an answer is "false," rewrite the sentence to make it true.

1. True or False? The practice of medicine began when we started keeping medical records.

____

____

2. True or False? Plants used to be the basis of all medications but are not anymore.

____

____

3. True or False? Cultural differences do not and should not influence the way we treat our patients.

____

____

4. True or False? Magic was practiced because it was considered an essential ingredient in chasing evil spirits away.

____

____

5. True or False? Ancient Eastern treatments included curing the spirit and nourishing the body.

____

____

6. True or False? Acupuncture uses the placement of needles in thousands of points on the body.

____

____

7. True or False? Women were not accepted as medical doctors in Western culture until the 1800s.

____

____

8. True or False? The "father of preventive medicine" was Louis Pasteur.

____

____

9. True or False? Edward Jenner developed the smallpox vaccine in the late 1700s.

____

____

10. True or False? The Oath of Hippocrates mentions mischief, sexual misconduct, and slaves.

____

____

VOCABULARY BUILDER

Misspelled Words

Find the words below that are misspelled; circle them, and correctly spell them in the spaces provided. Then insert the correct vocabulary terms from the list that best fit the descriptions below.

acepsis	malaria	septacemia
acupuncture	opiods	typhis
alopathic	pharmacopoies	yellow fever
bubonic plague	pluralistic	
____________	____________	____________
____________	____________	____________

1. In our ______________________ society, we rely on several philosophies of medicine that serve an individual's needs by respecting ethnic, cultural, and religious traditions while providing the best standard of care to patients and their families.

2. The piercing of the skin by long needles into any of 365 points along 12 meridians that traverse the body and transmit an active life force called qi is the practice of ______________________, an ancient Chinese technique thought by many today to be effective in the treatment of chronic pain.

3. That bacteria can enter the bloodstream to cause infection, ______________________, was observed in the nineteenth century by Hungarian physician and obstetrician Ignaz Philipp Semmelweiss.

4. Since the twentieth century, the discovery of antibiotics, the development of vaccines, and the institution of proper health and sanitation measures have largely contributed to the containment of many infectious diseases, including ______________________, ______________________, and ______________.

5. ______________________ physicians treat illness and disease with medical and surgical interventions intended to alleviate the condition or effect a cure.

6. A ______________________ is a book that describes drugs and their preparation and details plant, animal, and mineral substances as essential ingredients in effecting cures.

7. In the nineteenth century, ______________________, the process of sterilizing surgical environments to discourage the growth of bacteria, and anesthesia, the process of alleviating pain during surgery, revolutionized surgical practices throughout the world.

LEARNING REVIEW

Short Answer

1. Religion, magic, and science all play a vital part in the history of medicine. Describe each.

   Religion ______________________________

   ____

   Magic ______________________________

   ____

   Science ______________________________

   ____

   ____

2. Name the five methods of treatment important to the practice of medicine according to ancient Chinese tradition. How are these methods relevant for allopathic physicians today?

   ____

   ____

   ____

   ____

   ____

   ____

   ____

   ____

   ____

3. Individual cultures and people throughout history have conferred different, and often changing, status upon women in medicine. For each of the five cultures below, describe the status of women in medicine.

   (1) Primitive societies:

   ____

   ____

   ____

   (2) Chinese:

   ____

   ____

   (3) Muslim:

   ____

   ____

   (4) Italian:

   ____

   ____

(5) American:

4. Trace the progression of medical education by listing the important advances, discoveries, or medical philosophies for each period or century listed. What do you expect for the twenty-first century?

(1) Prehistoric times:

(2) Ancient times:

(3) Seventh century:

(4) Ninth century:

(5) Renaissance:

(6) Nineteenth century:

(7) Twentieth century:

(8) Twenty-first century:

5. Attitudes toward illness have changed throughout the history of medicine and also often differ among cultures. For each situation listed, give both historical and current attitudes toward the sick person. Discuss how attitudes toward illness may, or may not, have changed through history.

(1) Elderly and infirm people are encouraged to end their own lives or are outcast from society.

(2) Individuals with a frightening illness, for which there is no cure, are shunned or quarantined.

(3) Sickness is seen as a moral or spiritual failing of an individual.

(4) Survivors of illness are viewed as heroic individuals.

(5) People with disabilities are valued as individuals and receive care that allows them to function in mainstream society.

6. Name 15 infectious or epidemic diseases that have been controlled in the twentieth century through medical advances and discoveries such as antibiotics, vaccines, asepsis, and insulin.

7. The Hippocratic Oath, which originated in ancient Greece, embodies within it many ethical standards of treatment and care that providers espouse to this day. In contemporary layperson's language, name the five basic standards contained in the oath.

8. Fill in the blanks below with the three epidemics discussed in the chapter, along with descriptions of each and treatment options.

Epidemic	**Description, Causes, Treatment**

Matching I

For each of the following, write an R *if the statement describes a belief in religion, an* M *if the statement describes a belief in magic, or an* S *if the statement describes a belief in science.*

_________ 1. A recent research study involved two groups of patients with AIDS: One group received daily prayers from an anonymous prayer group hundreds of miles away, and the other received no prayers. The group receiving the prayers responded better to treatment.

_________ 2. Trephination was used by prehistoric cultures to release evil spirits responsible for illness.

_________ 3. Chinese acupuncture techniques are used to control pain or treat drug dependency.

_________ 4. Botanicals are effective in treating certain conditions. The Chinese pharmacopoeia is rich in the use of herbs.

_________ 5. Some Native Americans believe that someone recovering from a serious illness might hold extraordinary powers.

_________ 6. Some practitioners throughout history have held to the belief that healing involves not just medical treatment, but attention to the purity of the patient's soul and to the faith of the individual as well.

Matching II

Match the individuals listed below with each of their contributions to the history of medicine.

_________	1. Andreas Vesalius	A. Developed a vaccine for poliomyelitis
_________	2. Sir Alexander Fleming	B. "Father of medicine"
_________	3. W. T. G. Morton	C. Developed smallpox vaccine
_________	4. Moses	D. Discovered penicillin
_________	5. Edward Jenner	E. "Father of bacteriology"
_________	6. Clara Barton	F. Advocate of health rules in Hebrew religion
_________	7. Louis Pasteur	G. Invented the stethoscope
_________	8. Elizabeth Blackwell	H. First female physician in the United States
_________	9. Hippocrates	I. Rendered accurate anatomical drawings of body systems
_________	10. René Laënnec	J. Wrote first anatomical studies
_________	11. Robert Koch	K. Laid the groundwork for asepsis
_________	12. Florence Nightingale	L. Started the American Red Cross
_________	13. Anton van Leeuwenhoek	M. Founder of modern nursing
_________	14. Wilhelm von Roentgen	N. Introduced ether as an anesthetic
_________	15. John Hunter	O. Discovered lens magnification
_________	16. Elizabeth G. Anderson	P. Discovered X-rays
_________	17. Leonardo da Vinci	Q. Founder of scientific surgery
_________	18. Joseph Lister	R. Developed culture-plate method
_________	19. Jonas Salk	S. Discovered insulin
_________	20. Frederick G. Banting	T. First female physician

CERTIFICATION REVIEW

These questions are designed to mimic the certification examination. Select the best response.

1. Who of the following was not a scientist who contributed to the study of bacteriology?
   a. Louis Pasteur
   b. Robert Koch
   c. Joseph Lister
   d. John Hunter

2. The first female physician in the United States was:
   a. Clara Barton
   b. Elizabeth Blackwell
   c. Florence Nightingale
   d. Joan of Arc

3. The Oath of Hippocrates:
   a. establishes guidelines for all health care providers
   b. establishes guidelines for the practice of medicine
   c. is a well-known document about the ethics of ancient medicine
   d. was the first scientific journal of significance

4. The ancient culture that believed that illness was a punishment by the gods for violations of moral codes was the:
   a. Chinese
   b. Egyptian
   c. Mesopotamian
   d. Indian

5. Ancient healing priests performed many functions that involved the welfare of the entire community or village and were referred to as:
   a. shamans
   b. chi
   c. lipuria
   d. polypenia

6. Medical education in established universities began in what century?
   a. Second
   b. Fifteenth
   c. Eighteenth
   d. Ninth

7. What country today quarantines everyone who tests positive for HIV, even if they show no signs of the disease?
   a. Africa
   b. Cuba
   c. Korea
   d. Canada
8. In 1922, insulin was established as a treatment for diabetes by:
   a. Lister
   b. Pasteur
   c. Salk and Sabin
   d. Banting and Best

LEARNING APPLICATION

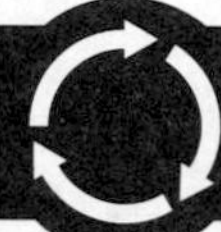

CASE STUDY

When 52-year-old Margaret Thomas, Martin Gordon's younger sister, begins to experience mild hand tremors and balance problems, Martin suggests that Margaret go see Dr. Winston Lewis. Dr. Lewis is Martin's primary care provider, who had provided treatment for Martin's prostate cancer. Feeling more comfortable with a female physician, Margaret chooses to make an appointment with Dr. Lewis's associate in the group practice, Dr. Elizabeth King. On the day of the examination, she brings her 25-year-old daughter with her to the clinic.

After taking a detailed patient history and undertaking a thorough physical examination of Margaret, Dr. King makes note of signs and symptoms, including a resting tremor, shuffling gait, muscle rigidity, and difficulty in swallowing and speaking. Margaret also complains of a "hot feeling" and odd, uncharacteristic moments of defective judgment when "she just can't keep things straight." Dr. King suspects Parkinson's disease and tells Margaret and her daughter that she would like to refer Margaret to a neurologist for more specific examination and medical tests. Dr. King explains that there are effective drug therapies for controlling the disease, although it has no known cure, and that the neurologist will outline Margaret's treatment options if a diagnosis of Parkinson's is made. Margaret seems to be shaken but takes Dr. King's words in stride.

Dr. King leaves Margaret and her daughter in the examination room with Audrey Jones, CMA (AAMA), who has assisted Dr. King throughout the examination and asks Audrey to be sure to give Margaret the referral to the neurologist. Margaret's daughter asks Audrey if Parkinson's is the disease that has shown promise in fetal tissue research and if her mother might be a candidate. Before Audrey can answer, Margaret becomes visibly distressed. "We're a good Catholic family, I could never consider that. Me—a grandmother." Looking to Audrey, she adds, "Please tell me I won't be involved with such a thing."

continues

CASE STUDY REVIEW QUESTIONS

1. What part does the role of women in medicine and in society play in this situation?

2. How should Audrey, the medical assistant, reply to Margaret and her daughter? What course of action, if any, should she take?

3. How do religious beliefs make an impact on the attitude toward illness held by the patient? How might these beliefs affect a treatment plan?

4. Discuss the issues that arise when a potential medical breakthrough involves controversial or radical ideas that challenge long-held cultural viewpoints and beliefs.

CHAPTER POST-TEST

Perform this test without looking at your book. If an answer is "false," rewrite the sentence to make it true.

1. True or False? The practice of medicine began long before we started keeping medical records.

2. True or False? Plants remain the basis of many medications.

3. True or False? Cultural differences do and should influence the way we treat our patients.

4. True or False? Magic has never played a role in medicine.

5. True or False? Ancient Eastern treatments did not include working with the human spirit.

6. True or False? Acupuncture uses the placement of needles in 365 points on the body.

7. True or False? Women were accepted as medical doctors in Chinese culture long before Western cultures.

8. True or False? The "father of preventive medicine" was Joseph Lister.

9. True or False? Edward Jenner developed the smallpox vaccine in the late 1800s.

SELF-ASSESSMENT

1. Make a list of the various ethnic, religious, and cultural groups you and your family members participate in or are descended from.

2. Interview family members to determine how their ethnic, religious, or cultural beliefs make an impact on the kind of medical care and treatment they expect to receive and how attitudes may have changed or evolved from generation to generation. Write a brief summary of your family's beliefs.

3. Write down any folk or home remedies used by your parents or grandparents that may or may not still be used by your family today. Why might these remedies have been more widely relied on by previous generations? Is there a scientific basis for each remedy?

4. An experimental treatment may be the only alternative available for your patient. How would this particular situation affect you, the medical assistant, if it is against your cultural or religious beliefs?

Name ______________________ Date __________ Score ______

CHAPTER 4

Therapeutic Communication Skills

CHAPTER PRE-TEST

Perform this test without looking at your book. If an answer is "false," rewrite the sentence to make it true.

1. True or False? Gestures and expressions have nothing to do with what a person is thinking or feeling.

2. True or False? You can make sick patients "feel better" just by the way you communicate with them.

3. True or False? Everyone enjoys a hug.

4. True or False? Patients should not be encouraged to verbalize their feelings and concerns.

5. True or False? Therapeutic communication can take place without considering the cultural and religious background of the patient.

6. True or False? Personal space is the distance at which we feel comfortable with others while communicating.

7. True or False? It is not necessary to accept the uniqueness in each person.

____

____

8. True or False? It is important for the patient to know that the provider will take the time to listen, answer any questions, and talk with the patient openly.

____

____

VOCABULARY BUILDER

Misspelled Words

Find the words below that are misspelled; circle them, and correctly spell them in the spaces provided. Then, insert the correct vocabulary terms from the list that best fits the descriptions below.

active listening	defense mechanisms	perseption
biases	denial	prejidices
body language	encode	rationalization
closed questions	hierarcky of needs	regression
cluster	indirect statements	repression
compinsation	interview technikes	roadblocks
congruancy	kinesics	therapuetic communication
cultural brokering	masking	time focus
decode	open-ended questions	

______________ ______________ ______________

______________ ______________

______________ ______________

______________ 1. Allows patients to feel comfortable, even when receiving difficult or unpleasant information, achieved through use of specific and well-defined professional communication skills

______________ 2. The person seems to experience temporary amnesia; forgetting or wiping things out of the conscious memory

______________ 3. Knowing how to encourage the best communication between the health care provider and the patient

______________ 4. Human needs grouped into five levels, each level being satisfied first before moving on to the next

______________ 5. Types of questions that require only a yes or no answer

______________ 6. Verbal or nonverbal messages that prevent patients from expressing themselves

______________ 7. The study of nonverbal communication, which includes unconscious body movements, gestures, and facial expressions

_______________ 8. Statements that turn a question into a topic of interest that allows the patient to speak without feeling directly questioned

_______________ 9. Being aware of what the patient is not saying or the ability to pick up on hints by the patient's body language regarding the real message

_______________ 10. Personal preferences slanting toward a particular belief

_______________ 11. An opinion or judgment that is formed before all the facts are known

_______________ 12. Nonverbal communication that conveys expression or feelings

_______________ 13. Types of questions that require more than a yes or no answer, the patient being required to verbalize more information

_______________ 14. An attempt to conceal or repress one's true feelings or real message

_______________ 15. Nonverbal messages grouped together to form a statement or conclusion

_______________ 16. When a person's nonverbal message agrees with that person's verbal message

_______________ 17. Interpreting the meaning of the message to understand it

_______________ 18. Creation of a carefully crafted message by a sender to match the receiver's ability to receive and interpret it properly

_______________ 19. Conscious awareness of one's own feelings and the feelings of others

_______________ 20. Substituting a strength for a weakness

_______________ 21. The mind's way of making unacceptable behavior or events acceptable by devising a rational reason for it

_______________ 22. Refusal to accept painful information that is apparent to others

_______________ 23. Attempt to withdraw from an unpleasant circumstance by retreating to a more secure state of life

_______________ 24. Act of bridging, linking, or mediating between groups or persons through the process of reducing conflict or producing change

_______________ 25. Statements eliciting a response from the patient without the patient's feeling questioned

_______________ 26. Unconscious behavior used to protect the ego from guilt, anxiety, or loss of esteem

Crossword Puzzle

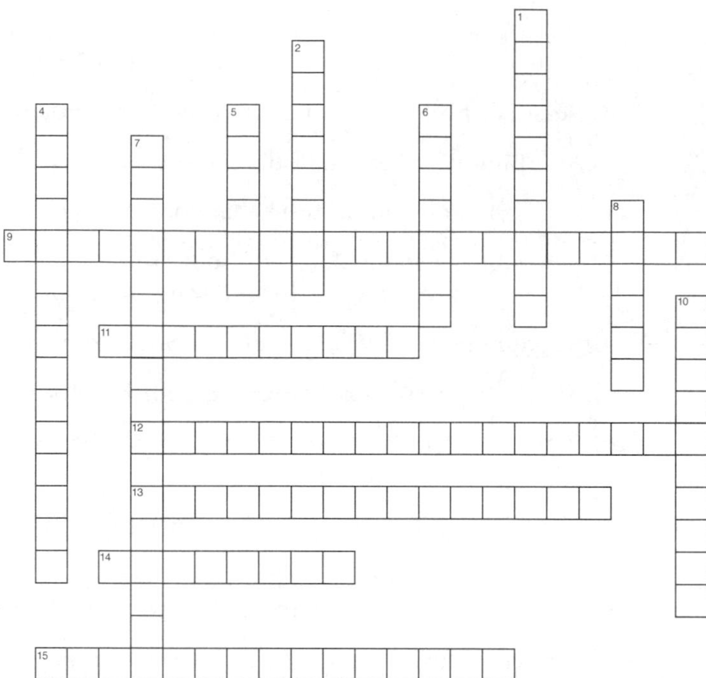

Across

9. Gestures and expressions together with body poses (two words)
11. Moving back to a former stage to escape conflict
12. This "cycle" involves sending and receiving messages, verbal and nonverbal (two words)
13. The art of really hearing another person's message and sometimes verifying with that person what you are hearing
14. The study of body movements
15. Questions that can be answered with a simple yes or no response

Down

1. Opinions or judgments formed before all the facts are known
2. Giving the speaker information about what you are hearing
3. The act of justification, usually illogically, that people use to keep from facing the truth
4. The rejection of or refusal to acknowledge information
5. The position of the body and parts of the body
6. Behavior that protects people from feelings of guilt, anxiety, and shame
7. A slant toward a particular belief
8. Sometimes referred to as temporary amnesia

LEARNING REVIEW

Short Answer

1. List the three listening goals of the health care professional.

____

____

____

2. The four modes of communication most pertinent in our everyday exchange are:

____

____

3. Circle the five correct responses. The five Cs of communication are:

clear	coherent	concise
constant	complete	curious
credible	courteous	comment
curt	cooperative	cohesive

4. Understanding Maslow's hierarchy will help medical assistants assess patients' needs and facilitate therapeutic communication. For each level, list a minimum of three needs that meet it.

____

____

____

____

5. Identify eight significant roadblocks to communication.

____

____

____

6. In order for any type of communication to take place, the patient must trust the health care provider. List the necessary steps in building the patient's trust.

____

____

____

____

____

7. How does therapeutic communication differ from normal communication?

____

____

8. List and explain the four basic elements included in the communication cycle.

____

____

____

____

____

____

9. Edith Leonard arrives at the clinic for a routine six-month follow-up examination. At her last visit, she had been referred to an ophthalmologist for removal of a cataract in her right eye. Compose (1) a closed question, (2) an open-ended question, and (3) an indirect statement regarding Ms. Leonard's condition.

   Closed question:

   ____

   ____

   Open-ended question:

   ____

   ____

   Indirect statement:

   ____

   ____

10. Time focus relates to whether the patient's attitude toward life is future, present, or past. Fill in the blanks below by explaining what each of these categories mean and list cultures or religions that are oriented to each.

Time focus	Meaning	Cultural or religious groups
Future time focus	______________	______________
	______________	______________
	______________	______________
	______________	______________
Present time focus	______________	______________
	______________	______________
	______________	______________
	______________	______________
Past time focus	______________	______________
	______________	______________
	______________	______________

Matching I

Identify each of the following as high-context communication (H) or low-context communication (L).

____ 1. African-American, Western culture

____ 2. Relies on highly detailed language to communicate ideas

____ 3. Asian culture

____ 4. Native American

____ 5. Relies on relevant phraseology to communicate ideas

____ 6. Caucasian, Western culture

____ 7. Hispanic and Latino cultures

____ 8. Islam

____ 9. Relies on body language to communicate ideas

Matching II

Biases and prejudices common in today's society have the potential to create hostility. Match each difficult situation below to the corresponding bias or prejudice that motivates it. Put a letter in the space provided.

A. A preference for Western-style medicine

B. The tendency to choose female rather than male providers

C. Prejudice related to a person's sexual preference

D. Discrimination based on race or religion

E. Hostile attitudes toward persons with a value system opposite to your own

F. A belief that persons who cannot afford health care should receive less care than those who can pay for full services

____ 1. Mr. Gordon refuses to accept a referral to an acupuncturist to help alleviate the chronic pain of advancing prostate cancer.

____ 2. Medical assistant Bruce Goldman mistakenly assumes that patient Bill Schwartz has AIDS when he arrives at the clinic with a gentleman friend, seeking attention for a recurring black mole on his calf.

____ 3. Rhoda and Lee Au fear they will not receive adequate medical care because they use Chinese as their first language and speak only broken English.

____ 4. Corey Boyer resists his gym teacher's efforts to get him to the clinic to check out a recurring rash on his arm because his family has no health insurance.

____ 5. Mary O'Keefe is relieved to find that the practice's OB/GYN is a female physician, Dr. Elizabeth King.

____ 6. Edith Leonard, a widow in her 70s, counsels medical assistant Liz Corbin that she should settle down and get married instead of pursuing a dream to attend medical school and become a pediatrician.

CERTIFICATION REVIEW

These questions are designed to mimic the certification examination. Select the best response.

1. Which of the following is not part of communication?
   a. Speech
   b. Facial expression
   c. Gestures
   d. Attitude
   e. Body positioning
2. Which is the most basic need in Maslow's hierarchy?
   a. Food
   b. Safety
   c. Status and self-esteem
   d. Need for knowledge
   e. Self-actualization

3. Your patient refuses to accept a diagnosis, claiming the doctor "must be mistaken." Assuming the doctor is correct, which self-defense mechanism is the patient using?

   a. Repression

   b. Denial

   c. Projection

   d. Compensation

   e. Rationalization

4. Congruency in communication can be described as when:

   a. the verbal message matches the body language

   b. the verbal message does not match the gestures

   c. the verbal message can be interpreted in two or more different ways

   d. two different messages are interpreted as the same

5. The conscious awareness of one's own feelings and the feelings of others is:

   a. congruency

   b. perception

   c. bias

   d. masking

6. The founder of humanistic psychology is:

   a. Jacobi

   b. Freud

   c. Erikson

   d. Maslow

7. The grouping of nonverbal messages into statements or conclusions is known as:

   a. assimilating

   b. feedback

   c. clustering

   d. introjection

8. The goal of therapeutic communication at the point of care is:

   a. to collect a blood specimen

   b. to determine the reason for the visit

   c. to explain the treatment plan for the patient

   d. all of the above

LEARNING APPLICATION

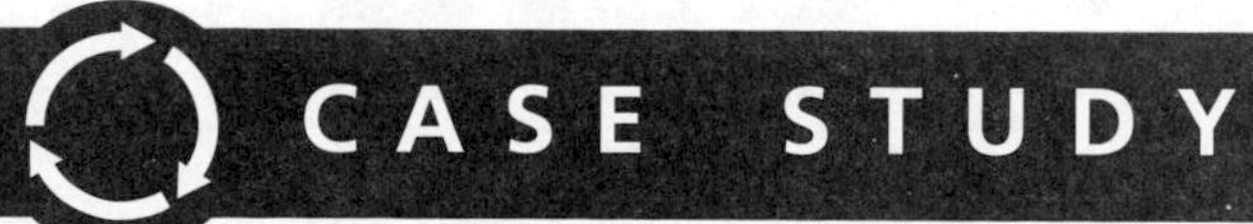

Wayne Elder arrives at the clinic for an examination to check on a recurrent ear infection that has been treated with antibiotics. Wayne, who is slightly retarded and lives in a group home, is still reporting dizziness and pain in his right ear. He has come to the clinic by himself, taking a bus from his job as a part-time dishwasher. Wayne's boss asked him to return to the clinic because Wayne could not concentrate at work.

Wanda Slawson, who is the medical assistant at the clinic, discovers from Wayne that he has not been taking his medication properly; he stopped taking his pills once his ear began to feel better. She must politely ask Wayne to repeat himself several times before she can clearly understand his slurred speech, and she has difficulty holding his attention or maintaining eye contact.

Wanda conveys Wayne's situation to Dr. Ray Reynolds, who examines Wayne and gives him a new prescription for antibiotics, gently explaining the need to finish the entire prescription to get well. After Dr. Reynolds leaves the examination room, however, it is clear to Wanda that Wayne is still confused about why he must take the medication even after he begins to feel better. Wanda carefully explains to Wayne that the infection will continue to heal even though he no longer feels sick. To be sure he understands, Wanda asks Wayne to repeat to her what he must do and why; she then asks Dr. Reynolds to step in briefly to remind Wayne once more to complete the prescription.

CASE STUDY REVIEW QUESTIONS

1. How does the unequal relationship that exists between patients and health care professionals have an impact on the therapeutic communication between provider, medical assistant, and patient?

2. How must medical assistant Wanda Slawson tailor her verbal and nonverbal messages to meet the abilities of her receivers: the provider and the patient?

continues

3. How does Wanda use active listening? Which interview techniques are the most effective in facilitating therapeutic communication? Does nonverbal communication play a role?

4. Using Maslow's hierarchy of needs, discuss how the health care team meets Wayne's special needs resulting from his disability.

5. Do you think the medical assistant acted appropriately? What else could she have done? What should she not do in this situation?

Role-Play Exercises

Active listening is an important element of therapeutic communication. To practice active listening skills, role-play as a patient and a medical assistant. Have the "patient" say each of the phrases below. The "medical assistant" should then rephrase each of the messages listed for verification from the sender and also include a therapeutic response. When you are finished role-playing, write what you have said in response to each statement below.

1. "I don't know what to do. My father takes so many pills he can't remember which is the right one, so he ends up refusing to take any of them."

2. "I can't give you my insurance card because I lost it and I can't remember the name of the company, either. You've always taken care of this before."

3. "I can't help being worried. The doctor just suggested a referral for treatment at that hospital where somebody had their wrong foot operated on. What do you think?"

4. "I feel dizzy just thinking about having my blood taken. Do you really need to do it?"

CHAPTER POST-TEST

Perform this test without looking at your book. If an answer is "false," rewrite the sentence to make it true.

1. True or False? Gestures and expressions can always tell you what a person is thinking or feeling.

2. True or False? You can make a sick patient "feel worse" just by the way you communicate with her.

3. True or False? Hugs are universally acceptable as a means of communicating.

4. True or False? Patients should not be allowed to say how they feel or what they are concerned about.

5. True or False? In therapeutic communication, it is not necessary to take into consideration the cultural and religious background of the patient.

6. True or False? The distance at which we feel comfortable while communicating with others is called personal space.

7. True or False? The health care provider should not accept the uniqueness of the patient.

8. True or False? Patients must realize that providers are taking the time to listen to them, answer any of their questions, and speak with them openly.

SELF-ASSESSMENT

Think about your own facial expressions and body language. Are you always portraying the message you want to send? List two situations in which you have been misinterpreted through your nonverbal communication, or situations in which you have misinterpreted someone else's message. Then think of what would have been a verbal message to help make the situation more accurate. That is, explain what you could have said to the person to determine if he or she was really hearing the message you meant to send.

Name ______________________ Date ____________ Score ______

CHAPTER 5

Coping Skills for the Medical Assistant

CHAPTER PRE-TEST

Perform this test without looking at your book. If an answer is "false," rewrite the sentence to make it true.

1. True or False? Stress is always something bad.

____

____

2. True or False? Stress is something we cannot prevent.

____

____

3. True or False? If you have a lot of responsibility in your job, you cannot avoid burnout.

____

____

4. True or False? Setting goals helps relieve stress.

____

____

5. True or False? Goal-oriented employees are more effective than those with no goals or future objectives.

____

____

6. True or False? Revitalization outside the workplace is not necessary when preventing burnout.

____

____

7. True or False? Worry causes stress but does nothing to resolve the problem that is causing the worry.

____

____

VOCABULARY BUILDER

Misspelled Words

Find the words below that are misspelled; circle them, and correctly spell them in the spaces provided. Then insert the vocabulary terms from the list next to their definitions below.

burnout	long-range goal	short-range goal
goal	outer-directed people	stress
inter-directed peepel	self-actualzation	stressers
______________	______________	______________

______________ 1. Achievements that may take several years to accomplish

______________ 2. Fatigue and exhaustion which results from stress and frustration

______________ 3. The body's response to change, which may be manifested in a variety of ways, such as increased blood pressure, heart rate, or headache

______________ 4. People who decide what to do based on events, environmental factors, or other people

______________ 5. Demands to change that cause stress

______________ 6. People who decide for themselves what they want to do

______________ 7. Achievement toward which effort has been directed

______________ 8. Interim goal that helps to achieve a larger goal over a longer period of time

______________ 9. Developing your full potential and experiencing fulfillment

Word Search

Find the words in the grid below. They may go in any direction.

T A K E C A R E O F Y O U R N S E L E F
S R O S S E R T S X K L E G O J D M L Y
L L J C K L K K C Y F L G M I E X R P T
T R T F O L F J R G O P W J T X D R O B
K H T P H P S G M R T X E Z A H R S E H
L W G R R T I X X Y N M J M T A F H P H
T T F I R I F N T R I G L J P U H O D S
H G C E L C O U G T F M L T A S L R E L
R R S I R F O R G S F F Z X D T B T T A
M S R R L N R N I R K J K D A I M R C O
N C B M R F I O U T L I Q R T O K A E G
N G T U X G N S T Q I X L L Y N P N R E
Y Q B V A C T O R H R Z H L K Q Z G I G
T W J N D R Z C C P G L I Z S M Z E D N
C R A J A H F F Z E R I Z N T H K G R A
W M T T J G D V T V L Q F T G B Y O E R
H Y I C O N T R O L T O T H N M R A N G
Z O R R S L A O G Q N T R C M P T L N N
N Z R T J Z K H N L C V K Y N M V S I O
O U T E R D I R E C T E D P E O P L E L

adaptation
burnout
control
coping skills
exhaustion
fight or flight
frustration
goals
inner-directed people
long-range goals
managing time
outer-directed people
prioritizing
role
role conflict
short-range goals
stress
stressors

LEARNING REVIEW

Short Answer

1. Han Selye's general adaptation syndrome (GAS) theory proposes that adaptation to stress occurs in four stages. Identify each stage in the order in which it is manifested and describe the physiologic changes that occur during each stage.

____

____

____

____

____

____

____

____

____

____

2. Identify six changes in your approach to your work environment and lifestyle that will help you to avoid burnout.

____
____
____
____
____
____

3. List and define the five considerations important in determining a goal.

____
____
____
____
____

4. Stressors are divided into three categories. List and describe them.

____
____
____
____

Matching

Burnout is stress-related energy depletion that takes place in the working world. Burnout occurs gradually over a period of continued stress. Place a P *next to those items that promote burnout and an* R *next to those that reduce the risk for burnout.*

___ 1. Keep work separate from your home life.

___ 2. Have regular physical examinations.

___ 3. Work harder than anyone else in the office.

___ 4. Feel a greater need than others to do a job well for its own sake.

___ 5. Prioritize tasks and perform the most difficult ones first.

___ 6. Prefer to tackle projects yourself rather than consult a supervisor.

___ 7. Never stop until you achieve your goals, regardless of the personal cost to yourself or loved ones.

___ 8. Postpone vacation time.

___ 9. Give up unrealistic goals and expectations.

___ 10. Maintain a positive self-image and your self-esteem.

___ 11. Develop interests outside your profession.

___ 12. Procrastinate.

___ 13. Wear loose-fitting, comfortable clothes and shoes.

___ 14. Stretch or change positions. Walk around and deliver charts or laboratory specimens.

___ 15. Know your limits and be aware of your body's needs.

Labeling

Hans Selye's General Adaptation Syndrome (GAS) theory proposes that four stages are involved in adapting to stress. Identify the four stages on the figure, and then explain each stage in the space below.

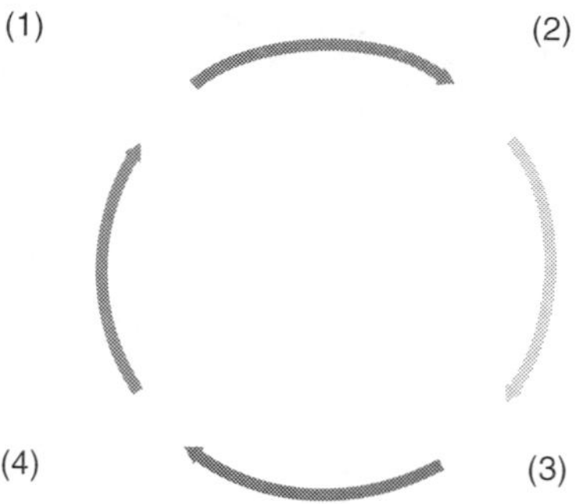

1. ______________________________

____

2. ______________________________

____

3. ______________________________

____

4. ______________________________

____

CERTIFICATION REVIEW

These questions are designed to mimic the certification examination. Select the best response.

1. The body's response to mental or physical change is called:
   a. stress
   b. adaptation
   c. denial
   d. burnout
2. Which of the following is not part of Hans Selye's general adaptation syndrome?
   a. Exhaustion
   b. Alarm
   c. Fear
   d. Fight or flight
   e. Return to normal

3. The four parts of the process leading to burnout are the honeymoon stage, the reality stage, the dissatisfaction stage, and the:

   a. sad stage

   b. angry stage

   c. retaliation stage

   d. giving up stage

4. In order for the body to survive, the sympathetic nervous system prepares the body for:

   a. fight or flight

   b. sleep

   c. developing a good appetite

   d. exercises

5. Time segments for short-range goals may be:

   a. monthly

   b. quarterly

   c. yearly

   d. all of the above

6. The result of long duration stress could be:

   a. making quick judgments

   b. job related

   c. immune system disorders

   d. an adrenaline rush

7. Stressors can be divided into which category(ies)?

   a. Frustration

   b. Conflicts

   c. Pressure

   d. All of the above

8. Needlessly worrying is an example of which type of stress?

   a. Short-term stress

   b. Episodic stress

   c. Long-term stress

   d. Intermediate stress

9. A common cause of stress in an organization would be:

   a. too much time spent on the telephone

   b. lack of motivation

   c. poor time management skills

   d. no smoke breaks

10. Discipline, perseverance, determination, and hard work are necessary in accomplishing:

    a. short-range goals

    b. long-range goals

    c. self-actualization

    d. prevention of burnout

11. The "wear and tear" our bodies experience as we continually adjust to a changing environment is called:

    a. adaptation

    b. stress

    c. prioritizing

    d. conditioning

12. The fight-or-flight response includes all but which one of the following reactions?

    a. Respirations and heart rate increase.

    b. Digestion is activated.

    c. Hormones are released into the bloodstream.

    d. Blood supply is increased to the muscles.

13. One of the characteristics associated with burnout is that the employee does not know what is expected and how to accomplish it. This is often called:

    a. role conflict

    b. role overload

    c. role ambiguity

    d. role reversal

14. When individuals with a high need to achieve do not reach their goals, they are apt to feel:

    a. angry and frustrated

    b. tired and lonely

    c. distrustful and leery

    d. motivated and enthusiastic

15. The best way to treat burnout is to:

    a. cover it up

    b. get a prescription to help you cope

    c. prevent it

    d. encourage it

LEARNING APPLICATION

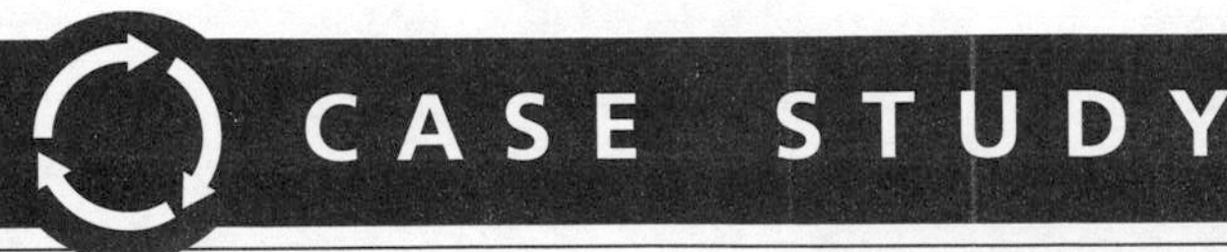

Dr. Angie Esposito is a provider at Inner City Health Care. It was her dream, even as a child, to become a physician and work in an environment where she could help people and benefit the community as well. Proud of her accomplishments, she is the first woman in her family to attend college, and she got herself through medical school with scholarships and student loans. Dr. Esposito works hard, often pulling double shifts. Liz Corbin, CMA (AAMA), has a similar dream and is working to save money to attend medical school to become a pediatrician. Dr. Esposito does her best to encourage Liz's ambitions and has taken Liz under her wing.

Late one night, Liz assists Dr. Esposito in treating three difficult emergency patients in a row. "That's it," Dr. Esposito says. "We're taking a fifteen-minute break. Ask Dr. Woo if he can cover for a short time." When Liz catches up with Dr. Esposito in the employee lounge, she finds her frustrated and in tears. "These double shifts," she says. "I'm so tired. And the patients just keep coming. I want to help them all," she sighs, and her voice trails off, "I just can't help them all. . . ."

CASE STUDY REVIEW QUESTIONS

1. Dr. Angie Esposito is experiencing burnout. What personality traits are promoting her burnout? Identify the stressors in Angie's life.

___
___
___
___
___
___
___

2. Liz Corbin sees her mentor breaking down under stress. Should Liz reevaluate her own long-range goals?

___
___
___
___
___
___

continues

3. Discuss the importance of keeping goals in perspective.

4. What would be Liz's best therapeutic response to Dr. Esposito?

CHAPTER POST-TEST

Perform this test without looking at your book. If an answer is "false," rewrite the sentence to make it true.

1. True or False? Stress is never a good thing.

2. True or False? Stress is something we can always prevent.

3. True or False? Even if you have a lot of responsibility at work, you can still avoid burnout.

4. True or False? Setting goals eliminates stress.

5. True or False? Those employees who are goal oriented are more effective than those employees who do not have a goal or future objective.

6. True or False? Revitalization outside the workplace is not a contributing factor to burnout.

____

____

7. True or False? Worry contributes to stress and does not resolve the problem that is the cause of the worry.

____

____

SELF-ASSESSMENT

Determining how well you now handle stress will help you to identify personal strengths and weaknesses and point you toward the skills you will need to develop to be successful on the job as a medical assistant. Complete the following stress self-test. For each question, circle the response that best describes you.

1. I exercise:
   a. three times a week
   b. less than three times a week
   c. only if I am forced to
2. When something stressful happens in my life, I:
   a. eat too much
   b. make sure I eat regular meals
   c. stop eating for days
3. If I am struggling with a problem or project, I am most likely to:
   a. consult someone who may be able to help
   b. become determined to solve the problem or finish the project on my own
   c. abandon the project or just hope the problem goes away
4. When I encounter difficult personalities, I:
   a. leave the scene and avoid the person in the future
   b. lose my temper and get into arguments
   c. practice the art of the diplomatic response
5. When offered a new challenge or responsibility that requires obtaining new skills or training, I:
   a. get tension headaches
   b. respond with enthusiasm and an open mind
   c. express concern about taking on a new duty
6. In emergency situations, I:
   a. react calmly and efficiently
   b. feel paralyzed
   c. wait for someone else to take charge
7. I feel confident and competent in group situations:
   a. only when I know everyone present
   b. most of the time
   c. hardly ever; conversations with others make me uncomfortable

8. I think meditating or taking time to be quiet and calm during a busy day is:
   a. a terrific waste of time; I always have to be doing something
   b. good for other people; I've tried it more than once, but I can't seem to get into meditation
   c. a great way to relax and refocus my mind
9. The key to handling stressful situations lies in:
   a. staying out of stressful situations
   b. examining my view of the situation from a new perspective
   c. insisting that everyone agree with my point of view
10. To accomplish my personal goals, I:
    a. am willing to get up an hour earlier each day
    b. will give up sleep altogether
    c. find myself losing sleep because I am worrying about how I am going to get everything done
11. I usually complete projects:
    a. on time
    b. at the last minute
    c. late—but only by a day
12. As I prepare for a day's activities, I:
    a. prioritize and use time management skills to budget time carefully
    b. do not prepare; I like to be spontaneous
    c. find myself overwhelmed and unable to complete anything
13. When I focus on setting a long-range goal, I:
    a. think through the short-range goals necessary to achieve it
    b. become impatient
    c. talk constantly about the goal without making plans to achieve it
14. I volunteer to take on:
    a. more tasks than any one person can easily accomplish—then amaze everyone by pulling them off
    b. only what I know I can reasonably accomplish
    c. only what is required to get the job done
15. After a stressful day, the best way to unwind is to:
    a. talk all night with family or friends about what happened
    b. rent a funny movie
    c. work late to prepare for tomorrow
16. People think of me as:
    a. a person who is unpredictable. No one knows what I will do next.
    b. someone fixed in life roles
    c. someone who is confident about who I am but who also is willing to grow and change as worthy opportunities arise

Scoring: In the "My Score" column, record the number of points earned for each of your answers. The higher your score, the less you are prone to stress. The highest possible score is 160 points. If your score is low, consider the areas you need to focus on to reduce stress in your life.

MY SCORE

1. a. 10 points b. 5 points c. 0 points ___________
   Regular exercise reduces stress.
2. a. 0 points b. 10 points c. 0 points ___________
   Eating regular meals reduces stress.
3. a. 10 points b. 5 points c. 0 points ___________
   Problems rarely just go away; ask for help before struggling on your own.
4. a. 5 points b. 0 points c. 10 points ___________
   You will not always be able to avoid a difficult person, and argument leads to stress. Tact and grace are needed.
5. a. 0 points b. 10 points c. 5 points ___________
   Worrying to the point of causing physical symptoms is not productive. Closed-mindedness could keep you from enjoying something new and cause stressful reactions.
6. a. 10 points b. 0 points c. 5 points ___________
   Feelings of helplessness increase stress.
7. a. 5 points b. 10 points c. 0 points ___________
   The ability to interact comfortably with others in group situations reduces stress.
8. a. 0 points b. 5 points c. 10 points ___________
   The more you can separate your sense of well-being from daily events by taking time to relax and refocus, the less stress you will experience.
9. a. 0 points b. 10 points c. 0 points ___________
   Stressful situations cannot always be avoided; keeping a flexible instead of a rigid viewpoint will reduce stress.
10. a. 10 points b. 0 points c. 0 points ___________
    Sleep is important in reducing stress. However, making time by getting up earlier is a good time management technique.
11. a. 10 points b. 5 points c. 0 points ___________
    Lateness causes stress for everyone.
12. a. 10 points b. 0 points c. 0 points ___________
    Unexpected things can always happen, but prioritizing and budgeting time can help keep a handle on the day's events and reduce stress.
13. a. 10 points b. 5 points c. 0 points ___________
    Achieving long-range goals takes perseverance and determination. Being realistic about goals reduces stress.
14. a. 0 points b. 10 points c. 5 points ___________
    Taking on too much responsibility leads to stress.
15. a. 0 points b. 10 points c. 0 points ___________
    Humor is an effective stress reducer—so is separating work from your home life.
16. a. 0 points b. 0 points c. 10 points ___________
    Being grounded but open to new experiences reduces stress.

TOTAL: ___________

Areas I need to focus on to reduce stress in my life:

Name ______________________ Date ____________ Score ________

CHAPTER **6**

The Therapeutic Approach to the Patient with a Life-Threatening Illness

CHAPTER PRE-TEST

Perform this test without looking at your book. If an answer is "false," rewrite the sentence to make it true.

1. True or False? Patients from different cultures will view death and life-threatening illnesses in different ways.

____

____

2. True or False? The strongest influences in managing life-threatening illnesses in the life of the patient comes from the medical team.

____

____

3. True or False? Health care professionals are responsible for making sure that patients have all their legal documents in order when diagnosed with a life-threatening illness.

____

____

4. True or False? Alternative methods of treatment should be discussed with the patient, as well as no treatment at all.

____

____

5. True or False? When facing a life-threatening illness, setting goals is no longer important.

____

____

6. True or False? According to Dr. Kübler-Ross, patients go through each of the five states of grief.

____

____

VOCABULARY BUILDER

Misspelled Words

Find the words below that are misspelled; circle them, and correctly spell them in the space provided. Then insert the correct vocabulary terms from the list that best fit the descriptions below.

durible power of attorney for health care	living will
health care directive	sychomotor retardation

______________________ ______________________

1. ______________________ allows the surrogate to make decisions related to health care when the patient is no longer able to do so.
2. A ______________________ allows patients to make decisions (before becoming incapacitated) of whether life-prolonging medical or surgical procedures are to continue or be withheld.
3. ______________________ is the slowing of mental responses, decreased alertness, and apathy.
4. A ______________________ is a legal document that allows a person to make choices related to treatment in a life-threatening illness.

Crossword Puzzle

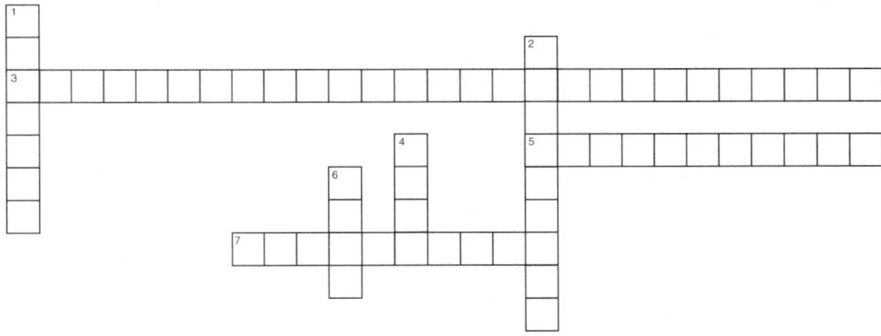

Across

3. This 1990 Act gave all patients in institutions that were Medicare or Medicaid funded certain rights.
5. Aiding health, healthful
7. This emotion is common in patients dealing with life-threatening illnesses.

Down

1. Recognition of another person's feelings by entering into those feelings
2. This type of support is vital when dealing with a life-threatening illness.
4. Late stages of HIV infection (abbreviation)
6. Abbreviation for end-stage renal disease

LEARNING REVIEW

Short Answer

1. List five issues that are appropriate to discuss with a patient facing a life-threatening illness.

____

____

____

2. Discuss the pros and cons of using the words *terminal illness* or *life-threatening illness*. Which term seems more comfortable to you? Defend your rationale.

____

____

3. The federal government passed the Patient Self-Determination Act in __________, giving all patients receiving care in institutions that receive payments from Medicare and Medicaid written information about their right to accept or refuse medical or surgical treatment.

4. Explain what each of the letters in the acronym TEAR means as it relates to the grieving process.

   T = _______________

   E = _______________

   A = _______________

   R = _______________

5. What is the best therapeutic response to the patient with a life-threatening disease?

____

____

____

____

True or False

Mark a true statement with a T *and a false statement with an* F. *If an answer is "false," rewrite the sentence to make it true.*

___ 1. It is important for those patients who are suffering from cancer to know that the provider is willing to relieve and treat the symptoms associated with the disease.

____

____

___ 2. When a person is faced with a life-threatening illness, he or she will go through certain stages of grieving.

____

____

___ 3. It is not necessary for the health care professional to encourage patients to set goals for themselves.

____

____

___ 4. It is not necessary to offer nonmedical forms of assistance to patients suffering from a life-threatening illness.

___

___

___ 5. All patients go through the five stages of grief.

___

___

CERTIFICATION REVIEW

These questions are designed to mimic the certification examination. Select the best response.

1. Your patient's culture influences:
   a. his or her views about illness
   b. his or her views about treatment
   c. his or her views about death
   d. all of the above

2. Your patient has just been diagnosed with a life-threatening illness. She tells you that she would much rather die quickly than to suffer through this disease. She asks you not to say anything about her comment to the doctor. What is your best response?
   a. You have had quite a shock. Dr. King would like to talk to you about those feelings. I'll go get him for you.
   b. You, above anyone else, know what is best for your life.
   c. I know what you mean, I would feel the same way.
   d. Don't worry about that right now. Dr. King will give you medication to help with the pain.

3. The health care directive and power of attorney for health care documents are legal in how many states?
   a. 10
   b. 25
   c. 5
   d. 50

4. The slowing of physical and mental responses, decreased alertness, withdrawal, apathy, and diminished interest in work are referred to as:
   a. passive-aggressive behavior
   b. fight or flight
   c. psychomotor retardation
   d. mood swings

5. The strongest influence in managing the life-threatening illness of a patient is the:
   a. health care team
   b. family and those closest to the patient
   c. social worker
   d. hospice

6. The range of psychological suffering a patient may experience can lead to:
   a. tachycardia
   b. anorexia
   c. agitation
   d. all of the above
7. What patients fear more than anything else when facing a life-threatening illness is:
   a. pain and loss of independence
   b. dementia
   c. financial issues
   d. becoming addicted to some medications
8. In caring for individuals with life-threatening illnesses, it can be helpful to remember:
   a. that family members have the strongest influence on patients
   b. that pain must be considered within a cultural perspective
   c. that choices and decisions regarding treatment belong to the patient
   d. all of the above
9. One of the most common problems that a patient with a life-threatening illness may exhibit is:
   a. displacement
   b. denial
   c. depression
   d. assimilation
10. Referrals to community-based agencies or service groups may include:
    a. health departments
    b. social workers
    c. hospices
    d. all of the above

LEARNING APPLICATION

Role Playing Exercises

With another student, role play the following scenarios as medical assistant and patient. What is the medical assistant's appropriate therapeutic response or action?

1. The patient's husband has just found out that her husband has end-stage renal disease. She tells the medical assistant under no circumstances should her husband be informed about the prognosis.

   ____

   ____

2. The patient has been diagnosed with HIV. The medical assistant knows the patient is estranged from his or her family.

   ____

   ____

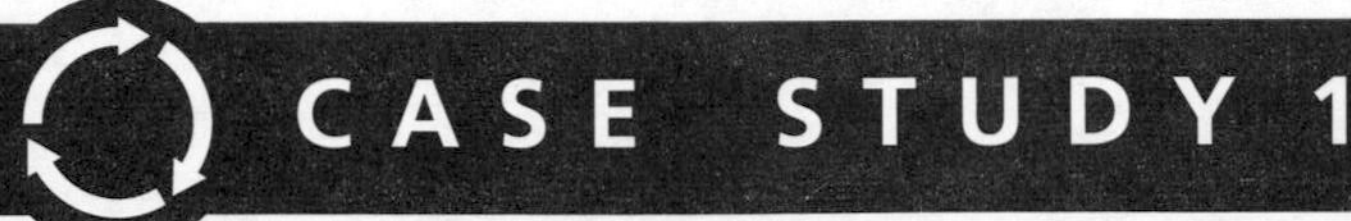

CASE STUDY 1

Jaime Carrera, a Hispanic man in his late 20s, is brought to Inner City Health Care, an urgent care center, by coworkers when he injures his head in an accident at a construction site where he is working. His head is bleeding profusely. As Jaime's coworkers watch the health care team implement Standard Precautions for infection control, one of them, his own shirt and hands covered with Jaime's blood, pulls the medical assistant aside and whispers frantically, "What are you doing? Does he have AIDS?"

CASE STUDY REVIEW QUESTIONS

1. What is the best therapeutic response of the medical assistant?

2. On what criteria do you base this response as the best therapeutic approach?

CASE STUDY 2

John Dukane, a longtime and much loved patient of the clinic, has end-stage renal disease. A kidney transplant is not appropriate due to his age, and John will not agree to receiving renal dialysis as treatment. That decision has been made clear in the provider's directive and the durable power of attorney for health care. He is healthy otherwise, and his family members feel he should try the dialysis, in hopes of extending his life by a few weeks or possibly even a few months. Discuss the arguments on both sides of the decision.

CHAPTER POST-TEST

1. True or False? Patients view death and life-threatening illnesses in different ways depending on their culture.

____

____

2. True or False? The strongest influences in the management of life-threatening illnesses in the life of the patient comes from the health care team.

____

____

3. True or False? Validating that patients have all their legal documentation in order when diagnosed with life-threatening illness is the responsibility of the health care provider.

____

____

4. True or False? Alternative methods of treatment, as well as the option of no treatment at all, should be discussed with the patient.

____

____

5. True or False? When facing a life-threatening illness, setting goals is not important.

____

____

6. True or False? Patients go through all five of the stages of grief as researched by Dr. Elisabeth Kübler-Ross.

____

____

SELF-ASSESSMENT

If you were faced with a life-threatening illness, would you choose to sustain your life regardless of the probable outcome? How far would you go with treatments? What four factors would enter into your decision? Have you discussed these issues with your family and physician?

Name ______________________ Date ____________ Score ______

CHAPTER 7

Legal Considerations

CHAPTER PRE-TEST

Perform this test without looking at your book. If an answer is "false," rewrite the sentence to make it true.

1. True or False? You may discuss a person's confidential medical information as long as you do not say the patient's name.

____

____

2. True or False? Your provider does not have a contract with the patient until he or she treats the patient.

____

____

3. True or False? A provider is not obligated to care for a patient even though the patient's condition may require treatment.

____

____

4. True or False? Medical assistants do not have to worry about a "standard of care" because their employers are ultimately responsible for everything the medical assistant does under their direction.

____

____

VOCABULARY BUILDER

Misspelled Words

Find the words below that are misspelled; circle them, and correctly spell them in the spaces provided. Then insert the correct vocabulary terms from the list that best fit the descriptions below.

administrative law
agents
civil law
constitutional law
defendents
doctrines
durable power of attorney for health care
emanciated minor
expert witness
expressed contract
implied consent
incompetent
invation of privacy
lible
litigation
malfeasance
malpractice
miner
neglegance
noncompliant
plaintiffs
risk management
slander
statutes
subpoena
tort

________________ ________________ ________________
________________ ________________ ________________
________________ ________________

________________ 1. Establishes agencies that are given power to enact regulations having the force of law

________________ 2. Law that includes 27 amendments, 10 of which are the Bill of Rights

________________ 3. A 17-year-old person serving in the U.S. armed forces

________________ 4. Medical practice acts, or laws, that regulate the practice of medicine, such as licensure and standards of care

________________ 5. A patient who refuses needed care, such as a cancer patient who will not complete a series of chemotherapy treatments

________________ 6. A provider or health care professional who testifies in court to establish a reasonable and expected standard of care with respect to a specific medical situation so that jurors can understand the nature of medical information

________________ 7. The failure to exercise the standard of care that a reasonable person would exercise in similar circumstances

________________ 8. Persons who bring charges in a civil case

________________ 9. Medical assistants are __________ of their employers.

________________ 10. A patient tilts her head back and opens her eyes wide for instillation of medicated eye drops from a medical assistant without any verbal instructions to do so.

________________ 11. Professional negligence

________________ 12. *Respondeat superior* and *res ipsa loquitur*

________________ 13. Court order

________________ 14. Persons against whom charges are brought

________________ 15. A medical assistant writes in the patient's record, "Jim Marshall is a ruthless, rude man who is very full of himself. Be careful around him."

________________ 16. A patient says loudly in the reception area of Inner City Health Care, filled to capacity with waiting patients, "Dr. Reynolds should retire. I know he's not up on the latest medical techniques."

_______________ 17. A 17-year-old student who lives with his or her parents

_______________ 18. Actions that make the medical assistant and the employer less vulnerable to litigation

_______________ 19. Lawsuit

_______________ 20. Written or verbal contract that describes exactly what each party in the contract will do

Crossword Puzzle

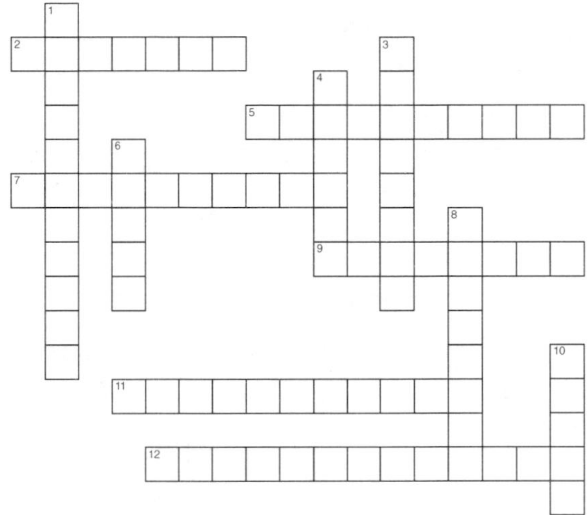

Across

2. The type of consent that is given when a patient is unconscious
5. When a doctor should have treated a patient, but did not, it can sometimes be called this.
7. Another word for lawsuit
9. Another word for laws
11. A type of lawsuit in which the doctor is accused of harming a patient
12. When a patient does not follow the doctor's orders, such as not taking medication that is prescribed

Down

1. Minors (under 18 years old) who are no longer under parental authority
3. Law that governs criminal acts
4. Person who represents another
6. Law that governs issues between persons
8. This document is a legal force with which you must comply
10. When someone harms another person's reputation by saying something untrue

LEARNING REVIEW

Identifying Civil and Criminal Law

Identify whether the following actions fall under the domain of civil law (CV) or criminal law (CM).

____ A. A provider is siphoning off narcotics from an urgent care center's locked drug cabinet and continuing to treat patients while under the influence of the drugs.

____ B. A woman in the advanced stages of breast cancer sues her insurer when it refuses to provide benefits for a bone marrow transplant.

____ C. An office manager steals, or embezzles, funds from the medical practice.

Short Answer

1. List and define the four Ds of negligence.

____

____

____

2. List at least 11 strategies for risk management in an ambulatory care setting that will lessen the potential for litigation.

____

____

____

____

____

____

____

____

____

____

____

____

3. Before any invasive or surgical procedure is performed, patients are asked to sign consent forms, which become a permanent part of the medical record. What four things must the patient know to give informed consent?

____

____

____

4. The unauthorized touching of one person by another is called ______________.

5. The federal government established laws in 1968 to allow people to make a gift of all or part of their body; it is known as the ______________________________.

6. The law mandates that the proper authorities be informed of certain harms and injuries, such as *(circle all that apply):*

   A. rape
   B. gunshot and knife wounds
   C. child abuse
   D. elder abuse

7. What term is used now in place of "domestic violence" and what does it mean? Why was this change made?

____

____

____

____

____

8. What is the difference between an advance directive and a POLST form?

____

____

____

____

____

____

CERTIFICATION REVIEW

These questions are designed to mimic the certification examination. Select the best response.

1. The Patient Self-Determination Act, which includes health care directives, ensures that patients are able to:
   a. choose their own providers
   b. control their own health care decisions
   c. have guaranteed confidentiality
   d. have health care benefits
2. Which of the following covers the relationship between providers and their patients?
   a. Informed consent
   b. Locum tenens
   c. Medical ethics
   d. Criminal law
3. *Res ipsa loquitur* means:
   a. the thing speaks for itself
   b. the physician is ultimately responsible
   c. the record must be opened in court
   d. patients have a right to their records
4. The 4 Ds of negligence are:
   a. duty, derelict, danger, damage
   b. danger, duty, direct cause, disaster
   c. duty, derelict, direct cause, damage
   d. disaster, damage, direct cause, danger
5. A 17-year-old individual who is in the Navy is considered to be:
   a. *respondeat superior*
   b. an emancipated minor
   c. privileged
   d. a naval dependent

6. *Respondeat superior* is the Latin word that means

   a. providers are responsible for their employees' actions

   b. the thing speaks for itself

   c. obey your superior

   d. breach of duty of care

7. What must the inventory of controlled substances include?

   a. List of the name, addresses, and DEA registration number of the provider

   b. Date and time of inventory

   c. Signature of the individual taking inventory

   d. All of the above

8. A provider is legally bound to treat a patient until the patient:

   a. breaks an appointment

   b. does not have health insurance

   c. cannot get a referral

   d. no longer needs treatment

9. If suspicion of child abuse is aroused, the health care provider should:

   a. send the patient home

   b. treat the child's injuries

   c. inform the parents of the child's diagnosis and that it will be reported to the police and social services agency

   d. b. and c.

10. When a patient is asked to walk across the hall to the treatment room while wearing only a patient gown and is in full view of other patients, this is considered:

    a. a HIPAA violation

    b. implied consent

    c. invasion of privacy

    d. defamation of character

11. Protection of health care professionals who may provide medical care in emergencies without fear of being sued comes under:

    a. Good Samaritan laws

    b. provider's directives

    c. durable power of attorney for health care

    d. litigation

12. An order for a physician to appear in court with a medical record is:

    a. *res ipsa loquitur*

    b. *subpoena duces tecum*

    c. *respondeat superior*

    d. an interrogatory

13. When a patient reports a sore throat and the provider takes a swab for a throat culture to diagnose and treat the ailment, this act is considered:
    a. an expressed contract
    b. implied consent
    c. informed consent
    d. an implied contract

LEARNING APPLICATION

CASE STUDY 1

On a busy afternoon at Inner City Health Care, the reception area is filled with walk-in patients, and the staff struggles to keep up with the patient load. Administrative medical assistant Liz Corbin gives the patient file for Edith Leonard to clinical medical assistant Bruce Goldman. "Dr. Reynolds wants a CBC done stat on the older adult woman in exam room 1," she tells Bruce, handing him the file. Bruce proceeds to examination room 1. Without identifying the patient, he performs a venipuncture on Cele Little, who has come to the clinic for a hearing problem. Cele asks Bruce why the procedure needs to be performed and that she does not want to have it. Bruce insists that Dr. Reynolds has ordered the procedure and performs the venipuncture anyway. The procedure frightens Cele, and she begins to fear that her hearing loss is indicative of a more serious illness.

CASE STUDY REVIEW QUESTIONS

1. What errors were made that could leave the medical assistants and provider vulnerable to litigation?

____

____

____

____

2. How might the errors leave the health care professionals open to potential lawsuits?

____

____

____

____

3. How could the errors have been avoided through effective risk management techniques?

____

____

____

____

____

CASE STUDY 2

Dr. Elizabeth King has just completed a routine physical examination of Abigail Johnson. Elizabeth asks Anna Preciado, RMA, to administer a flu shot to Abigail before the patient leaves the office. Abigail, an older African American woman, is accompanied by her daughter. When Anna attempts to administer the flu vaccine, Abigail says, "Is that a flu shot? They make me sick; I don't want it." Abigail's daughter says, "Yes, she does want it. Go ahead and give it to her." Abigail begins to laugh. "Okay," Anna says, "may I give you the vaccinations?" Abigail says nothing, but she rolls up her sleeve. As Anna administers the parenteral injection, the older woman looks up at her seriously and says, "I didn't want any flu shot. My daughter makes me get it every year." However, Abigail does not withdraw physically.

CASE STUDY REVIEW QUESTIONS

1. What errors were made that could leave the medical assistant and provider vulnerable to litigation?

____

____

____

____

2. How might the errors leave the health care professionals open to potential lawsuits?

____

____

____

____

3. How could the errors have been avoided through effective risk management techniques?

____

____

____

____

____

____

____

____

CASE STUDY 3

Dr. Elizabeth King is going over the daily list of scheduled patients with Ellen Armstrong, CMAS. They are standing at the front desk close to the reception area, and several patients are waiting for the first appointments of the day. Elizabeth's eyes move down the list and stops over the name Mary O'Keefe. "Mary O'Keefe," she mutters, "she's so neurotic and pestering. It's a small wonder her husband hasn't left her yet; just wait till they have that third child. . . . I don't think I have the patience for Mary today."

CASE STUDY REVIEW QUESTIONS

1. What errors were made that could leave the medical assistant and provider vulnerable to litigation?

2. How might the errors leave the health care professionals open to potential lawsuits?

3. How could the errors have been avoided through effective risk management techniques?

CASE STUDY 4

Lydia Renzi, a deaf woman with some residual hearing, comes to Inner City Health Care and has waived her right to a certified sign language interpreter as provided under ADA. She is at the clinic today with a recurrent vaginal discharge. Lydia is diagnosed by Dr. Angie Esposito with candidiasis, a yeast infection caused by the fungus *Candida albicans*. Angie prescribes a vaginal suppository and asks Wanda Slawson, CMA (AAMA), to give Lydia instructions for using the prescription. Lydia wears a hearing aid and has trouble understanding Wanda, who is soft spoken. Wanda is also standing against a brightly lit window, and Lydia has trouble seeing her face. Lydia writes on a pad she has brought with her, "Is this a sexually transmitted illness?" In frustration, Wanda begins shouting, "You just have a yeast infection; it's not like you have herpes or anything." At that moment, another medical assistant, Bruce Goldman, is escorting a male patient past the open door of the examination room. Both men turn their heads away, though it is clear that they have overheard.

CASE STUDY REVIEW QUESTIONS

1. What errors were made that could leave the medical assistants and provider vulnerable to litigation?

____
____
____
____

2. How might the errors leave the health care professionals open to potential lawsuits?

____
____
____
____

3. How could the errors have been avoided through effective risk management techniques?

____
____
____
____
____
____

CASE STUDY 5

Construction workers Jaime Carrera and Ralph Samson are required to take a reemployment drug screening test before they can be hired to work on a new site to which they have applied. Jaime and Ralph come to Inner City Health Care, where urine specimens are collected for examination. The test comes back positive for Jaime, and his potential employer does not give him the job. Ralph tests negative. Two weeks later, Ralph returns to Inner City Health Care for a routine physical examination. "Whatever happened to Jaime Carrera?" Ralph asks Bruce Goldman, CMA (AAMA). "I haven't seen him around the site." "Oh," Bruce replies, "he tested positive for chemical substance abuse, and now he's in a rehab program that Dr. Whitney suggested."

CASE STUDY REVIEW QUESTIONS

1. What errors were made that could leave the medical assistant and provider vulnerable to litigation?

2. How might the errors leave the health care professionals open to potential lawsuits?

3. How could the errors have been avoided through effective risk management techniques?

CHAPTER POST-TEST

Perform this test without looking at your book. If an answer is "false," rewrite the sentence to make it true.

1. True or False? As long as you do not say the patient's name, you may discuss the patient's illnesses and treatments with anyone.

 ____

 ____

2. True or False? The patient–provider contract begins when the patient makes the appointment.

 ____

 ____

3. True or False? If the patient's condition should be treated, the provider is not obligated to care for the patient.

 ____

 ____

4. True or False? Because provider-employers are ultimately responsible for everything medical assistants do under their direction, medical assistants do not have to worry about a "standard of care."

 ____

 ____

SELF-ASSESSMENT

1. Have you ever been in a situation in which you were asked to disclose information about another person that might have been considered confidential? Or have you ever been told confidential information? If this has happened (or if it happens in the future), what should you have done or said? What will you do/say in the future?

 ____

 ____

 ____

 ____

 ____

Name ______________________ Date __________ Score ______

CHAPTER 8

Ethical Considerations

CHAPTER PRE-TEST

Perform this test without looking at your book. If an answer is "false," rewrite the sentence to make it true.

1. True or False? Ethics has to do with what is right and wrong.

____

____

2. True or False? Bioethics has to do with ethical issues dealing with human life.

____

____

3. True or False? When abuse is suspected, the provider and medical assistant have ethical responsibilities to report it.

____

____

4. True or False? When a patient has HIV, the provider may refuse to treat the patient.

____

____

5. True or False? A provider and a medical assistant can refuse to perform abortions.

____

____

VOCABULARY BUILDER

Misspelled Words

Find the words below that are misspelled; circle them, and correctly spell them in the spaces provided. Then insert correct vocabulary terms from the list that best fit into the descriptions below.

bioethics	genetic enginering	microallocation
code of ethics	macroallocation	serrogate
criopreservation		

_______________ _______________ _______________

_______________ 1. Someone who substitutes for another

_______________ 2. Biotechnology dealing with sophisticated medical research regarding the prevention of genetic disorders

_______________ 3. Medical decisions made by Congress, health systems, agencies, and insurance companies

_______________ 4. Set of principles and guidelines usually found in professional organizations

_______________ 5. Medical decisions made individually by providers and the health care team at the local level

_______________ 6. Applying biological systems to technological advances for disease diagnosis, production of medicine, and research

_______________ 7. Ethical issues dealing with life

Word Search

Find the words in the grid below. They may go in any direction.

```
S T R R E S O U R C E S I S V E T
O Y M D C E O W H A T I C S M M E
O G I R O S R E W O P I A A L L N
L O C Y D U A L W S T N C D G E G
A L R T E B A R E E C R H N I C I
C O O S S A O L N A O I I A L L N
I N A P N N Y E L A D S H R I M E
H H L R G O G G L O I E S T O H E
T C L O T L I L G T C A R R E Y R
E E O T N N O S R R M A A S G Q I
O T C E K C T E I M I L T P H W N
I O A C A L V P E C L G L I Y I G
B I T T V D P L R Y E N H P O R P
T B I I A Z I Y M V V D G T N N W
M O O N N D L Y R E S E A R C H R
N X N G E T A G O R R U S N K D D
P C O N F I D E N T I A L I T Y G
```

abuse
advertising
allocation
bioethical
biotechnology
codes
confidentiality
decisions
dilemmas
engineering
ethics
genetics
leadership
macroallocation
microallocation
morally
power
protecting
research
resources
right
surrogate
wrong

LEARNING REVIEW

Code of Ethics Matching

The AAMA Code of Ethics presents five basic principles that medical assistants must pledge to honor as members of the medical assisting profession. For each situation presented, identify the AAMA ethical principle that applies.

A. Render service with full respect for the dignity of humanity
B. Respect confidential information
C. Uphold the honor and integrity of the profession
D. Pursue continuing education activities and improve knowledge and skills
E. Participate in community service and education

____ 1. Marilyn Johnson, CMA (AAMA), in conversation with co–office manager Shirley Brooks, CMA (AAMA), refuses to speculate about whether a diagnosis of AIDS will be confirmed for patient Maria Jover.

____ 2. Administrative medical assistant Karen Ritter joins a study group to prepare for the CMA (AAMA) certification examination as a method of securing her certification credentials, which must be updated every 5 years.

____ 3. Clinical medical assistant Anna Preciado, RMA, agrees to speak to a group of high school students who are interested in pursuing a career in the medical assisting profession.

____ 4. Liz Corbin, CMA (AAMA), politely reminds older adult patient Edith Leonard that she is a certified medical assistant, not a nurse, but assures Edith that she is qualified to perform the instillation of medicated eye drops ordered by Dr. Susan Rice.

____ 5. When patient Dottie Tate makes an appointment at Inner City Health Care for follow-up treatment of chronic back pain and a recent history of frequent falls, Bruce Goldman, CMA (AAMA), arranges for a wheelchair to accommodate Dottie's office visit.

____ 6. Karen Ritter volunteers at the local community office of Planned Parenthood on weekends.

____ 7. Jane O'Hara gently and kindly guides patient Wayne Elder, whose mild retardation often causes him to become confused in unfamiliar settings, back to the proper examination room after she finds him wandering down the hallway in search of Dr. Ray Reynolds.

____ 8. When filing a group of recent laboratory reports into the correct patient files, Ellen Armstrong, CMA (AAMA), takes care to complete the task quickly and efficiently. She performs the task at a private office station away from the general reception area and does not leave the charts open or unattended as she works.

____ 9. Audrey Jones approaches office manager Shirley Brooks, CMA (AAMA), about opportunities for obtaining advanced training to become qualified to perform a wider array of clinical procedures in the ambulatory care setting.

____ 10. Clinical medical assistant Wanda Slawson assists Dr. Mark Woo in the treatment of patient Rhoda Au, who is diagnosed with lupus erythematosus. Wendy believes the patient is foolhardy when she rejects Dr. Woo's treatment plan of Western drug therapy in favor of an approach that integrates traditional Chinese medicine. However, she respects the patient's heritage and right to choose her own health care.

Short Answer

1. According to the *Current Opinions of the Council on Ethical and Judicial Affairs of the AMA,* advertising by health care providers is considered ethical if the ad follows certain requirements. Which of the following are appropriate types of advertisements? Circle the correct responses.

   A. Testimonials from patients cured of serious illnesses or whose conditions were reversed or controlled under the care and treatment of the provider

   B. Providers' credentials and their hospital or community affiliations

   C. A description of the practice, facility hours of operation, and the types of services available to health care consumers

   D. Guarantees of cure promised within a specific time frame

2. Patient medical records are confidential legal documents. Name three instances, however, in which health professionals are allowed or required to reveal confidential patient information by law.

   ____

   ____

   ____

   ____

   ____

3. Issues of bioethics common to every medical clinic are *(circle all that apply):*

   a. allocation of scarce medical resources

   b. genetic engineering or manipulation

   c. many choices surrounding life and death

4. Individuals who are truly aware of their ethical power are able to *(circle all that apply):*

   a. not compromise any procedure or technique

   b. not put the patient at risk

   c. hide the truth regarding a possible error

5. Allocation of scarce resources may refer to *(circle all that apply):*

   a. rationing of health care

   b. denied services

   c. advertising by health care professionals

6. In the case of suspected child abuse, the medical professional should *(circle all that apply):*

   a. report the case

   b. protect and care for the abused

   c. treat the abuser, if known, as a victim also

7. List the five Ps of ethical power.

   ____

   ____

8. List the eight questions adapted from Stephen Covey's book that can be used as guidelines for making ethical decisions.

____

____

____

____

9. List three factors that constitute intimate partner violence. Does your state require that intimate partner violence be reported?

____

____

____

____

____

____

CERTIFICATION REVIEW

These questions are designed to mimic the certification examination. Select the best response.

1. The AAMA Code of Ethics includes all but which one of the following?
   a. We should render service with respect for the dignity of our patients.
   b. We should be paid an equitable salary/wage.
   c. We should respect confidential information.
   d. We should accept the disciplines of the profession.
   e. We should seek to improve our knowledge and skills.
2. Providers may choose who to treat but may not refuse treatment based on certain criteria. Which of the following is untrue?
   a. Providers may not refuse to treat patients based on race, color, religion, or national origin.
   b. It is unethical for a provider to refuse to treat a patient who is HIV-positive.
   c. Providers must inform a patient's family of a patient's death and not delegate that responsibility to others.
   d. Providers who know they are HIV-positive should tell their patients.
   e. Providers should report unethical behaviors committed by other providers.
3. Medical records and information in them are the property of the:
   a. patient
   b. patient and family
   c. provider and patient
   d. provider

4. Once a provider takes a case, the patient cannot be neglected or refused treatment unless:
   a. she did not pay for her last visit
   b. official notice is given from the provider to withdraw from the case
   c. the patient was a no-show
   d. the patient did not keep her last appointment
5. If a provider suspects that an HIV-seropositive patient is infecting an unsuspecting individual:
   a. every attempt should be made to protect the individual at risk
   b. the case should be reported to the CDC
   c. the patient should be dismissed from the practice
   d. the provider should notify the Department of Health
6. When a breach of ethics is about to occur, the health care provider should:
   a. rationalize her actions
   b. disregard the outcome
   c. be encouraged to step back and review his or her actions and their likely consequences
   d. not ask for help
7. Providers who know they are HIV-positive should:
   a. refrain from any activity that would risk transmission of the virus to others
   b. wear a mask
   c. inform the patients
   d. retire
8. Revealing information about patients without consent unless otherwise required to do so by law is:
   a. a breach of confidentiality
   b. bioethics
   c. a conflict of interest
   d. genetic manipulation
9. *Roe v. Wade* refers to guidelines for:
   a. artificial insemination
   b. surrogacy
   c. abortion
   d. fetal tissue transplant

LEARNING APPLICATION

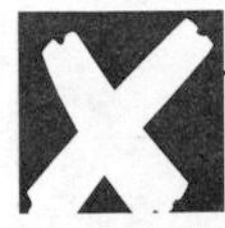

Critical Thinking Discussion

In small groups, explore these questions that were presented in Figure 8-1 and in the text, and present your findings to the class.

1. An increasing number of children live within dysfunctional families where one or more parent is absent, is a substance abuser, or has little time to spend with them. Many children have multiple parents or caregivers. Many spend large parts of the day in a day care environment. Child abuse is a concern. Children must be protected, but can be caught in a web of social services so overloaded and understaffed that only the most severe concerns receive attention. How do health professionals protect these children?
2. Adolescents as young as 14 to 18 years of age may seek treatment for substance abuse, birth control, even abortion without parental consent. Does this violate a parents' right to medical information regarding their children? Should the adolescent, often fearful of parental reaction, have a right to treatment?
3. Adequate and quality health care is a problem. Some adults have no health care coverage; others are part of managed care programs that keep changing as employers seek lower health care premiums. Many adults do not have an ongoing provider–patient relationship. Do medical providers have a responsibility to ensure that the needs of those without medical coverage are met? How can providers care for those without medical coverage in their communities?
4. Scientists have cloned mice, sheep, rabbits, goats, pigs, and a dog. Where does cloning stop? Will human beings be cloned if science moves forward in research with stem cells?

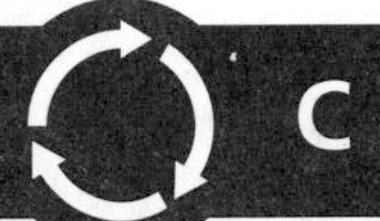

CASE STUDY

Lourdes Austen arrives at the offices of Drs. Lewis and King for her annual physical examination. It has been one year since Lourdes had surgery to remove a tumor in her breast by lumpectomy with axillary lymph node dissection, followed by a course of radiation. Lourdes's one-year mammogram and follow-up examination with her surgeon and radiologist find no evidence of a recurrence of the cancer. Lourdes is a single woman in her late 30s. As Dr. King begins the routine physical examination, assisted by Anna Preciado, RMA, Lourdes begins to cry. "I'm so happy to be alive," Lourdes says. "And so afraid of the cancer coming back. But I want to celebrate life. I've talked to my boyfriend about it and we want to get pregnant. What should I do?" Dr. King takes Lourdes's hand. "I know that living with cancer is hard. You are doing well. There are many things to consider…."

CASE STUDY REVIEW QUESTIONS

1. What bioethical dilemma exists in Lourdes's situation? In your opinion, is Lourdes's choice to become pregnant an ethical one?

____

____

____

____

continues

2. How do deeply held beliefs and attitudes about parenthood and the role of women in our society have an impact on the patient's decision? How could these beliefs have an impact on the health care team's response to Lourdes?

3. What is Dr. King's best therapeutic response to Lourdes? What medical issues should the health care team consider if Lourdes becomes pregnant?

4. What is the role of the medical assistant in this situation?

CHAPTER POST-TEST

Perform this test without looking at your book. If an answer is "false," rewrite the sentence to make it true.

1. True or False? Doing what is right is called ethical behavior.

2. True or False? Ethical issues dealing with human life are called bioethics.

3. True or False? The provider and medical assistant have ethical responsibilities to report suspected abuse.

4. True or False? A provider may refuse to treat an HIV-positive patient.

5. True or False? Whether to perform abortions is a choice each provider and medical assistant can make for themselves.

SELF-ASSESSMENT

1. Identify how you are able to demonstrate the five Ps of ethical power in your own life.

2. There are eight questions adapted from Stephen Covey's book that can be used as guidelines for making ethical decisions. Identify how your life fits into these guidelines and where/if you are striving to do better.

Name ______________________ Date ____________ Score ________

CHAPTER 9

Emergency Procedures and First Aid

CHAPTER PRE-TEST

Perform this test without looking at your book. If an answer is "false," rewrite the sentence to make it true.

1. Of the following, which is the most important in an emergency?
   a. Whether the patient has medical insurance
   b. Whether the patient is HIV-positive
   c. Whether the patient is taking any medication
   d. Whether the patient is breathing
2. The abbreviation ABC stands for:
   a. airway, biodynamics, circulation
   b. airway, bleeding, circulation
   c. airway, breathing, circulation
   d. airway, bleeding, cardiac
3. True or False? As a medical assistant, it is important to know how to respond in emergency situations.

   ____

   ____

4. True or False? A first-degree burn is the worst because it has damaged deeper tissues.

   ____

   ____

5. True or False? Whenever a person has a penetrating object embedded in his or her body, it is important that you remove it as soon as possible so you can treat the wound.

   ____

   ____

VOCABULARY BUILDER

Misspelled Words

Find the key vocabulary words below that are misspelled; circle them, and then correctly spell them in the spaces provided.

anaphalaxis
automated external defibillator
cardioversion
crepidation
explicit
hypothermia
occlusion
sprane
syncopy

______________________ ______________________ ______________________

______________________ ______________________

Word Search

Find the words in the grid below. They may go in any direction.

B E A W A R E E O F Y O U R O W N S A F
E T T R I A G E U Y A S S Y O U C A G Y
R E F O R O T S H C P E R S I N A S R C
N E M E R G P E N R S C Y X X M D T E N
S Y T M L I P R A Z Z E C Q L E Y R E E
Q P H V R Q P I B K K C R H T L S A N G
D C L A R C N W S G Y V O U D M H I S R
N F L I T C O R K Y N G N M Q K O N T E
E D V G N U R V K R N I M X P Q C K I M
G K V N N T V R W I M C H Q X O K T C E
A K L D H M N L S M R D O T W L U D K M
D L S F L M Z S O R J I J P A B T N L Z
N H T T Z C E C P T J A D R E E R D D L
A V G D P R C B R N T T Y Q P R R L K D
B W L R D N D F M Y R S Z T Q K R B D Z
C A R D I A C G W C P R G N I D E E L B
V G E R U T C A R F H I J L N V T Q N N
N O I S S E R P E D L F N K Z J M F M W
F A N A P H Y L A X I S W L N H B N T N
Z D T H Y P O T H E R M I A K T H B K P

anaphylaxis
bandage
bleeding
breathing
cardiac
comminuted
compound
CPR
depression
dressing
emergency
first aid
fracture
greenstick
hypothermia
rescue
shock
spiral
splint
sprain
strain
syncope
wounds

LEARNING REVIEW

Matching I

Identify each of the following terms as an emergency condition (EC), an emergency or first aid procedure performed by health care professionals (EP), emergency equipment (EQ), or an emergency service provided to assist in emergency situations (ES).

___ A. First aid

___ B. Screening

___ C. Syncope

___ D. Shock

___ E. Wounds

___ F. Crash cart

___ G. Occlusion

___ H. Universal emergency medical identification symbol and card

___ I. Hypothermia

___ J. Chest Compressions

___ K. CPR

___ L. Sprain

___ M. Emergency medical service (EMS)

___ N. Fracture

___ O. Splints

___ P. Strain

___ Q. Rescue breathing

Matching II

Match each of the terms in Matching I with its definition below.

___ 1. A break in a bone. There are several types, but all are classified as open or closed.

___ 2. A tray or portable cart that contains medications and supplies needed for emergency and first aid procedures

___ 3. An injury to the soft tissue between joints that involves the tearing of muscles or tendons and occurs often in the neck, back, or thigh muscles

___ 4. A break in the skin or underlying tissues, categorized as open or closed

___ 5. Closure of a passage

___ 6. An injury to a joint, often an ankle, knee, or wrist, that involves a tearing of the ligaments. Most are minor and heal quickly; others are more severe, include swelling, and may not heal properly if the patient continues to put stress on the affected joint.

___ 7. A local network of police, fire, and medical personnel trained to respond to emergency situations. In most communities, the system is activated by calling 911.

___ 8. Identification sometimes carried by individuals to alert to any health problems they might have

___ 9. Any device used to immobilize a body part. Often used by EMS personnel

___ 10. An extremely dangerous cold-related condition that can result in death if the individual does not receive care and if the progression of the condition is not reversed. Symptoms include shivering, cold skin, and confusion.

___ 11. Fainting

___ 12. The immediate care provided to persons who are suddenly ill or injured, typically followed by more comprehensive care and treatment

___ 13. A condition in which the circulatory system is not providing enough blood to all parts of the body, causing the body's organs to fail to function properly

___ 14. The combination of rescue breathing and chest compressions performed by a trained individual on a patient experiencing cardiac arrest

___ 15. To assess patients' conditions and prioritize the need for care

___ 16. Performed on individuals in respiratory arrest, this is a mouth-to-mouth (using appropriate protective equipment) or mouth-to-nose procedure that provides oxygen to the patient until emergency personnel arrive.

___ 17. The combination of rescue breathing and this is known as CPR.

Short Answer

1. To identify the nature of the emergency and respond effectively, what five things must the medical assistant do to screen, or assess, the patient's situation?

____

____

____

____

____

2. What five infection control measures can health care professionals follow to greatly reduce the risk for transmitting infectious disease when providing emergency care?

____

____

____

____

____

3. For each of the patient symptoms or conditions below, identify the type of shock that is most likely.

Patient Symptom/Condition	Type of Shock
Patient suffers heart attack	____________
Patient experiences severe infection after colon surgery	____________
Patient experiences syncope after witnessing a traumatic event	____________
Patient experiences reaction to food allergy	____________
Choking patient has extreme difficulty breathing	____________
Diabetic patient lapses into a coma	____________
Patient has serious head trauma	____________
Accident victim experiences extreme loss of blood	____________

4. A common procedure for treating closed wounds is to RICE them. What do the letters of this acronym stand for?

____

____

5. Match each type of open wound (incision, puncture, laceration, avulsion, abrasion) to its defining characteristics.

Characteristics	**Type of Open Wound**
A wound that pierces and penetrates the skin. This wound may appear insignificant, but actually can go quite deep.	____________
These wounds commonly occur at exposed body parts such as the fingers, toes, and nose. Tissue is torn off and wounds may bleed profusely.	____________
A wound that results from a sharp object such as a scalpel blade.	____________
A painful wound. The epidermal layer of the skin is scraped away.	____________
A wound that results in a jagged tear of body tissues and may contain debris.	____________

6. For each type of wound, describe proper emergency concerns, care, and treatment.

____

____

____

____

____

____

____

____

____

____

____

____

____

____

____

7. Name three sources, other than heat, that can cause burns. For each, describe the proper emergency concerns, care, and treatment.

8. Musculoskeletal injuries, or injuries to muscles, bones, and joints, can be difficult to screen, especially for closed fractures. List five assessment techniques that health care professionals can use to determine the seriousness of musculoskeletal injuries.

9. For each set of symptoms that follows, identify the most likely emergency condition and describe emergency concerns, care, and treatment.

Symptom	Likely Emergency Condition	Emergency Concerns, Care, and Treatment
Off-color, cold skin with a waxy appearance		
Hives, itching, lightheadedness		

Cold, clammy skin; profuse sweating; abdominal cramps; headache; general weakness ____________________ ____

Lightheadedness, weakness, nausea, unsteadiness ____________________ ____

Moist, pale skin; drooling; lack of appetite; diplopia; full pulse ____________________ ____

Numbness in face, arm, and leg on one side of body; slurred speech; nausea and vomiting, loss of vision, severe headache, mental confusion, difficulty breathing and swallowing ____________________ ____

Convulsions, clenched teeth ____________________ ____

Cold, clammy skin; rapid, weak pulse; low blood pressure, shallow breathing; dizziness, faintness, thirst, restlessness, feeling of anxiety; abdomen may be stiff and hard to the touch ____________ ____________

____
____
____
____
____
____

10. Identify the method of entry into the body for each of the following poisons:

____________ 1. Carbon monoxide

____________ 2. Insect stingers

____________ 3. Chemical pesticides used in the garden

____________ 4. Spoiled food

____________ 5. Poison oak

____________ 6. Cleaning fluid fumes

CERTIFICATION REVIEW

These questions are designed to mimic the certification examination. Select the best response.

1. Which of the following is not an appropriate treatment for hypothermia?
   a. Give the victim warm liquids to drink.
   b. Remove any wet clothing.
   c. Rub the victim's skin vigorously to increase circulation.
   d. Use warm water to warm the person if possible.
2. In anaphylactic shock, the patient will:
   a. feel a constriction in the throat and chest
   b. have difficulty breathing
   c. have swelling and tingling of the lips and tongue
   d. All of the above
3. While waiting for EMS to arrive, what should be checked?
   a. Degree of responsiveness
   b. Airway, breathing
   c. Heartbeat (rate and rhythm)
   d. All of the above
4. Closed wounds that are painful and swollen require that a cold compress be applied:
   a. until the victim feels tingling
   b. for 10 minutes, then off for 40 minutes
   c. for 20 minutes, then off for 20 minutes
   d. for at least 1 hour, then off for 2 hours

5. To control nosebleeds, the patient should be seated, the patient's head elevated, and nostrils pinched for:
   a. 10 minutes
   b. 20 minutes
   c. 30 minutes
   d. 40 minutes
6. When a patient calls regarding a poisoning or suspicion of poisoning, the advice to give is to:
   a. call the poison control center
   b. give the patient charcoal
   c. tell the patient to drink milk
   d. flush the mouth with water
7. The best treatment for patients who are experiencing a seizure is to:
   a. restrain them
   b. stick a tongue depressor in their mouth
   c. protect from injury and care for them with understanding
   d. stop the seizure
8. Shock that occurs as a result of overwhelming emotional factors such as fear, anger, or grief is called:
   a. neurogenic
   b. psychogenic
   c. anaphylactic
   d. septic
9. The type of burn that may occur resulting in an entrance and exit burn wound area is:
   a. chemical
   b. electrical
   c. solar radiation
   d. explosion
10. In burn depth classifications, third-degree burns are also called:
   a. superficial
   b. full thickness
   c. partial thickness
   d. sunburns
11. The type of fracture often caused by falling on an outstretched hand that involves the distal end of the radius is called:
   a. greenstick
   b. spiral
   c. Colles
   d. implicated

12. Jaw and left shoulder pain; a rapid, weak pulse; excessive perspiration; and cold, clammy skin may be symptomatic of:
    a. seizure
    b. heart attack
    c. stroke
    d. sepsis

LEARNING APPLICATION

Screening Activity

In an urgent care setting, two or more patients may present with emergency symptoms. The order in which emergency patients will receive care depends on the health care professionals' abilities to screen patients' symptoms to determine who needs care most urgently. The following five patients present simultaneously on New Year's Eve at Inner City Health Care, an urgent care center. Office manager Walter Seals, CMA (AAMA), is working the evening shift with Dr. Mark Woo. In what order will Walter and Mark screen the priority of treatment? Number the patients 1 (most urgent) through 5 to correspond to the urgency of their conditions.

Patient	Urgency
Patient A presents with a gunshot wound to the leg that is bleeding severely. The patient is conscious but his pupils are dilated and he is unable to answer simple questions put to him by Walter and Dr. Woo. He cradles his right arm and will not let anyone touch it, although there is no immediate evidence of an open wound to the arm.	_______
Patient B, an elderly man, is brought in by his grandson. He describes debilitating chest pains, difficulty breathing, and nausea after eating a large family dinner. The patient's medical record indicates that he has a hiatal hernia, slipped disks, high blood pressure, and mild angina. The man is walking and speaking with moderate distress and is extremely anxious.	_______
Patient C, a young woman, presents with her boyfriend. She appears to have multiple abrasions on her right palm and knee, with damage to the right knee and ankle joints sustained after a fall while on in-line skates. Both joints are swollen and painful.	_______
Patient D, a man in his mid-30s, presents with the cotton tip of a swab stuck in his ear canal. Although the man feels a dull consistent pain in the ear, he says he has no trouble hearing. The outside of the ear appears normal, there is no bleeding evident, and the man appears annoyed but not distressed.	_______
Patient E, a young woman, presents with a group of friends, all college students, with an eye injury sustained by a champagne cork. The cork, which had a metal covering over its tip, hit the patient's eye. The young woman's eye is red and tearing and she is experiencing severe pain in the eye.	_______

CASE STUDY 1

Mary O'Keefe calls Dr. King's office in a panic. Ellen Armstrong, CMA (AAMA), answers the telephone.

Mary: "Oh my God, help me. I need Dr. King."
Ellen: "This is Ellen Armstrong. Who is this calling? What is the situation?"
Mary: "It's my baby, oh God, get Dr. King."
Ellen: "Dr. King is unavailable, but we can help you. Now, tell me your name."
Mary: "It's Mary O'Keefe. Help me, I think my baby is dead."
Ellen: "Are you at home?"
Mary: "Yes."
Ellen: "Good. Tell me what's happened."
Mary: "My son Chris pried the plug off an outlet and he's electrocuted himself!" Mary cries. "He's just lying there. I'm so scared, if I touch him, will I electrocute myself? Oh my God, my baby, my baby. What should I do?"

Ellen, who has been writing down the details on a piece of paper, motions to Joe Guerrero, another CMA (AAMA) in the office, and hands him her notes. Joe immediately accesses the O'Keefe address from the patient database and uses another telephone to call EMS with the nature of the emergency situation and directions to the O'Keefe residence. Meanwhile, Ellen remains on the line with Mary. Dr. King is on rounds at the hospital this morning and will not be in the office for at least another hour.

Ellen: "Mary, we are calling EMS, and they will be there as soon as possible. In the meantime, I'm going to need you to focus and answer my questions, okay?"

CASE STUDY REVIEW QUESTIONS

1. What steps did the medical assistant take to screen the emergency situation?

____

____

____

____

____

____

2. What questions should Ellen ask Mary regarding the emergency situation?

____

____

____

____

____

continues

3. What should the medical assistant do after EMS arrives and takes over emergency care? What follow-up procedures are necessary?

CASE STUDY 2

Lenore McDonell, a wheelchair-bound woman in her early 30s, experiences a serious laceration to the right arm sustained from a fall while performing an independent transfer from the examination table to her wheelchair. Joe Guerrero, CMA (AAMA), assists Dr. Winston Lewis in administering emergency care.

CASE STUDY REVIEW QUESTIONS

1. What Standard Precautions must the health care professionals follow before administering emergency treatment?

2. Joe and Dr. Lewis attempt to control Lenore's bleeding by applying a dressing and pressing firmly. When the bleeding does not stop, what two actions should the health care professionals perform?

continues

3. In the unlikely event that bleeding continues, what piece of medical equipment will the health care team use in substitution for a tourniquet? Why is this alternative equipment effective and widely used today?

4. The bleeding stops, and Joe applies a pressure bandage over the dressing. This patient is prone to fractures, and a radiograph will need to be taken. What is the next emergency procedure Dr. Lewis will perform? Why is this procedure necessary, and what equipment will the provider and medical assistant require?

5. Before applying a sling, what do the health care professionals check to be sure that the medical equipment used has not been too tightly applied?

6. What Standard Precautions will the health care team follow after the emergency treatment of the patient is successfully completed?

7. What information will the health care team include in documenting the procedure for the patient's medical record?

Research Activity

Using a medical encyclopedia or reference such as the *Physician's Desk Reference* (PDR), describe the following emergency medications and identify potential uses for each. Remember that only a provider can order medications or treatment.

Lidocaine: ______________________________

____

Verapamil: ______________________________

____

Atropine: ______________________________

____

____

____

Insulin: ______________________________

____

Nitroglycerin: ______________________________

____

Marcaine: ______________________________

____

Diphenhydramine: ______________________________

____

Diazepam: ______________________________

____

CHAPTER POST-TEST

Perform this test without looking at your book. If an answer is "false," rewrite the sentence to make it true.

1. Of the following, which is the most important in an emergency?
   a. Whether the patient has medical insurance
   b. Whether the patient is HIV-positive
   c. Whether the patient is taking any medication
   d. Whether the patient is breathing
2. ABC stands for:
   a. airway, biodynamics, circulation
   b. airway, bleeding, circulation
   c. airway, breathing, circulation
   d. airway, bleeding, cardiac

3. True or False? As a medical assistant, you should be prepared to respond to small-scale and large-scale emergency situations.

____

____

4. True or False? A first-degree burn is the worst because it has damaged deeper tissues.

____

____

5. True or False? Whenever a penetrating object has been embedded in a person's body, it is important that you remove it as soon as possible so you can treat the wound.

____

____

SELF-ASSESSMENT

1. A. On a scale of 1 to 5, rate your personal comfort in regard to the following emergency situations that medical assistants may find themselves involved with in an ambulatory or urgent care setting.

   1 = extremely uncomfortable   4 = comfortable

   2 = uncomfortable   5 = very comfortable

   3 = somewhat comfortable

   ______ Assisting in treatment of patients with injuries clearly sustained by an act of violence or abuse

   ______ Administering back blows and thrusts to a conscious infant

   ______ Performing rescue breathing on someone who has poor personal hygiene

   ______ Bandaging the open wound of an HIV-infected person

   ______ Caring for a person experiencing a seizure

   ______ Administering care to a patient who faints after venipuncture

   ______ Administering care to a patient in extreme pain

   ______ Administering care to a patient who is verbally abusive or uncooperative

2. On a scale of 1 to 5, rate your level of agreement with the statements that follow.

1 = never   4 = most of the time

2 = occasionally   5 = all of the time

3 = sometimes

_____ Life-threatening emergencies frighten me.

_____ I respond well under pressure.

_____ I am bothered by the sight of blood.

_____ I lose my temper easily, becoming openly frustrated and angry.

_____ I become frustrated and overwhelmed by feelings of helplessness in emergency situations.

_____ I remain calm and clearheaded in emergency situations.

_____ I forget about myself completely and focus on the emergency victim.

_____ I am concerned about administering care in emergency situations in which danger to myself may exist when giving such care.

_____ I am comfortable speaking to the family or friends of emergency victims.

Name ______________________ Date __________ Score ______

CHAPTER **10**

Infection Control and Medical Asepsis

CHAPTER PRE-TEST

Perform this test without looking at your book. If an answer is "false," rewrite the sentence to make it true.

1. The single most important action you can take to avoid acquiring communicable diseases is to:

   a. not mingle with people in crowded areas

   b. wear a mask when in public

   c. wear gloves at all times

   d. wash hands frequently

2. To sanitize something means literally to:

   a. wash and rinse well

   b. sterilize it

   c. disinfect it

   d. wipe it off

3. True or False? The difference between sterilizing and disinfecting is that sterilization gets rid of all microbes and their spores, whereas disinfection gets rid of surface microbes, but not their spores.

   ____

   ____

4. Epidemiology is the study of:

   a. communicable diseases only

   b. diseases and other conditions and their patterns

   c. *epi-*, or surfaces

   d. bugs

5. The word *pathogen* means:

   a. all "germs" or microorganisms

   b. bacteria and viruses only

   c. only those microorganisms that cause diseases

   d. all of the above

VOCABULARY BUILDER

Misspelled Words

Find the words below that are misspelled; circle them, and correctly spell them in the spaces provided. Then insert one of the correct vocabulary terms into the sentences below. Each word will be used once.

contaminated	infection control	sanitization
ecoriated	medical asepsis	transmision
epidemology	microorganisms	

_______________ _______________ _______________

1. ___________________________ is the study of the history, cause, and patterns of infectious diseases.

2. Microscopic living creatures, also known as ___________________________, that are capable of causing disease are called pathogens. The spread of infectious diseases can occur through direct contact, indirect contact, inhalation, ingestion, or bloodborne contact.

3. ___________________________ refers to various methods, including the CDC's Standard Precautions, that health care professionals use to eliminate or reduce the risk of spreading disease.

4. Spreading disease is another way of describing the ___________________________ of infectious microorganisms from one person to another.

5. ___________________________ involves specific techniques that are designed to destroy pathogens after they leave the body and to decrease the risk for spreading infection to others.

6. To reduce the risk that any item, including equipment, surgical trays, and instruments, could be ____________ or exposed to microorganisms or infectious material, various sterilization techniques are used.

7. Before instruments or other fomites are disinfected or sterilized, they must be scrubbed or cleaned and rinsed to remove tissue, debris, or other impurities that may harbor pathogens, a process called __________________.

8. Medically aseptic hand washing techniques should be performed on a regular basis to ensure the reduction of pathogens spread by the hands. To reduce the risk for chapped, ___________________________ skin, medical assistants can apply water-based antibacterial lotion to the hands after washing.

Matching

Match the following terms with the correct definitions.

amoebic dysentery
bloodborne pathogen
fomites
infectious agent
malaria
palliative
pathogen
scabies
trichomoniasis

_______________ 1. Infection with a *Trichomonas* parasite, which can be transmitted through sexual intercourse

_______________ 2. Infectious skin disease caused by the itch mite, *Sarcoptes scabiei,* which is transmitted by direct contact with infected persons

_______________ 3. An agent that relieves only symptoms of the disease instead of curing the infection

_______________ 4. A pathogen responsible for a specific infectious disease

_______________ 5. Infectious intestinal disease characterized by inflammation of the mucous membrane of the colon and diarrhea

_______________ 6. Any microorganism capable of causing disease found in blood or components of blood

_______________ 7. Infectious disease caused by protozoan parasites within red blood cells; transmitted to humans by female mosquitoes

_______________ 8. Substances that absorb and transmit infectious material, that is, contaminated items such as equipment

_______________ 9. Any disease-producing microorganism

Definitions

Write a brief definition for each correct vocabulary term.

1. Resistance:

____

____

2. Vaccine:

____

____

3. Antibody:

____

____

4. Immunoglobulins:

____

____

5. Immunity:

____

____

6. Disinfection:

____

____

7. Antigen:

____

____

Word Search

Find the words in the grid below. They may go in any direction.

```
H P B F H X V L N O I T A Z I T I N A S S P
V A L N V C H N P K D C K D R B N L F W T R
T N I D I S I N F E C T I O N L M M P J E E
J T N D D G T K F L L P Q P N Y Y V K M R V
N I F E N R O B D O O L B G O S A L X M I E
O B L T J T K L D I S E A S E C P H M D L N
I I A A P A T H O G E N J T C K S R G L I T
T O M N T C O N T R O L B I L M Y O E K Z I
C T M I A Y S U R I V M N M K H H N R A E O
E I A M Y I R R T J K E I V A P O L V C D N
T C T A C T R V Y C S C B N N I K S N L I W
O S I T T V T E I G R Y D Q S G S U O N M M
R H O N T X Q T T O O W D S L N Y R I J M S
P L N O M A P A O C A L I N O L S G T H U U
X Z H C T E S R U S A M O I X R Z I C K N G
B P G N S T G E H T S B T I E L X C E B I N
R X X I P A R I P N O U H I M R T A F R Z U
L K T J N G N P A S A C R L D E M L N J A F
T N Z I P G Q R Q C I R L R W H D W I K T F
A P S J M H T H E L A S M A X M Z I D M I Y
B M L Y N H F R N B R L Z B V V M T P D O K
S T X R H G P Y Q K L G L M X E H V M E N Z
```

antibiotics
antiseptic
asepsis
autoclave
bacteria
barriers
bloodborne
contaminated
control
disease
disinfection
epidemiology
fungus
hand washing
immunization
infection
inflammation
microorganisms
microscopic
pathogen
precautions
prevention
protection
sanitization
spread
sterilize
transmission
vaccines
virus

LEARNING REVIEW

Fill in the Blanks

Immunity is defined as the ability of the body to resist disease. Identify the correct terms or the specific form of immunity that may occur in response to specific antigens.

1. The immune response that involves T cells and B cells to attack viruses, fungi, organ transplants, or cancer cells is called ______________________________.

2. The immune response that produces antibodies to kill pathogens and recognize them in the future is called ______________________________.

3. The immunity that follows the administration of vaccines is called ______________________________.

4. The short-term immunity provided to a newborn that occurs when antibodies pass to a fetus from the mother is called ______________________________.

5. The immunity that results from contracting an infectious agent and experiencing either an acute or a subclinical infectious disease is called ______________________________.

6. The immunity achieved through administration of ready-made antibodies, such as gamma-globulin, is called ______________________________.

Short Answer

1. The following are the five common stages of many infectious diseases: acute, prodromal, declining, convalescent, incubation. Place the stages in the proper order in the table below, starting with initial infection with a pathogen, and then describe the identifying characteristics and symptoms associated with each.

Order	Stage	Characteristics and Symptoms
1	__________	______________________________
2	__________	______________________________
3	__________	______________________________

4 ______ ______

5 ______ ______

2. For each vaccine listed below, identify the disease for which the vaccine provides immunity.

Vaccine	Disease
DTaP	______
HBV	______
MMR	______
Hib	______
IPV	______

3. A susceptible host is a person who is not resistant or immune to a pathogenic organism and is, therefore, able to contract the pathogenic organism and experience development of an infection. List the five reasons a person may be susceptible.

______

4. Susceptibility of a person depends on several factors, such as occupation or lifestyle environment, youth or advanced age, poor psychological health, poor physical condition, presence of underlying disease, the number of pathogens exposed to, and the duration of exposure. For each example given, identify the correct factor of susceptibility.

Example	Susceptibility Factor
A. Dr. Angie Esposito is physically worn down by working double shifts at Inner City Health Care. Although she loves the excitement of working intensely with patients in an urgent care setting, flu season is coming and Dr. Esposito is worried that she will become ill.	______
B. Significantly overweight and a heavy smoker, Herb Fowler is prone to colds that just will not go away; Dr. Winston Lewis is treating Herb for a case of chronic bronchitis.	______
C. Mary O'Keefe's 3-year-old son, Chris, and several other members of his play group come down with chickenpox after playing with a child infected with the disease, caused by the varicella zoster virus.	______
D. Pneumocystis pneumonia is an infection common to patients who have full-blown cases of AIDS.	______
E. Jim Marshall, stressed out by the pressure to complete an architectural design ahead of schedule and on a tight budget, is depressed and angry when he gets laid up with the flu and misses two days of work.	______

F. Margaret Thomas's college-age niece is caught in an epidemic of scabies that sweeps through her dorm floor and places the students in temporary isolation until the outbreak is controlled. ______________________________

G. While vacationing at a remote spot in Mexico, Bill Schwartz eats almost a pound of shrimp at a local restaurant; the next day, he experiences severe diarrhea and vomiting. He is diagnosed with cholera, caused by the *Vibrio cholerae* bacterium harbored in the shellfish he ate. ______________________________

5. For each infectious disease listed below, identify the agent of transmission (virus, bacteria, fungus, etc.), at least one route of transmission, and common symptoms.

Disease	Agent	Route	Symptoms
AIDS			
TB			
Gastroenteritis			
Hepatitis B			
Chickenpox			
Influenza			

6. Describe three methods of medical asepsis used to reduce the presence of pathogens in an ambulatory care setting.

____
____
____
____
____
____
____

7. Place an X next to each statement below that represents the appropriate use of medical asepsis in the ambulatory care setting.

____ Joe Guerrero, CMA (AAMA), washes his hands before performing the transfer of patient Lenore McDonell from the wheelchair to the examination table.

____ Wanda Slawson, CMA (AAMA), runs a clean sheet of disposable paper over the examination table to prepare the room for the next patient. She picks up the cloth gown that she does not think patient Lydia Renzi used and places it on the examination table for the next patient to use.

____ After performing a venipuncture procedure on patient Leo McKay, Bruce Goldman, CMA (AAMA), tells Leo he can just dispose of the gauze pad he has been holding on the venipuncture site in the trash can.

____ Anna Preciado, CMA (AAMA), moving quickly to assist a patient who may be about to faint, accidentally bumps into a sterile tray of instruments, knocking some of them to the floor. The patient, who is bent over in front of Anna, picks the instruments up off the floor and places them back on the tray in the sterile field. "You dropped these," he says.

____ After assisting in the removal of an infected sebaceous cyst from a patient, clinical medical assistant Audrey Jones cleans, dresses, and bandages the wound as directed by Dr. Winston Lewis. She then disposes of all contaminated items following Standard Precautions and OSHA guidelines, and properly removes personal protective equipment (PPE), removes her gloves, and washes her hands.

8. For each item in Question 7 that does not reflect proper techniques of medical asepsis, explain what went wrong and how the error should be corrected.

____
____
____
____
____
____
____
____
____
____
____

CERTIFICATION REVIEW

These questions are designed to mimic the certification examination. Select the best response.

1. Susceptibility to an infectious microorganism depends on all of the following *except:*
   a. number and specific types of pathogens
   b. duration of exposure to the pathogen
   c. indirect contact
   d. general physical condition
2. The body's natural way of responding when invaded by a pathogen is:
   a. inflammation
   b. septicemia
   c. immunosuppression
   d. immunization
3. The greatest natural barrier is:
   a. intact skin
   b. cilia
   c. hydrochloric acid
   d. mucous membranes
4. Specialized antibodies that can render a pathogen unable to reproduce or continue to grow are called:
   a. antigens
   b. immunoglobulins
   c. pathogenic toxins
   d. spores

LEARNING APPLICATIONS

Hands-on Activities

Complete the following forms with the indicated information.

1. You tested the eyewash station on the first of this month. Complete the Eyewash Testing Log below in the next space.

Tested by:	Date	Assessment Action taken
Janie Carter, RN	August 14, 20xx	Flushed until clear, working appropriately.
B. Abbott, RMA	September 16, 20xx	Flushed until clear, working properly.
Joe Guerrero, CMA (AAMA)	October 10, 20xx	Flushed until clear, working appropriately.

2. You checked the emergency cleanup spill kits in all your exam rooms and in the clinical laboratory. You made sure they were complete, had not expired, were intact without tears, and were ready to use when needed. Make notation of your checks on the following form.

Location	Checked by	Date	Assessment - Action Taken
Exam Room #1			
Exam Room #2			
Exam Room #3			
Lab Staion #1			
Lab Kit #2			

3. You were exposed to a patient's blood through an accidental needlestick. Fill out the following form.

OSHA's Form 301
Injury and Illness Incident Report

Attention: This form contains information relating to employee health and must be used in a manner that protects the confidentiality of employees to the extent possible while the information is being used for occupational safety and health purposes.

U.S. Department of Labor
Occupational Safety and Health Administration

Form approved OMB no. 1218-0176

This *Injury and Illness Incident Report* is one of the first forms you must fill out when a recordable work-related injury or illness has occurred. Together with the *Log of Work-Related Injuries and Illnesses* and the accompanying *Summary*, these forms help the employer and OSHA develop a picture of the extent and severity of work-related incidents.

Within 7 calendar days after you receive information that a recordable work-related injury or illness has occurred, you must fill out this form or an equivalent. Some state workers' compensation, insurance, or other reports may be acceptable substitutes. To be considered an equivalent form, any substitute must contain all the information asked for on this form.

According to Public Law 91-596 and 29 CFR 1904, OSHA's recordkeeping rule, you must keep this form on file for 5 years following the year to which it pertains.

If you need additional copies of this form, you may photocopy and use as many as you need.

Completed by ______________________

Title ______________________

Phone (______)______-________ Date ____/____/____

Information about the employee

1) Full name ______________________

2) Street ______________________

City ______________ State ______ ZIP ______

3) Date of birth ____/____/____

4) Date hired ____/____/____

5) ☐ Male
☐ Female

Information about the physician or other health care professional

6) Name of physician or other health care professional ______________________

7) If treatment was given away from the worksite, where was it given?

Facility ______________________

Street ______________________

City ______________ State ______ ZIP ______

8) Was employee treated in an emergency room?
☐ Yes
☐ No

9) Was employee hospitalized overnight as an in-patient?
☐ Yes
☐ No

Information about the case

10) Case number from the *Log* ______________ *(Transfer the case number from the Log after you record the case.)*

11) Date of injury or illness ____/____/____

12) Time employee began work ______________ AM / PM

13) Time of event ______________ AM / PM ☐ Check if time cannot be determined

14) ***What was the employee doing just before the incident occurred?*** Describe the activity, as well as the tools, equipment, or material the employee was using. Be specific. *Examples:* "climbing a ladder while carrying roofing materials"; "spraying chlorine from hand sprayer"; "daily computer key-entry."

15) ***What happened?*** Tell us how the injury occurred. *Examples:* "When ladder slipped on wet floor, worker fell 20 feet"; "Worker was sprayed with chlorine when gasket broke during replacement"; "Worker developed soreness in wrist over time."

16) ***What was the injury or illness?*** Tell us the part of the body that was affected and how it was affected; be more specific than "hurt," "pain," or sore." *Examples:* "strained back"; "chemical burn, hand"; "carpal tunnel syndrome."

17) ***What object or substance directly harmed the employee?*** *Examples:* "concrete floor"; "chlorine"; "radial arm saw." *If this question does not apply to the incident, leave it blank.*

18) ***If the employee died, when did death occur?*** Date of death ____/____/____

Public reporting burden for this collection of information is estimated to average 22 minutes per response, including time for reviewing instructions, searching existing data sources, gathering and maintaining the data needed, and completing and reviewing the collection of information. Persons are not required to respond to the collection of information unless it displays a current valid OMB control number. If you have any comments about this estimate or any other aspects of this data collection, including suggestions for reducing this burden, contact: US Department of Labor, OSHA Office of Statistical Analysis, Room N-3644, 200 Constitution Avenue, NW, Washington, DC 20210. Do not send the completed forms to this office.

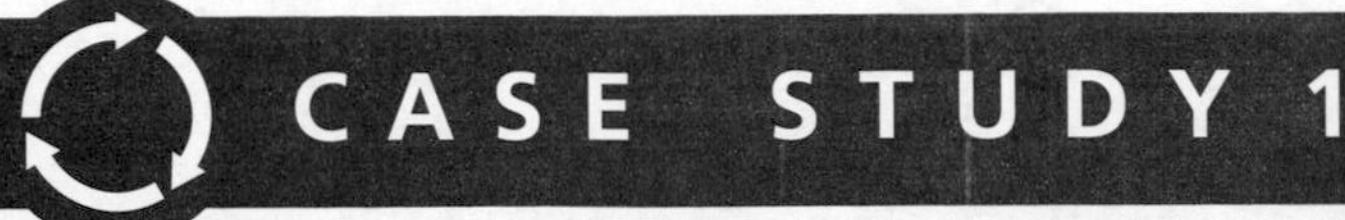

CASE STUDY 1

Veronica Hernandez, a medical assisting intern at the Northborough Family Medical Group of Drs. Winston Lewis and Elizabeth King, attends to patient procedures and examinations under the supervision of office manager Jacquie Cavanaugh, CMA (AAMA). Although Veronica is careful to follow all infection control methods during patient care, severe dermatitis has developed on her hands. She is concerned that this condition, which has not responded to creams and lotions, is related to the latex gloves she wears during procedures.

CASE STUDY REVIEW QUESTIONS

1. Discuss the possible causes of Veronica's symptoms.

____

____

____

____

____

2. Suggest a course of action that both addresses Veronica's condition and maintains the proper degree of asepsis.

____

____

____

____

____

CASE STUDY 2

One-year-old Marissa O'Keefe is a patient at the practice of Drs. Lewis and King. During her well-baby check, Joe Guerrero, CMA (AAMA), gives Marissa an MMR vaccination and is about to administer the DTaP when Marissa's mother voices concerns about the safety of the vaccinations.

CASE STUDY REVIEW QUESTIONS

1. Should Joe continue to administer the DTaP even though the mother is concerned?

____

____

____

____

____

continues

2. What is Joe's best therapeutic response?

____

____

____

____

____

____

____

CHAPTER POST-TEST

Perform this test without looking at your book. If an answer is "false," rewrite the sentence to make it true.

1. The single most important action you can take to avoid contracting a communicable disease is to:
   a. mingle with people in crowded areas so you create immunities
   b. wear a mask when in public
   c. wear gloves at all times
   d. wash hands frequently
2. Disinfection is a way to:
   a. clean hands
   b. prepare the patient's skin for surgery
   c. clean inanimate objects, such as countertops
   d. sterilize
3. True or False? The difference between sterilizing and disinfecting is that disinfection gets rid of all microbes and their spores, whereas sterilization gets rid of all surface microbes, but not their spores.

   ____

   ____
4. Epidemiology is:
   a. the study of communicable diseases only
   b. the study of diseases and other conditions and their patterns
   c. the study of *epi-*, or surfaces
   d. the study of bugs
5. The word *pathogen* means:
   a. all "germs" or microorganisms
   b. viruses only
   c. only those microorganisms that cause diseases
   d. all of the above

SELF-ASSESSMENT

As you answer the following questions, think about how you have changed your awareness of disease prevention because of what you have learned in this chapter.

1. Are you always 100% careful to wash your hands after using the restroom?

2. How does it make you feel when you see others leaving a public restroom without washing their hands?

3. Are you always careful to wash your hands just before eating? Even if you are in a car and there is not a sink handy? What can you do in that case?

4. Besides washing your hands and avoiding direct contact with sick people, what do you suppose is the other single most important action you can take to stay healthy?

5. Do you think stress can make you sick? If so, how do you suppose that happens?

Name ______________________ Date __________ Score ______

CHAPTER 11

The Patient History and Documentation

CHAPTER PRE-TEST

Perform this test without looking at your book. If an answer is "false," rewrite the sentence to make it true.

1. True or False? To "diagnose" is to give a name to the condition or disease a patient has.

____

____

2. True or False? Subjective statements can be described as "opinion."

____

____

3. When a patient "complains" of something, he or she is:

   a. just whining

   b. filing a lawsuit

   c. explaining his or her symptoms

   d. gossiping

4. True or False? Once a medical assistant has asked a patient whether he or she has any allergies, and the information has been recorded, the medical assistant does not need to keep asking.

____

____

5. True or False? If a disease is familial, that means it is communicable to close family members living in the same house.

____

____

VOCABULARY BUILDER

Misspelled Words

Find the words below that are misspelled; circle them, and correctly spell them in the spaces provided. Then, insert one of the correct vocabulary terms into the sentences below. Each word will be used once.

allergy's	clinical diagnosus	SOAP
chart	famileal	SOMR
CHEDDAR	objective	subjective
chief complaint	POMR	

______________ ______________ ______________

1. The ________________________ is the main reason the patient has come to the doctor.
2. ________________________ diseases are those diseases or conditions with genetic links such as breast and colon cancers, coronary artery disease, diabetes mellitus, and hypertension.
3. Mary O'Keefe calls Dr. King's office to schedule an emergency appointment and tells Ellen Armstrong, CMA (AAMA), that her 3-year-old son Chris awakened during the night with extreme pain in his right ear. This is a ________________________ complaint, as it is known by the patient but cannot be seen or measured by the provider.
4. Dr. King examines 3-year-old Chris O'Keefe's right ear with an otoscope and observes that the ear is inflamed; the ear is also draining. Since these conditions can be visualized, they are called ________________________ signs.
5. When a 19-year-old young woman comes into Inner City Health Care with extreme abdominal pain localized to the lower right quadrant, vomiting, slight fever, and loss of appetite, Dr. Whitney orders a CBC, a urinalysis, and an abdominal ultrasound to determine a ________________________ between possible diagnoses of acute appendicitis and an ovarian cyst.
6. Dr. Whitney confirms a ________________________ of acute appendicitis for the female emergency patient, based on subjective and objective information from the patient's history, the findings of the physical examination, and the results of the laboratory tests ordered.
7. A patient's file containing medical history and treatments kept by the provider is called the patient ________________________.
8. ________________________ is a traditional form of charting that consists of a chronological set of notes for each visit, beginning with the patient's first visit.
9. The charting method that lists patient data in the following order: subjective, objective, assessment, plan, is referred to as ________________________ charting.
10. Acquired abnormal immune responses to substances (allergens) that do not normally cause reactions are called ________________________.
11. The most efficient way of recording chart notes, especially in multiprovider clinics or practices, is ________________________.
12. ________________________ is another more comprehensive approach to charting, which encourages greater detail to SOAP/SOAPER.

LEARNING REVIEW

Reading Chart Notes

1/10/XX CC: NVD x 4 days. T: 100°F for 2 days. Loss of appetite.

1. Write what this chart note means.

____

____

____

2. A mistake has been made in the chart note above: three days should be listed instead of four. Using proper procedure for correcting a paper chart, correct the note.

____

____

3. To practice charting, translate the following statements (A through H) into medical terms as you would document it in a patient's medical record. Use the lines provided.

   A. The patient was examined on January 12, 20XX at Ten fifteen in the morning.

   ____

   ____

   B. The patient says she has had lower abdominal pain on the left side for a week and has been feeling more and more tired.

   ____

   ____

   C. Weight is 135 pounds. Height is 5 feet 4 inches. Temperature is 99.8°F, slightly elevated above normal. Respiration is 19 breaths per minute and is clear. Pulse is 78 beats per minute and is regular. Blood pressure reading is 134 (systolic)/82 (diastolic).

   ____

   ____

   D. The patient describes an increasing urge to urinate with a burning sensation upon urination; pressure in abdomen; lack of energy.

   ____

   ____

   E. The patient has a medical history that is positive for frequent urinary tract infections. The patient was diagnosed with type II diabetes mellitus in 1987 and takes a prescribed dosage of 3 mg of Glynase orally daily in tablet form. The patient quit smoking 20 years ago and has lost 10 pounds in the last 2 years.

   ____

   ____

   ____

F. The patient has no known allergies.

G. There is no change in family history.

H. The patient has less than two glasses of wine per week, does not smoke, and exercises regularly.

Short Answer

1. Every provider/patient interview is a cross-cultural one. List four questions a medical assistant might ask while taking a medical history that would help bridge social and cultural beliefs to obtain accurate information about a patient's condition that the provider will need to give proper care and treatment.

2. List eight possible characteristics of chief complaints.

3. After the history is taken by the medical assistant, the provider will perform a review of systems (ROS). In addition to the patient's general state of health, list 10 body systems the provider will assess during the ROS.

4. True or False? Charts (medical records) belong to the provider, and nobody has a right to see them without a court order.

5. True or False? Abbreviations of medical terms can be confusing from institution to institution, so the Joint Commission has actually created a list of "forbidden" abbreviations.

CERTIFICATION REVIEW

These questions are designed to mimic the certification examination. Select the best response.

1. Which is *not* a component of SOAP charting?
   a. Subjective information
   b. Assessment of symptoms
   c. Symptoms
   d. Plan for treatment
2. POMR stands for:
   a. privacy of medical records
   b. problem-oriented medical record
   c. payment of medical resources
   d. parts of medical records
3. The medical history form includes the social history, medical history, family history, review of systems, and:
   a. insurance information
   b. chief complaint
   c. provider's history
   d. diagnosis and prognosis
4. Primary administrative information includes the patient's full name, telephone numbers, insurance information, and:
   a. addresses
   b. date of birth
   c. vital signs
   d. a. and b.
5. The Continuity of Care Record (CCR):
   a. ensures that a minimum standard of information is to be shared with other providers
   b. will have no effect on the amount of errors made in the patient's chart
   c. is being established by the American Academy of Gerontologists
   d. can be completed only by providers
   e. All of the above

LEARNING APPLICATION

Hands-on Activities

1. Interview students from your school's English-as-a-Second-Language program or someone for whom English is not the primary language. Have them describe diseases or conditions that have bothered them in the past or are bothering them now. Discuss the following questions with classmates:

   a. Was there a problem with communication because of the language differences?

   ____

   ____

   ____

   b. What types of creative communication methods did you use?

   ____

   ____

   ____

   c. Did you find that some people can read another language better than they can "hear" it (or vice-versa)?

   ____

   ____

   ____

2. On a separate piece of paper decode each component of Figure 11-8 in your textbook. Put all the information in lay terms and write out all the abbreviations.

3. Pretend you are a patient and complete the following Health History Questionnaire. You should use "made up" information to protect your privacy, but be sure to put your real name on it for clarification. With another student, take turns role-playing as medical assistant and patient using the forms you have filled out.

CONFIDENTIAL HEALTH HISTORY

Name: ______________________ Date: __________

Birthdate: __________ Age: ______ Date of last physical examination: __________

Occupation: ______________________

Reason for visit today: ______________________

MEDICATIONS List all medications you are currently taking	**ALLERGIES** List all allergies

SYMPTOMS Check (✓) symptoms you currently have or have had in the past year.

GENERAL

- ☐ Chills
- ☐ Depression
- ☐ Dizziness
- ☐ Fainting
- ☐ Fever
- ☐ Forgetfulness
- ☐ Headache
- ☐ Loss of sleep
- ☐ Loss of weight
- ☐ Nervousness
- ☐ Numbness
- ☐ Sweats

MUSCLE/JOINT/BONE

Pain, weakness, numbness in:

- ☐ Arms
- ☐ Back
- ☐ Feet
- ☐ Hands
- ☐ Hips
- ☐ Legs
- ☐ Neck
- ☐ Shoulders

GENITO-URINARY

- ☐ Blood in urine
- ☐ Frequent urination
- ☐ Lack of bladder control
- ☐ Painful urination

GASTROINTESTINAL

- ☐ Appetite poor
- ☐ Bloating
- ☐ Bowel changes
- ☐ Constipation
- ☐ Diarrhea
- ☐ Excessive hunger
- ☐ Excessive thirst
- ☐ Gas
- ☐ Hemorrhoids
- ☐ Indigestion
- ☐ Nausea
- ☐ Rectal bleeding
- ☐ Stomach pain
- ☐ Vomiting
- ☐ Vomiting blood

CARDIOVASCULAR

- ☐ Chest pain
- ☐ High blood pressure
- ☐ Irregular heart beat
- ☐ Low blood pressure
- ☐ Poor circulation
- ☐ Rapid heart beat
- ☐ Swelling of ankles
- ☐ Varicose veins

EYE, EAR, NOSE, THROAT

- ☐ Bleeding gums
- ☐ Blurred vision
- ☐ Crossed eyes
- ☐ Difficulty swallowing
- ☐ Double vision
- ☐ Earache
- ☐ Ear discharge
- ☐ Hay fever
- ☐ Hoarseness
- ☐ Loss of hearing
- ☐ Nosebleeds
- ☐ Persistent cough
- ☐ Ringing in ears
- ☐ Sinus problems
- ☐ Vision - Flashes
- ☐ Vision - Halos

SKIN

- ☐ Bruise easily
- ☐ Hives
- ☐ Itching
- ☐ Change in moles
- ☐ Rash
- ☐ Scars
- ☐ Sores that won't heal

MEN only

- ☐ Breast lump
- ☐ Erection difficulties
- ☐ Lump in testicles
- ☐ Penis discharge
- ☐ Sore on penis
- ☐ Other

WOMEN only

- ☐ Abnormal Pap Smear
- ☐ Bleeding between periods
- ☐ Breast lump
- ☐ Extreme menstrual pain
- ☐ Hot flashes
- ☐ Nipple discharge
- ☐ Painful intercourse
- ☐ Vaginal discharge
- ☐ Other

Date of last menstrual period __________

Date of last Pap Smear __________

Have you had a mammogram? __________

Are you pregnant? __________

Number of children __________

MEDICAL HISTORY Check (✓) the medical conditions you have or have had in the past.

- ☐ AIDS
- ☐ Alcoholism
- ☐ Anemia
- ☐ Anorexia
- ☐ Appendicitis
- ☐ Arthritis
- ☐ Asthma
- ☐ Bleeding Disorders
- ☐ Breast Lump
- ☐ Bronchitis
- ☐ Bulimia
- ☐ Cancer
- ☐ Cataracts
- ☐ Chemical Dependency
- ☐ Chicken Pox
- ☐ Diabetes
- ☐ Emphysema
- ☐ Epilepsy
- ☐ Gall Bladder Disease
- ☐ Glaucoma
- ☐ Goiter
- ☐ Gonorrhea
- ☐ Gout
- ☐ Heart Disease
- ☐ Hepatitis
- ☐ Hernia
- ☐ Herpes
- ☐ High Cholesterol
- ☐ HIV Positive
- ☐ Kidney Disease
- ☐ Liver Disease
- ☐ Measles
- ☐ Migraine Headaches
- ☐ Miscarriage
- ☐ Mononucleosis
- ☐ Multiple Sclerosis
- ☐ Mumps
- ☐ Pacemaker
- ☐ Pneumonia
- ☐ Polio
- ☐ Prostate Problem
- ☐ Psychiatric Care
- ☐ Rheumatic Fever
- ☐ Scarlet Fever
- ☐ Stroke
- ☐ Suicide Attempt
- ☐ Thyroid Problems
- ☐ Tonsillitis
- ☐ Tuberculosis
- ☐ Typhoid Fever
- ☐ Ulcers
- ☐ Vaginal Infections
- ☐ Venereal Disease

CONFIDENTIAL HEALTH HISTORY

HOSPITALIZATIONS Year	Hospital	Reason for Hospitalization and Outcome

Have you ever had a blood transfusion? ☐ Yes ☐ No
If yes, please give approximate dates: ______

OCCUPATIONAL CONCERNS Check (✓) if your work exposes you to the following:	HEALTH HABITS Check (✓) which substances you use and indicate how much you use per day/week.	PREGNANCY HISTORY Year of Birth	Sex of Birth	Complications if any
☐ Stress	☐ Caffeine			
☐ Hazardous Substances	☐ Tobacco			
☐ Heavy Lifting	☐ Drugs			
☐ Other	☐ Alcohol			

SERIOUS ILLNESS/INJURIES	DATE	OUTCOME

FAMILY HISTORY Fill in health information about your family.

Relation	Age	State of Health	Age at Death	Cause of Death	Check (✓) if your blood relatives had any of the following Disease	Relationship to you
Father					☐ Arthritis, Gout	
Mother					☐ Asthma, Hay Fever	
Brothers					☐ Cancer	
					☐ Chemical Dependency	
					☐ Diabetes	
					☐ Heart Disease, Strokes	
Sisters					☐ High Blood Pressure	
					☐ Kidney Disease	
					☐ Tuberculosis	
					☐ Other	

I certify that the above information is correct to the best of my knowledge. I will not hold my doctor or any members of his/her staff responsible for any errors or ommisions that I may have made in the completion of this form.

______ Signature ______ Date

______ Reviewed By ______ Date

CASE STUDY

Yvonne Black is a new patient of Dr. Esposito's at Inner City Health Care. Yvonne is an 88-year-old Italian-born woman who comes to the doctor at the urging of her granddaughter, Kristine, who accompanies her to the clinic. Yvonne's primary care provider has just retired after being her family doctor for over 35 years, and she requested Dr. Esposito because he is of Italian descent. Yvonne has many health problems and wants to describe each of them in great detail, making the intake interview complicated and difficult to perform. To add to the challenge, she is a poor historian when relating dates and events and does not always agree with the records obtained from her former doctor. This upsets Kristine, who wants to correct her, and they end up arguing.

CASE STUDY REVIEW QUESTIONS

1. What communication skills will Liz, the CMA (AAMA), need to get the most accurate information from Yvonne?

2. What can the manner in which the patient relates the information reveal about her?

3. What effect does Kristine have on the process of getting intake information for the patient? Is Kristine helpful or disruptive? What can you do and say to direct the conversation most effectively and efficiently?

CHAPTER POST-TEST

Perform this test without looking at your book. If an answer is "false," rewrite the sentence to make it true.

1. True or False? To "diagnose" means to predict the outcome of a disease or condition.

2. True or False? Objective statements can be described as "opinion."

3. When a patient "denies" something, he or she is:
   a. just whining
   b. not being truthful
   c. explaining his or her symptoms
   d. trying to blame someone else

4. True or False? Once a medical assistant has asked a patient whether he or she has any allergies, and the information has been recorded, the medical assistant needs to keep asking that patient at every office visit.

5. True or False? If a disease is familial, that means it has a pattern of occurring within families and blood relations.

SELF-ASSESSMENT

Think about your own personal experiences when answering the following questions. Be as self-reflective as you can.

1. When you are asked to complete a Medical History form, what are some of the emotions that you experience? Do you dread the work (especially if you aren't feeling well)? Are you concerned that you will not know all the answers, have all the dates and numbers, and so on? Are you frustrated because you have filled out so many forms already? Are you ever embarrassed by some of the questions? Do you feel guilty that you will not answer some of the questions honestly? Do you feel stupid if you do not understand all the questions? Do you feel hindered because you did not bring your glasses or you have a sprained wrist or are too sick to fill out the form? Think of other feelings you have that are not listed here.

2. Whenever a patient sees a new doctor or has not been in to the doctor for a while, or even on a periodic basis, a new Medical History form needs to be filled out. There is always paperwork to complete. Can you think of a better/easier/more efficient way to update patient information? Could computers make the job easier? What do you think will happen in the future?

___

___

___

3. Remember your feelings when you ask your patients to fill out the Medical History forms, and be sensitive to their needs. How might you assist them, without dedicating time away from your other duties?

___

___

___

___

___

Name ______ Date ______ Score ______

CHAPTER 12

Vital Signs and Measurements

CHAPTER PRE-TEST

Perform this test without looking at your book. If an answer is "false," rewrite the sentence to make it true.

1. True or False? Patient weight is measured only to determine how much fat the patient has.

______

______

2. True or False? A normal pulse rate is between 60 and 120 beats per minute for adults.

______

______

3. True or False? A normal respiration rate for adults is between 12 and 20 breaths per minute.

______

______

4. True or False? Blood pressure is the amount of pressure the blood exerts on the inside of veins.

______

______

5. True or False? High blood pressure is also called hypertension.

______

______

6. True or False? High blood pressure is always caused by inactivity and diet.

______

______

VOCABULARY BUILDER

Misspelled Words

Find the words below that are misspelled; underline them, and correctly spell them in the space provided. Then, fill in the blanks below with the appropriate terms from the list.

apnea	emphasema	hypotention
arhythmia	eupnea	orthopnia
baseline	frenulum	rhonchi
bradycardia	hyperpnea	strider
bradypnea	hypertension	systolic
dyspnea	hyperventilation	wheese

______________ ______________ ______________

______________ ______________ ______________

1. Tiffany comes to the office of Drs. Lewis and King reporting that she cannot breathe well when she lies down. Joe Guerrero, CMA (AAMA), notes ______________________ in her chart.
2. Winston Lewis, MD, warns his patient, Herb, that he is in the early stages of ______________________, a chronic pulmonary condition that causes destruction of the air sacs in the lungs, caused by his smoking.
3. Liz Corbin, CMA (AAMA), writes ______________________ in Carolyn's chart after she counts her respirations at 45 breaths per minute.
4. Wanda Slawson, CMA (AAMA), is taking Edith's temperature orally and is careful to insert the digital thermometer under her tongue, next to the ______________________.
5. Marissa is rushed in to see Dr. King after swallowing a coin. Dr. King can clearly hear a crowing __________ whenever the toddler tries to inhale. This indicates to the doctor that the coin is lodged in the upper airway.
6. At a scheduled examination, Lenny's pulse is recorded at 40 beats per minute. This is called ______________ in medical terms.
7. Ludmilla has cut her hand and arrives at the Inner City Health Care clinic in an anxious state. She says she is feeling tingly and lightheaded. Bruce Goldman, CMA (AAMA), notes that her respiratory rate is 35 and that Ludmilla is taking deep, rapid breaths. Bruce suspects ______________________ and calmly has her breathe slowly into her cupped hands until the tingling goes away.
8. Wanda Slawson, CMA (AAMA), can hear a deep snoring sound in the patient's throat when he measures Leo's respirations. This sound is described as ______________________.
9. Jim's blood pressure is a high 180/98. The number 180 is called the ______________________ pressure.
10. Dr. Lewis takes careful note of Mr. Marshall's 160/100 blood pressure reading and discusses with him the dangers of ______________________ and the possible need for lifestyle changes and possible medication to control this condition.
11. Keisha's breathing is noticeably labored at one of her well-child checkups. Joe Guerrero, CMA (AAMA), notes this as ______________________ in her chart.
12. Three-year-old Chris has had a somewhat persistent chest cold for weeks but has a high-pitched __________ when he exhales, leading Dr. Lewis to consider asthma as a diagnosis.
13. Kareem has normal respirations. This could be described in the chart notes as ______________________.
14. Liping's breath sounds are normal, but her respiration rate is very slow, only 8 to 9 breaths a minute. This ______________________ worries Liz Corbin, CMA (AAMA), so she alerts Dr. King immediately.

15. While checking Robert's pulse, Joe Guerrero, CMA (AAMA), notices an obvious irregularity in the pulse. This is known as an ____________________________.

16. When Jamar shares that his wife sometimes stops breathing in her sleep for a couple of minutes, Dr. Lewis becomes concerned that she might be experiencing ___________________________ and recommends that a sleep study be performed.

17. Juanita's resting blood pressure is 60/44. This is ___________________________, and Dr. Rice is concerned about this being a side effect of the prescribed medication Juanita is taking.

18. Dr. Susan Rice orders an ECG on her patient Rebecca, just as a ___________________________ for future reference.

LEARNING REVIEW

Short Answer

1. Temperature, pulse, respiration, and blood pressure are collectively referred to as

____

____

2. How is heat produced within the body? What part of the brain maintains the balance between heat production and heat loss? What are ways the body cools itself in hot weather and heats itself in cold weather?

____

____

____

____

3. List the five ways in which the body loses heat next to each example below.

   a. Ellen climbs into a cold bed. ____________________

   b. Anara enjoys her aerobic workout, which causes her to sweat. ____________________

   c. On a trip to New York, Richard attends a live studio performance where the temperature in the room was kept at about 58 degrees. ____________________

   d. Christine uses a portable fan when she is working as a seamstress and all the sewing machines and irons tend to make the room too warm. ____________________

   e. Liz performs daily yoga breathing exercises. ____________________

4. What is another word for fever?

____

____

5. Explain the differences in the patterns of fevers in the list below.

   Remittent:

____

____

   Intermittent:

____

____

Continuous:

____

____

6. Circle the correct words to complete the sentences: A(n) (increase/decrease) in temperature may be caused by several factors, such as eating, medications that increase metabolism, exercise, bacterial infections and exposure to heat, pregnancy, stress, and age. A(n) (increase/decrease) in body temperature may result from fasting, inactivity, medications that decrease metabolism, exposure to cold, and age.
7. An aural temperature is taken where?

____

____

8. Write the normal ranges of blood pressures for the following age groups:

Child, age 10 ____________

Adolescent, age 16 ____________

Adult ____________

9. Define the following terms and explain what each factor has to do with blood pressure and how each affects the pressure.

Blood volume:

____

____

____

Elasticity of arterial walls:

____

____

____

____

Lumen of the arteries (peripheral resistance):

____

____

____

____

____

Strength of the heart muscle:

____

____

____

____

Viscosity of the blood:

____

____

____

10. List four other factors that influence blood pressure that are not listed in Question 9.

11. What is the name of the various sounds sometimes heard during blood pressure measurement?

12. When measuring blood pressure, it is important to not allow the gauge to move faster than

13. List five types of hypertension and explain each type, whether it is curable, and what its treatment(s) and caus(es) are. Then give an example of each.

Type	**Description and Example**

14. List and explain three possible causes of hypotension.

15. A very rapid pulse rate is described medically as ______________________.

16. A very slow pulse rate is described medically as ______________________.

17. The medical term meaning difficulty and/or painful breathing is ____________________.

18. Write the normal pulse ranges for the following age groups:

    Birth ________________

    Infants ________________

    Child, age 1 year ________________

    Child, age 7–14 years ________________

    Adult ________________

19. Identify the name of each common pulse site described below and match the site to its proper location on the body in the figure below by placing the correct letter in the space provided.

    a. The site most commonly used for BP reading: ______________________________

    b. The site for blood pressure measurements in the leg: ______________________________

    c. The site commonly used for infant pulse rates: ______________________________

    d. The site used in emergencies and when performing cardiopulmonary resuscitation (CPR): ____________

    e. The site used to check for circulation in the lower limbs: ______________________________

    f. The most commonly used site to measure pulse: ______________________________

    g. The site used in an emergency to control bleeding in the leg: ______________________________

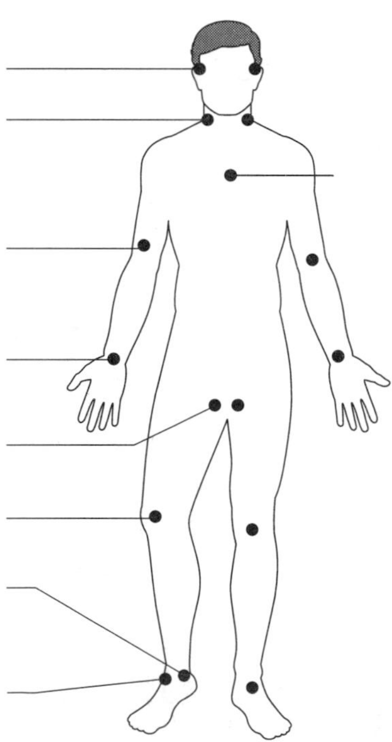

20. List and define four characteristics of the pulse.

____

____

____

____

21. Write the normal range of respiratory rates for each of the following ages.

Infant ______________________

Child, age 1–7 years ______________________

Adult ______________________

22. List and define three characteristics of respiration.

____

____

____

CERTIFICATION REVIEW

These questions are designed to mimic the certification examination. Select the best response.

1. Which of the following is *not* a routine body measurement?
   a. Chest circumference
   b. Head circumference
   c. Ankle circumference
   d. Height
2. In converting inches to feet, which of the following is true?
   a. 62 inches is 5 feet, 2 inches
   b. 62 inches is 6 feet, 2 inches
   c. 62 inches is 6 feet exactly
   d. 62 inches is 5 feet 6 inches
3. When converting Fahrenheit to Celsius, which of the following is the correct formula?
   a. Fahrenheit temperature minus 32 multiplied by 5/9
   b. Fahrenheit temperature multiplied by 5/9 minus 32
   c. Fahrenheit temperature plus 32 multiplied by 5/9
   d. Fahrenheit temperature multiplied by 9/5 plus 32
4. What is considered a normal pulse and respiration rate for an adult?
   a. Pulse of 76, respiration of 20
   b. Pulse of 80, respiration of 18
   c. Pulse of 56, respiration of 16
   d. Pulse of 20, respiration of 60
   e. Both a. and b. are correct.

5. Which of the following is *not* a requirement in order to obtain accurate blood pressure?
   a. The cuff should be the proper size.
   b. The cuff should be placed correctly over the radial artery.
   c. The arm should be above heart level.
   d. The deflation should not be faster than 2 mm/degrees per heartbeat.
   e. The patient should be seated with feet on the floor and back supported.
6. A pulse obtained at the intersection of the fifth intercostal space at the mid-clavicular line on the left chest is called the:
   a. femoral pulse
   b. temporal pulse
   c. brachial pulse
   d. apical pulse
7. Malignant hypertension:
   a. is borderline
   b. is below normal
   c. is life threatening
   d. spreads to other parts of the body

LEARNING APPLICATION

Charting Exercises

Chart the following patient vital signs in the corresponding paper chart record below:

1. On January 4, 20XX you checked Ludmilla in for her office visit at 2:30 PM. Her height was 64 inches, and she weighed 145 pounds. Her temperature taken orally was 99.2 degrees Fahrenheit. You took her pulse rate and respiration rate for 30 seconds and they were 44 and 10, respectively. Her blood pressure measured in her right arm while she was sitting down was 146 over 68. (Be sure to initial your charting.)

   ____

   ____

2. On March 22nd, you checked Abigail in for her checkup at 10:30 AM. Her height was 66½ inches and she weighed 212 pounds. Her temperature taken orally was 97.8 degrees Fahrenheit, her pulse rate was 90 and irregular twice within 60 seconds. Her respiration rate was 15 in 30 seconds and she was breathing with difficulty. Her blood pressure measured in her right arm while she was sitting down was 190 over 94. You notified Dr. King of her pulse and respirations and stayed with the patient to observe her. (Be sure to initial your charting.)

   ____

   ____

   ____

Hands-on Activities

Perform the following exercises and then measure your pulse and respirations. Chart the measurements in the spaces provided using proper documentation.

1. After three minutes of rest, sitting in a chair with your feet flat on the floor

____

____

2. After three minutes of marching in place at a comfortable rate

____

____

3. After three minutes of strong aerobic exercise such as jumping jacks or jogging in place

____

____

4. Note the variations in the characteristics of your pulse and respirations as you moved from rest to strong activity. Calculate the ratio of respiration to pulse for your resting, active, and aerobic rates listed earlier. Show your results below.

Resting ____

____

Active ____

____

Aerobic ____

____

CASE STUDY 1

Wayne lives near Inner City Health Care in a group home for developmentally delayed adults. Wayne has a history of frequent colds and ear infections. He visits the clinic one morning with pain in both ears. He is also drinking a cup of hot coffee.

CASE STUDY REVIEW QUESTIONS

1. What method would Wanda, the CMA (AAMA), use to take Wayne's temperature?

____

____

____

____

2. How might Wanda explain to Wayne why she is using the axillary method?

____

____

____

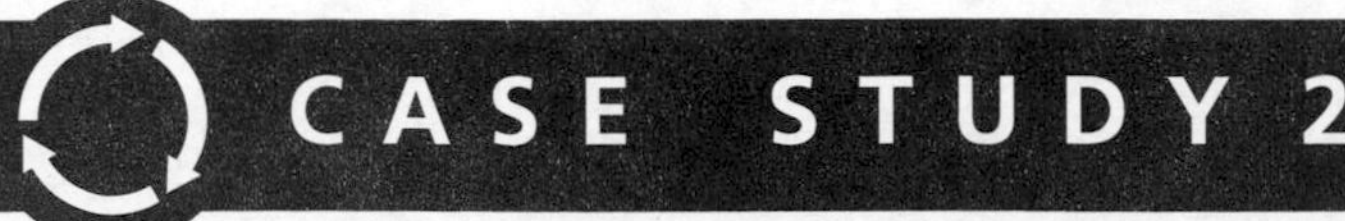

CASE STUDY 2

Henry, who is 4 years old, is rushed to Inner City Health Care. He is bleeding profusely from a cut on his head. "He fell down the stairs," sobs his mother, Juanita. Henry does not seem to be fully conscious and appears confused. Dr. James Whitney attends to Henry's laceration, applying direct pressure on the cut to stop the bleeding. He directs clinical assistant Bruce Goldman to call 911 for emergency services. Then Bruce takes Henry's pulse. "What are you doing?" Juanita asks Bruce. "Why doesn't he wake up?"

CASE STUDY REVIEW QUESTIONS

1. What site would Bruce use to take Henry's pulse?

2. How might Bruce answer Juanita's questions about what he is doing?

CASE STUDY 3

Abigail, who suffers from many problems related to her advanced age, also has type II diabetes. She is very friendly and has a good rapport with everyone in the clinic—all of whom she says are "just like family"—and she is very eager to please the staff. One winter day she comes to the clinic complaining of flu symptoms. When clinical assistant Audrey asks Abigail to step onto the scale to get her weight, Abigail says, "Oh, do we have to? I just don't feel up to it right now."

CASE STUDY REVIEW QUESTION

1. How might Audrey explain to Abigail about why her weight is important at every visit?

CHAPTER POST-TEST

1. True or False? Patient weight is measured sometimes to determine how much fluid the patient is retaining.

2. True or False? A normal pulse rate is between 80 and 100 for adults.

3. True or False? A normal respiration rate is between 16 and 20 for adults.

4. True or False? Blood pressure is the amount of pressure that is exerted on the inside of the arteries.

5. True or False? High blood pressure is also called hypotension.

6. High blood pressure can be lowered by regular exercise, dietary changes, losing weight, and medications.

SELF-ASSESSMENT

As you respond to the following questions, think of how your experiences will affect how you treat your patients.

1. Think of the last time you had your height and weight measured. Did you have enough privacy to make you comfortable?

2. When you had your blood pressure taken, did the medical assistant share your measurements with you? Did you feel comfortable asking questions?

3. Has any health care provider ever discussed any of your vital signs or body measurements with you? Have you been informed of the health factors related to your vital signs or body measurements?

4. Do you still have mercury thermometers in your home? If so, call the health department to find out where you can take them for disposal and then obtain an electronic or digital thermometer for future use at home. How do you think your patients will feel when you encourage them to do the same? Write out exactly what you will say to them to convince them of the importance of replacing all mercury thermometers with a safer alternative. Explain mercury poisoning to them.

Name ______________________ Date __________ Score ______

CHAPTER 13

The Physical Examination

CHAPTER PRE-TEST

Perform this test without looking at your book.

1. *(Circle the correct answer)* Palpation/Palpitation is when the patient can feel his or her heartbeat.
2. Which of the following is *not* a method used during a physical examination?
   a. Percussion
   b. Menstruation
   c. Manipulation
   d. Auscultation
3. Which is a component of a routine physical examination?
   a. What the patient looks like
   b. How the patient walks
   c. Whether the patient has bad breath
   d. All of the above
4. Which of the following is *not* a position used in physical examinations of patients?
   a. Lithotomy
   b. Supine
   c. Dorsal recumbent
   d. Reverse Trendelenburg
5. Choose the correct spelling of the instrument used to examine the inside of the eyeball.
   a. Opthalmoscope
   b. Optomescope
   c. Ophthalmoscope
   d. Otoscope

VOCABULARY BUILDER

Misspelled Words

Find the words below that are misspelled; circle them, and correctly spell them in the spaces provided. Then identify the correct vocabulary terms most appropriate for each example below from a patient's physical examination.

ataxia	labirynthitis	symmetry
bruits	pallor	tinnitus
cyanosis	piorrhea	vertigo
jaundice	schleroderma	vertiligo

_____________ _____________

_____________ _____________

1. During a physical examination of Louise Kipperley, a 48-year-old woman, Dr. Esposito notices that Louise's facial skin has become tight and atrophied, suggesting possible ________________________.
2. Leo McKay comes to Inner City Health Care with mouth pain. Dr. Reynolds examines Leo's mouth and discovers ________________________, which is discharge of pus from the gums around the teeth.
3. Medical assistant Liz Corbin observes the gait of Geraldine Potter, a 36-year-old woman diagnosed with multiple sclerosis. Geraldine's gait is lurching and unsteady, with her feet widely placed. Liz charts this as ________________________.
4. Annette Samuels is diagnosed with hepatitis B virus (HBV) by Dr. John Pettit. Among Annette's symptoms, noted by Dr. Pettit during the physical examination, was ________________________, a distinct yellowing of Annette's skin and the whites of her eyes.
5. Lenny Taylor, an older adult man with Alzheimer's disease, is brought to Inner City Health Care by his son George. Apparently, Lenny has had problems breathing. Dr. Whitney observes ________________________, a bluish color in Lenny's skin.
6. After performing a routine venipuncture procedure on patient Rhoda Au, Bruce Goldman, CMA (AAMA), notices that all color has drained from Rhoda's face. He assumes that her ________________________ is due to a psychological reaction to the venipuncture, so he has her lie down on the examination table for a few minutes until her color improves.
7. Abigail Johnson's 28-year-old granddaughter Lucy comes in for an examination with Dr. King after observing white patches of depigmentation, or ________________________, on her hand. "Is this what Michael Jackson had?" she asks Dr. King.
8. While performing a complete physical examination on patient Rowena Lawrence, Dr. King listens for abnormal sounds, or ________________________, from vital organs while auscultating her abdomen.
9. During a routine physical examination of Lenore McDonnell, a young woman confined to a wheelchair, Dr. Lewis checks for balance or ________________________ of size, shape, and position of body parts on opposite sides of her body.
10. Mary Tice comes in to see Dr King for ringing in her ears. Dr. King asks her if she is taking large doses of aspirin, which can cause ________________________.
11. Rowena Lawrence's 6-year-old daughter, Felicia, diagnosed with a case of the mumps, returns with her mother for a reexamination with Dr. Lewis when the child experiences a sensation that the room is spinning, caused by inflammation of the labyrinth, called ________________________.
12. While her blood was being taken, Susan O'Donnell described the room as spinning and felt lightheaded. This ____________________ quickly passes in a few minutes.

LEARNING REVIEW

Matching

Match the correct method of examination used by a physician in Column A to the entry in Column B that best describes it.

Column A

____ 1. Auscultation

____ 2. Observation or inspection

____ 3. Manipulation

____ 4. Mensuration

____ 5. Percussion

Column B

A. On his physical examination of Charles Williams, Dr. Winston Lewis looks at the patient to assess his general health, posture, body movements, skin, mannerisms, and care in grooming while verbally reviewing Charles's medical history with him.

B. Dr. Mark Woo uses a stethoscope to listen to the bowel sounds that accompany peristalsis.

C. Dr. King performs range of motion exercises on patient Margaret Thomas, who is suspected of having Parkinson's disease.

D. Dr. Rice taps Edith Leonard's chest to feel and hear the hollow quality expected from clear lungs.

E. During Marissa O'Keefe's well-baby visit, chest and head circumference measurements are recorded in the patient's medical record.

Short Answer

1. For each procedure listed below, identify the most likely examination position that will be required during the physician's examination. Use a medical encyclopedia for reference, if necessary.

Examination	Position
a. Urinary catheterization	____________
b. Auscultation for audible bowel sounds that are a normal part of the digestive process	____________
c. Colposcopy to observe the cervix under magnified illumination for evidence of precancerous cells, followed by a cone biopsy for laboratory analysis	____________
d. Internal hemorrhoids are examined through the use of a proctoscope	____________
e. Percutaneous renal biopsy to aid in diagnosis of suspected glomerulonephritis	____________
f. An ECG is performed on an older adult woman with angina pectoris	____________
g. A variation of this position is used for patients experiencing shock	____________
h. Proctoscopy to investigate a suspected case of proctitis, inflammation of the rectum	____________

2. Identify each entry below as a piece of medical equipment (ME), a laboratory procedure (LP), a body part (BP), or a patient illness or condition (PI). Then identify the correct component or sequence of the physical examination to which the entry relates. The first two entries have been completed for you as an example.

A. Sphygmomanometer	ME	Vital signs
B. Aphonia	PI	Speech
C. Lymph nodes	____	____________________
D. Edema	____	____________________
E. Anal fissures	____	____________________
F. Emphysema	____	____________________
G. Pharyngeal mirrors	____	____________________
H. Scrotum	____	____________________
I. Areola	____	____________________
J. Electrocardiography	____	____________________
K. Kyphosis	____	____________________
L. Dysphasia	____	____________________
M. Urinalysis	____	____________________
N. Achilles tendon	____	____________________
O. Tympanic membrane	____	____________________

3. Symmetry would be noted by using what method of assessment?

____

4. What is another term for the supine position or the position assumed when lying face up?

____

5. *(Circle the correct answer)* Orthostatic hypotension occurs as blood pressure decreases/increases/normalizes.

6. What is the preferred position for administration of an enema or rectal suppositories?

____

7. Determining the amount of flexion and extension of a patient's extremities would be which form of assessment?

____

Image Identification

Identify each of the positions shown in the photos below.

A.

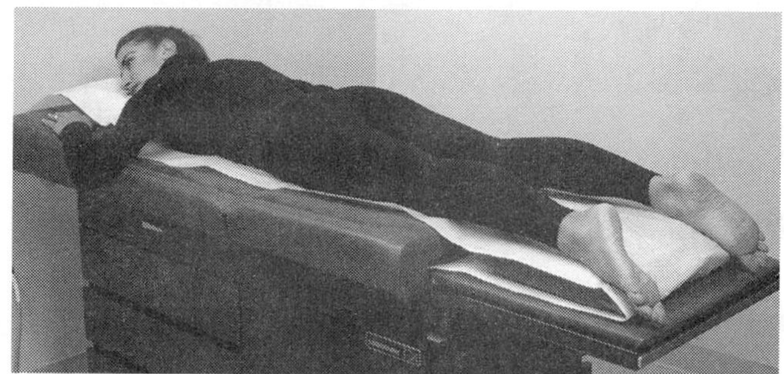

____

B.

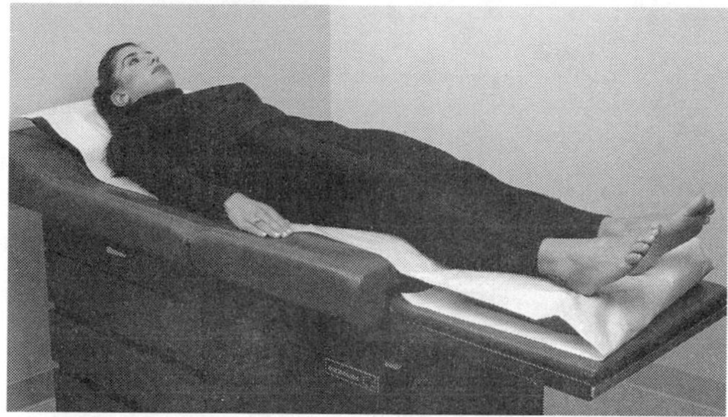

____

C.

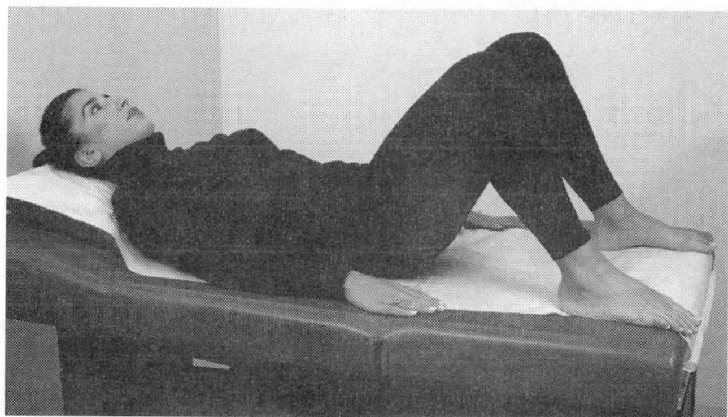

____

D.

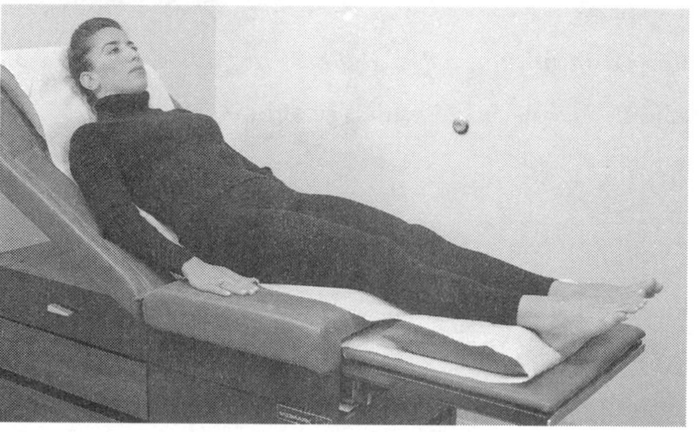

____

E.

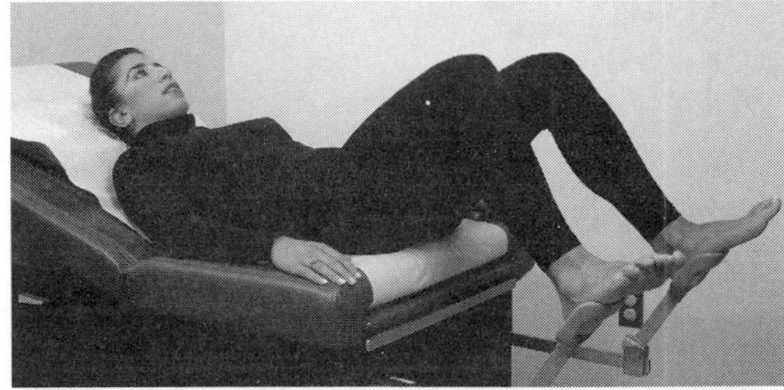

____

F.

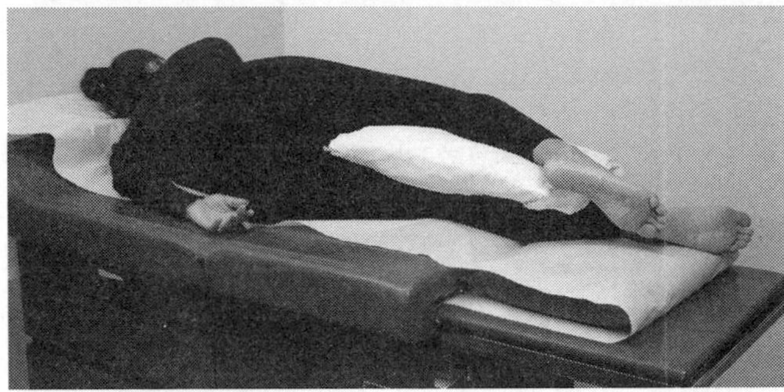

____

G.

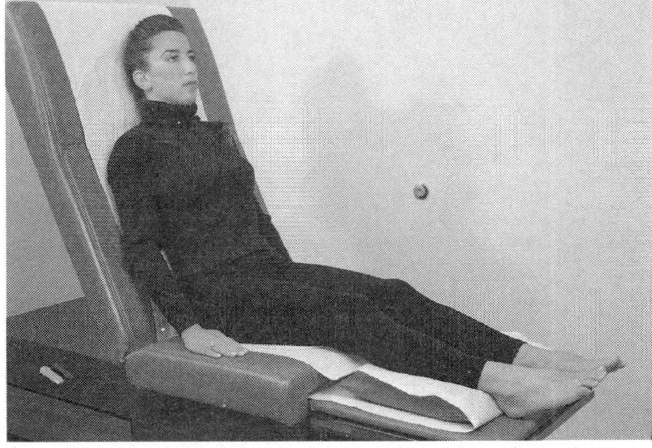

____

CERTIFICATION REVIEW

These questions are designed to mimic the certification examination. Select the best response.

1. A patient having an examination of the abdomen should be placed in which position?
   a. Supine
   b. Prone
   c. Lithotomy
   d. Sims'

2. Listening to the patient's chest as he or she breathes is called:
   a. auscultation
   b. percussion
   c. inspection
   d. palpation
3. The process of inspection is also called:
   a. percussion
   b. measuration
   c. observation
   d. palpitations
4. Which of the following is *not* a piece of equipment needed in the examination room?
   a. Goose-neck lamp
   b. Mayo tray
   c. Biohazard waste container
   d. Adjustable stool
5. Which of the following is *not* a word used to describe skin color?
   a. Jaundice
   b. Cyanosis
   c. Bruits
   d. Pallor

LEARNING APPLICATION

Role-Play Exercises

Using the list of patient positions from the book, practice placing your classmates into the various positions for examination. Pay special attention to knee and back problems and any physical limitations patients may have.

CASE STUDY

Kristine Bolt brings her young son Christopher to Inner City Health Care with a suspected case of mumps, which his older sister is just recovering from. As Bruce Goldman, CMA (AAMA), helps the child remove his shirt for the examination, Ian becomes increasingly fearful and begins to cry. Kristine's gentle reprimand to get him to relax is not working. It is obvious the child is feverish and not feeling well.

CASE STUDY REVIEW QUESTIONS

1. What can Bruce do to calm Christopher and make him more comfortable?

____

____

____

____

____

____

2. What should Bruce's therapeutic response be?

____

____

____

____

____

____

CHAPTER POST-TEST

Perform this test without looking at your book.

1. Fill in the blank: ____________________ is when the physician feels the patient's abdomen.
2. Which of the following is *not* a method used during a physical examination?
   a. Percussion
   b. Manipulation
   c. Auscultation
   d. Symmetry
3. Which is *not* a component of a routine physical examination?
   a. What the patient looks like
   b. How the patient walks
   c. Whether the patient has bad breath
   d. The patient's test results

4. Which of the following is *not* a position used in physical examinations of patients?
   a. Lithotomy
   b. Reverse Trendelenburg
   c. Prone
   d. Dorsal recumbent
5. Choose the correct spelling of the instrument used to examine the inside of the eyeball.
   a. Opthalmoscope
   b. Ophthalmoscope
   c. Optalmascope
   d. Otoscope

SELF-ASSESSMENT

Think about the last time you went to the doctor. As you answer the following questions and remember your personal experience(s), think about how your experience(s) will affect the way you treat your patients in the future. If you have no personal experiences, try to imagine how you would feel and react.

1. Did you have to undress at all? How did that feel? Did you get cold or feel a bit awkward?

____

____

____

____

2. When you had your blood pressure taken, did the cuff cause pain or discomfort as it got tighter? Did you say something to the medical assistant? Do you think most people speak up when they are uncomfortable?

____

____

____

____

3. Have you ever noticed a sick patient in a public place? What were the clues that told you the patient was sick? Do you think your skills of observation will be enhanced after you complete this chapter?

____

____

____

____

Name ______________________ Date __________ Score ______

CHAPTER **14**

Obstetrics and Gynecology

CHAPTER PRE-TEST

Perform this test without looking at your book. If an answer is "false," rewrite the sentence to make it true.

1. True or False? Obstetrics is the branch of medicine that concerns management of pregnancy, childbirth, and the puerperium, whereas gynecology is the study of the diseases of female reproductive organs.

   ____

   ____

2. Which of the following are addressed during the initial prenatal visit and examination?
   a. Genetic diseases/conditions in the family
   b. Kidney and heart diseases/conditions and diabetes
   c. Nutritional deficiencies
   d. All of the above
3. During pregnancy, which of the following is potentially dangerous?
   a. Rapid weight gain
   b. Visual changes
   c. Hypertension
   d. Chill, fever
   e. All of the above
4. True or False? It is recommended that pelvic examinations and Pap smears be performed on all women no later than 21 years of age (or at the onset of sexual activity).

   ____

   ____

5. True or False? Because the provider will perform a breast examination during the annual physical, it is not important for women to perform breast self-examinations on themselves.

   ____

   ____

6. The Pap smear is designed to detect which type of cancer?
   a. Cervical
   b. Vaginal
   c. Ovarian
   d. All of the above
   e. a. and b. only

VOCABULARY BUILDER

Misspelled Words

Find the words below that are misspelled; circle them, and correctly spell them in the spaces provided. Then fill in the blanks in the following sentences with the correct vocabulary terms from the list.

abortion	gestation	parturation
Braxton-Hicks	gonorrhea	pelvic inflammatory disease
cervical punch biopsy	human papillomavirus	placenta abruption
delation	hysterosalpingogram	placenta previa
dismenorrhea	lochia	preeclampsia
dyspareunia	multigravida	sickle cell anemia
ectopic	neonatal	Tay-Sachs
effacement	nullipara	trichomoniasis

____________________ ____________________ ____________________

1. Discharge from the uterus of blood, mucus, and tissue during the period after childbirth is called ____________________.
2. The period of development from conception to birth is called ____________________.
3. Any pregnancy that occurs outside of the uterus is called ____________________.
4. A ____________________ is a visual examination of vaginal and cervical tissues using a type of microscope with a magnifying lens and powerful lights.
5. ____________________ is an infection of the uterus, fallopian tubes, and adjacent pelvic structures.
6. A term that means "painful menses" is ____________________.
7. ____________________ occurs when the placenta implants itself low in the uterus and partially or completely covers the cervical os.
8. ____________________ is the term given to a woman who has not carried a pregnancy to birth.
9. Two types of sexually transmitted diseases are ____________________, which is caused by bacteria, and ____________________, which is caused by a virus.
10. ____________________ is an invasion of a protozoa, often transmitted through sexual contact.

Spelling Review

Choose the correctly spelled words in each row.

1. puerperium	purperium	puerpurium
2. La Maz	Lamaze	Lamase
3. eeclampsia	eclampsia	eclamsia
4. amneocentesis	amniocentisis	amniocentesis
5. coposcopy	colposcapy	colposcopy
6. cryosurgery	criosurgery	crysurgery
7. primogravida	primigravida	Primegravida

LEARNING REVIEW

Matching

Match each female condition or disease in Column A to its description in Column B.

	Column A	Column B
____	1. PID	A. Malignant cells found in the ovaries
____	2. Menopause	B. Painful menstruation
____	3. Endometriosis	C. The end of menstruation
____	4. Ovarian cancer	D. Inflammatory disease of the pelvis involving some or all of the reproductive organs
____	5. Ovarian cysts	E. Painful condition characterized by endometrial cells adhering to tissues and organs outside of the uterus
____	6. Dysmenorrhea	F. Cysts located on the ovaries

Labeling

Identify each part of the female reproductive system below. Describe each part and its function in the spaces provided. Use your medical dictionary if needed.

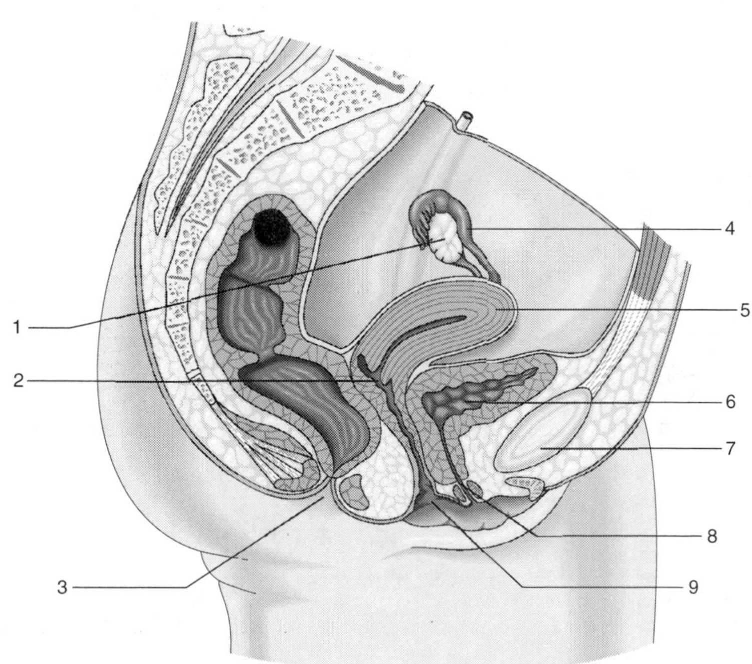

Part	Description and Function
1. ______________	______________
2. ______________	______________
3. ______________	______________
4. ______________	______________
5. ______________	______________
6. ______________	______________
7. ______________	______________
8. ______________	______________
9. ______________	______________

Short Answer

1. The obstetric history includes the total number of pregnancies and the number of live births. For each history, give the number of pregnancies and the number of live births.

Obstetric History	Pregnancies	Live Births	Abortions
A. Gravida 2 Para 1 Abortion 1	________	________	________
B. Gravida 6 Para 4 Abortion 2	________	________	________
C. Gravida 3 Para 1 Abortion 2	________	________	________

2. What branch of medicine treats the mother and fetus through all stages of labor, delivery, and postpartum?

____

____

3. List at least two signs/symptoms of preeclampsia.

____

____

4. A potentially life-threatening disorder during pregnancy that is characterized by hypertension, edema, and proteinuria and may put both mother and fetus in danger is known as what? ______________

5. Breast self-examination should be performed at least once every ______________.

6. The gynecologic disease in which an infection is caused by a microorganism that may lead to infertility or ectopic pregnancy if not treated is ______________.

7. Describe the six types of abortion (interruptions of pregnancy).

____

____

____

____

____

____

8. Fill in the Description, Symptom(s), and Treatment(s) columns below that correspond to the complications of pregnancy listed in the table.

Complication	Description	Symptom(s)	Treatment(s)
Eclampsia			
Preeclampsia			
Gestational diabetes			
Hyperemesis gravidarum			

Placenta previa

Placenta abruptio

CERTIFICATION REVIEW

These questions are designed to mimic the certification examination. Select the best response.

1. Which of the following are types of abortions?
   a. Spontaneous, complete, incomplete, interrupted, medical
   b. Miscarriage, threatened, induced, voluntary, medical
   c. Induced, spontaneous, postpartum, complete, medical
   d. Complete, threatened, incomplete, induced, missed, spontaneous
   e. Interrupted, complete, induced, medical, voluntary
2. During a prenatal visit, the urine is tested for which two substances?
   a. Drugs, including alcohol, and glucose
   b. Infection and glucose
   c. Glucose and protein
   d. Bilirubin and protein
3. Which of the following is *not* a routine test/procedure performed on pregnant women?
   a. Ultrasound
   b. Amniocentesis
   c. Chorionic villi sampling
   d. Alpha-fetoprotein
   e. Colonoscopy

4. LMP means:

   a. localized medical practices

   b. last menstrual period

   c. localized menstrual pain

   d. limited medical plan

   e. last medical prenatal (examination)

5. A prenatal condition that causes sudden weight gain, an increase in blood pressure, and proteinuria is called:

   a. Rh incompatibility

   b. preeclampsia

   c. hyperemesis gravidarum

   d. gestational diabetes

   e. a. and b.

6. A painful condition characterized by tissue from inside of the uterus adhering to the organs outside the uterus is called:

   a. preeclampsia

   b. endometriosis

   c. metrometriosis

   d. menopause

   e. pelvic inflammatory disease

7. Bartholin glands:

   a. contain mucus for lubrication of the vagina

   b. can become inflamed and infected

   c. are situated on both sides of the vaginal orifice

   d. are similar to the male's Cowper's glands

   e. All of the above

8. Chlamydia, condylomata, HIV, and gonorrhea are all:

   a. complications of pregnancy

   b. diagnosed during the Pap smear and pelvic examination

   c. sexually transmitted

   d. curable

   e. diagnosed through blood tests

LEARNING APPLICATION

CASE STUDY

CASE STUDY REVIEW QUESTION

1. In the office, the provider instructs you that a Pap smear and pelvic examination will be performed on Ms. Smith in Room 1. Describe your role in assisting with these procedures.

CHAPTER POST-TEST

Perform this test without looking at your book. If an answer is "false," rewrite the sentence to make it true.

1. True or False? Obstetrics has to do with female issues, and gynecology has to do with pregnancy.

2. Which of the following are addressed during the initial prenatal visit and examination?
   a. Genetic diseases/conditions in the family
   b. Kidney and heart diseases/conditions and diabetes
   c. Nutritional deficiencies
   d. All of the above

3. During pregnancy, which of the following is potentially dangerous?
   a. Rapid weight gain
   b. Visual changes
   c. Hypertension
   d. Chill, fever
   e. All of the above

4. True or False? It is recommended that pelvic examinations and Pap smears be performed on all women older than 25 years (or at the onset of sexual activity) on an annual basis.

____

____

5. True or False? Even though the provider will perform a breast examination during the annual physical, it is still important for women to perform breast self-examinations on themselves.

____

____

6. The Pap smear is designed to detect which type of cancer?

   a. Cervical

   b. Ovarian

   c. Vaginal

   d. Breast

   e. All of the above

   f. a. and c. only

SELF-ASSESSMENT

Think about the last time you went to your provider for an examination. As you answer the following questions and remember your personal experiences, think about how your experiences will affect the way you treat your patients in the future. If you have no personal experiences, try to imagine how you would feel and react. All of the following situations may be discussed in small groups with your classmates.

1. Which questions were you asked the last time you went to your provider for a pelvic examination? Try to think of five.

____

____

____

____

2. When the provider came into the room, were you dressed and in the examination room? Were you undressed and sitting on the examination table? Were you undressed and lying down? Were you undressed and lying down in the lithotomy position? Which of the previous scenarios would make you the most comfortable? Which would make you the most uncomfortable?

____

____

____

____

3. How comfortable are you with discussing private information with your provider? How about with your medical assistant? Are you more comfortable with one or the other? Why do you suppose you would be?

____

____

____

____

Name ______________________ Date ____________ Score ______

CHAPTER **15**

Pediatrics

CHAPTER PRE-TEST

Perform this test without looking at your book. If an answer is "false," rewrite the sentence to make it true.

1. True or False? Pediatrics is the branch of medicine that cares for newborns, infants, children, and adolescents.

____

____

2. Toddlers are:

   a. children from birth to 2 years old

   b. children from about 1 to about 3 years old

   c. children from the time they are able to walk until they are in kindergarten

   d. children from about 2 to 5 years old

3. True or False? Measurements of newborn infants consist of length, weight, chest circumference, and head circumference.

____

____

4. Normal childhood immunizations include which of the following?

   a. DTaP, MMR, Hib, and HIV

   b. Tetanus, DTaP, MMR, and IPV

   c. IPV, MMR, DTaP, Hib, and HBV

   d. HBV, Hib, pertussis, and HAV

   e. Both c. and d.

5. The preferred site for injections for a child younger than 2 years is:

   a. the vastus lateralis

   b. the gluteus medius

   c. the deltoid

   d. Any of the above is acceptable.

6. Normal pulse and respiration for an 8-year-old child is:
   a. pulse of 80, respiration of 30
   b. pulse of 80, respiration of 12
   c. pulse of 120, respiration of 20
   d. pulse of 86, respiration of 18
   e. none of the above

VOCABULARY BUILDER

Misspelled Words

Find the words below that are misspelled; circle them, and then correctly spell them in the spaces provided.

blood preasure	myringotomy	phynelketonuria
circumfrence	pediatrics	tonsilitis
fontanelle	pediculosis	vacination

_______________ _______________ _______________

_______________ _______________

Definitions

Define the following vocabulary terms.

1. Exudate ____

2. Myringotomy ____

3. Suppurative ____

4. Tympanostomy ____

5. Otitis media ____

6. Tonsillitis ____

7. Pediculosis ____

LEARNING REVIEW

Short Answer

1. Mary O'Keefe has called for an emergency appointment with Dr. King for her 3-year-old son, Chris, who awakened during the night with a high fever and severe pain in his right ear, which is draining. Ellen Armstrong, CMA (AAMA), must prepare the examination room for the patient. Based on Chris's symptoms, what equipment will Ellen want to assemble for Dr. King's physical examination of Chris? List the equipment in the order it will most likely be used in the examination.

2. When Mary O'Keefe arrives with her son, Ellen takes them to examination room 2 and prepares the patient for Dr. King's physical examination. Ellen takes and records the child's vital signs: T 102.1°F (Ax); P 115 (AP) bounding, sinus arrhythmia; R 28; 76/42/0, rt. arm, sitting. Ellen tells Mary that Dr. King will be examining Chris's ear and may want to take some laboratory tests.

   A. What method did Ellen use to take Chris's temperature?

   B. What method did Ellen use to measure Chris's pulse? Where on the body is this measured?

   C. Are Chris's vital signs normal?

   D. Chris is fussy and disagreeable, but not uncooperative, while Ellen takes his vital signs. What can a medical assistant do to facilitate the measurement of a fussy child's vital signs?

3. Ellen assists Dr. King with the physical examination of the patient. After assessing the vital sign measurements taken by the medical assistant, Dr. King examines Chris's ear and lungs. A swab of fluid discharge is taken from the patient's ear. What is the role of the medical assistant during the provider's examination of this patient?

4. Dr. King makes a clinical diagnosis of otitis media for this patient and orders laboratory testing to be performed on the patient's specimen. What criteria are necessary for a provider to make a clinical diagnosis?

5. What is otitis media? Why are children more likely at risk for this condition? How is otitis media commonly treated? What patient education can the health care team offer? (Consult a medical reference or encyclopedia for help in answering this question.)

CERTIFICATION REVIEW

These questions are designed to mimic the certification examination. Select the best response.

1. The head circumference of a newborn should range between:
   a. 12.5 and 14.5 inches
   b. 14.5 and 16.5 inches
   c. 16.5 and 18.5 inches
   d. 18.5 and 20.5 inches

2. The axillary temperature is taken in the:

   a. rectum

   b. mouth

   c. armpit

   d. ear

3. The respiratory rate of a 1-year-old child should range between ______ breaths per minute.

   a. 20 and 30

   b. 20 and 40

   c. 16 and 20

   d. 12 and 20

4. Otitis media is:

   a. an inflammation of the middle ear

   b. an infestation of parasitic lice

   c. a spasm of the bronchi

   d. an infection of the tonsils

LEARNING APPLICATION

CASE STUDY

The following is a true story of a young boy (about 8 years of age) who came in to the office with testicular torsion. This is when the testicle twists on its cord and often becomes ischemic, resulting in tissue death. The surgeon needs to explore the area to determine if the testicle can be saved or if it needs to be removed. The testicle is usually quite swollen and tender. When the child was told that he needed to go to the surgery center and that the doctor would take care of his problem and make him feel better, he began to cry. He was inconsolable. Why do you think he was so upset? Here are some options to discuss with fellow classmates:

1. He was afraid of the pain.
2. He was afraid of the surgery.
3. He was embarrassed.
4. Other?

CASE STUDY REVIEW QUESTION

1. Discuss what you could do as a medical assistant to help the boy and his parents with all of the above possible scenarios. The reason the child was afraid might surprise you and reminds us all to be careful not to assume we know what a patient is thinking.

   ____

   ____

   ____

   ____

CHAPTER POST-TEST

Perform this test without looking at your book. If an answer is "false," rewrite the sentence to make it true.

1. True or False? Pediatrics is the practice of medicine with children from birth through age 14.

____

____

2. Toddlers are children from:

   a. about 1 to 3 years old

   b. birth to 2 years old

   c. the time they are able to walk until they are in kindergarten

   d. about 2 to 5 years old

3. True or False? Measurements of babies consist of chest circumference, head circumference, length, and weight.

____

____

4. Normal childhood immunizations include which of the following?

   a. MMR, tetanus, DTaP, and IPV

   b. Hib, DTaP, MMR, and HIV

   c. IPV, MMR, DTaP, Hib, and HBV

   d. HBV, Hib, pertussis, and HAV

   e. Both c. and d.

5. The preferred site for injections for a child younger than 2 years is:

   a. the vastus lateralis

   b. the gluteus medius

   c. the deltoid

   d. Any of the above sites is acceptable.

6. Normal pulse and respiration for a child who is 8 years old is:

   a. respiration of 30, pulse of 80

   b. respiration of 18, pulse of 86

   c. respiration of 12, pulse of 80

   d. respiration of 20, pulse of 120

   e. none of the above

SELF-ASSESSMENT

As you respond to the following questions, think of how your experiences will affect how you treat your patients.

1. Think of your first memory of going to the doctor's office or getting any medical treatment. Think of how you felt from what you can remember. You may have more than one vivid memory, or you may have to think really hard to come up with any memories. Maybe your memories are not from a hospital or doctor's office; that is, maybe you received medical care from your parents, grandparents, or a neighbor. Your memories might not be exactly accurate, but they are a child's perception, and the feelings are real. This awareness can help you interact well with your young patients. Circle all of the words from the following list that come to mind as you take this mental journey back in time (if you have more than one incident to remember, use different colored inks to circle the words). You may even add a couple of your own descriptors if necessary.

helpless	pain	invaded
embarrassed	guilty	angry
alone	afraid of being punished	afraid of what was happening
afraid of pain	happy with the attention	dizzy
relieved	loved	powerless
excited	safe	afraid of the blood
stupid	other: ________________	other: ____________________

Each of our memories will be different, and we will all have different feelings about them. Try to keep this in mind as you treat your young patients. Try to respect what feelings they have and strive to make them comfortable. Reassure them as much as you can.

____

____

____

____

Name ______________________ Date __________ Score ______

CHAPTER 16

Male Reproductive System

CHAPTER PRE-TEST

Perform this test without looking at your book. If an answer is "false," rewrite the sentence to make it true.

1. The most common disease afflicting men older than 50 years is:
   a. prostate cancer
   b. benign prostatic hypertrophy (BPH)
   c. epididymitis
   d. testicular cancer
2. ED stands for:
   a. erectile disorder
   b. erectile dysfunction
   c. elemental disease
   d. epididymal disorder
3. Which of the following is *not* a sexually transmitted disease (STD) that afflicts men?
   a. Genital herpes
   b. Chlamydia
   c. Gonorrhea
   d. Epididymis
4. Vasectomy consists of:
   a. dissection of the seminal vesicles
   b. dissection of the vas deferens
   c. dissection of the testicles
   d. removal of the epididymis
5. True or False? Because of the latest discoveries in medications, ED can always be cured.

   ____

   ____

VOCABULARY BUILDER

Misspelled Words and Definitions

Find the words in Column A below that are misspelled; circle them, and correctly spell them in the space provided. Then match the following correct vocabulary terms listed in Column A with their corresponding definitions listed in Column B.

	Column A	Correct Spelling
____	1. Chriptorchidism	____________________
____	2. Intervenous pyelogram	____________________
____	3. Orchectomy	____________________
____	4. Residual	____________________
____	5. Retention	____________________
____	6. Transluminator	____________________
____	7. Transureteral resection	____________________

Column B

A. Urine held in the bladder; inability to empty the bladder

B. Amount of urine remaining in bladder immediately after voiding; seen with hyperplasia of prostate

C. Undescended testicle

D. X-ray of the kidneys, ureter, and bladder using a contrast medium

E. Instrument used to inspect a cavity or organ by passing a light through the walls

F. Removal of prostate tissue using a device inserted through the urethra

G. Surgical excision of a testicle

LEARNING REVIEW

Short Answer

1. Identify each part of the male reproductive system below. Describe each part and its function in the space provided. Then, using the textbook, a medical dictionary, or the Internet, list at least one common disorder that would adversely affect the part described.

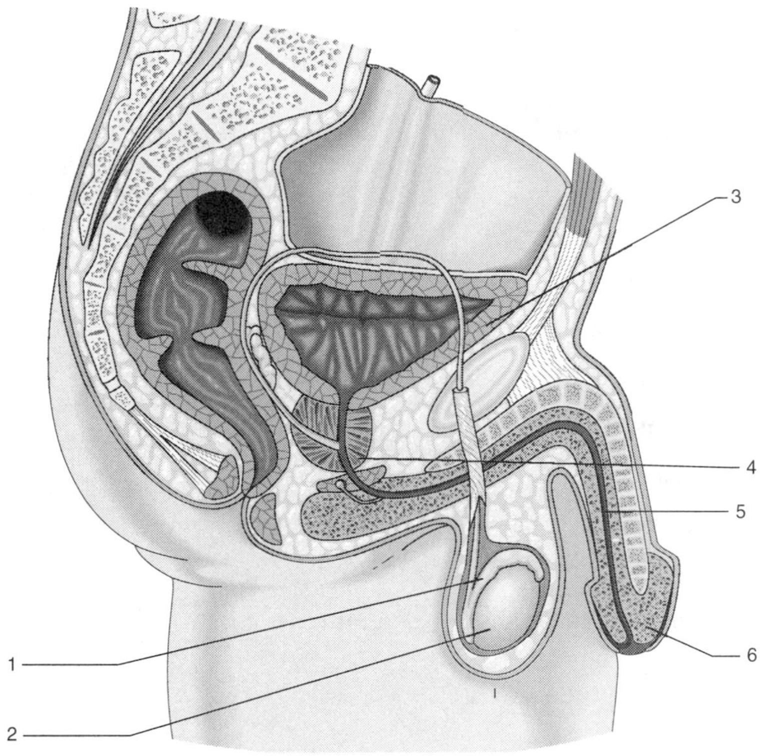

	Part	Common Disorder(s)
1.	______________	______________________________
2.	______________	______________________________
3.	______________	______________________________
4.	______________	______________________________
5.	______________	______________________________
6.	______________	______________________________

2. List at least two symptoms of a benign hypertrophic prostate gland.

____

____

____

3. The third leading cause of cancer deaths among men is ______________________.

4. Name at least two sexually transmitted diseases.

____

____

5. PSA tests should be performed ______________________ beginning at age 40.

CERTIFICATION REVIEW

These questions are designed to mimic the certification examination. Select the best response.

1. Testicular cancer is one of the leading causes of death in men younger than:
   a. 25
   b. 60
   c. 40
   d. 50
2. Male individuals from the onset of puberty should examine their testicles every:
   a. 6 months
   b. year
   c. month
   d. 3 months
3. BPH is a condition of the prostate. It stands for:
   a. benign prostatic hypertrophy
   b. benign prostatic hyperplasia
   c. beginning prostate hyperactivity
   d. benign prostate hyperactivity
4. The best way to determine that a patient has prostate cancer is by a(n):
   a. biopsy of the prostate
   b. PSA blood test
   c. rectal examination
   d. X-ray
5. Which of the following STDs is *not* treated with antibiotics?
   a. Chlamydia
   b. Gonorrhea
   c. Syphilis
   d. Genital herpes
   e. None of the above

LEARNING APPLICATION

CASE STUDY

CASE STUDY REVIEW QUESTION

1. Mr. Jones, a 75-year-old patient, has just been diagnosed with prostatic cancer. The provider has explained what is to be expected, but Mr. Jones is upset and asks you for your help in understanding the disease and treatment. How will you help him?

____

____

____

____

____

____

____

CHAPTER POST-TEST

Perform this test without looking at your book.

1. In men older than 50 years, a common disease condition is:
   a. prostate cancer
   b. BPH
   c. epididymitis
   d. testicular cancer
2. ED stands for:
   a. erectile dysfunction
   b. erectile disorder
   c. erectile disease
   d. epididymal disorder
3. Which of the following is an STD that can afflict men?
   a. Chlamydia
   b. Balanitis
   c. Peyronie's
   d. Epididymis

4. The dissection of the vas deferens is called a:
   a. vas-deferenectomy
   b. vasotomy
   c. vasectomy
   d. deferenectomy

SELF-ASSESSMENT

How do you think you will feel when assisting with a genitourinary examination or procedure on a male patient? Do you think it will be easier if the patient is much younger or much older than you are? Do you think older medical assistants feel more comfortable assisting with these types of examinations, regardless of their professional experience? Do you think you will become more comfortable with time? Do you think your male patient is also uncomfortable? After giving these questions some thought, answer the following questions. Discuss your ideas with other students. Discuss your ideas with male friends, family members, or classmates to gain more perspectives.

1. Do you think your behavior or attitude will have anything to do with your patients' comfort level?

   ____

   ____

   ____

   ____

2. What might you do to make yourself more comfortable during a male genitourinary examination/procedure?

   ____

   ____

   ____

   ____

3. What might you do to make your patient more comfortable?

   ____

   ____

   ____

   ____

Name ______________________ Date __________ Score ______

CHAPTER 17

Gerontology

CHAPTER PRE-TEST

Perform this test without looking at your book. If an answer is "false," rewrite the sentence to make it true.

1. True or False? Older adults are healthier today than they were a generation ago.

____

____

2. True or False? Chronic diseases are just a part of what will happen as we age.

____

____

3. True or False? To be old is to be sick, weak, and confused.

____

____

4. True or False? Every system in the body undergoes changes as people age.

____

____

5. True or False? The senses of sight, hearing, taste, and smell diminish with age.

____

____

VOCABULARY BUILDER

Misspelled Words and Definitions

Find the words in Column A below that are misspelled; circle them, and correctly spell them in the space provided. Then match the following correct vocabulary terms listed in Column A with their corresponding definitions listed in Column B.

	Column A	Correct Spelling
____	1. Arterialsclerosis	____________
____	2. Dementia	____________
____	3. Geriatrics	____________
____	4. Incontinance	____________
____	5. Macular degeneration	____________
____	6. Pernicous anemia	____________
____	7. Presbycusis	____________
____	8. Residule urine	____________
____	9. Transient ischemic attack	____________

Column B

A. The branch of medicine that is concerned with the problems of older adults

B. Disease marked by degeneration of the macular area of the retina of the eye

C. Progressive loss of hearing ability caused by the normal aging process

D. Temporary loss of blood to the brain, causing stroke-like symptoms

E. Urine remaining in the bladder after urination

F. Loss of the ability to retain urine in the bladder

G. Disorder involving the stomach that causes a deficiency of red blood cells

H. Decrease in cognitive abilities, especially memory impairment, often associated with Alzheimer's and Parkinson's diseases

I. Disease that leads to thickening, hardening, and loss of elasticity of the arteries

LEARNING REVIEW

True or False?

Tell whether each statement below is true or false. If an answer is "false," rewrite the sentence to make it true.

____ 1. When going over medications with geriatric patients, it is helpful for them to bring all their medications with them in their original containers.

____

____

____ 2. If you suggest memory joggers (such as use of a calendar for appointments and making lists) to your geriatric patients, you will insult their intelligence.

____

____

___ 3. Every system in the body is going to be affected by aging.

___ 4. Older adult patients have a heightened sense of pain compared with younger patients.

___ 5. True or False? There is not much a person can do to counteract the effects of aging.

Short Answer

1. List at least five ways to improve communication with the geriatric patient.

2. Why is gerontology becoming more recognized?

3. Why does food become less appealing as one ages, often decreasing the desire to eat and causing weight loss?

4. Fill in the chart below, listing two problems that might occur with each system as people age. The first row has been filled out as an example for you.

A. Vision and hearing	Dry, red, irritated eyes; sensitivity to light; inability to see clearly; inability to tell colors apart; inability to see small print; loss of hearing
B. Taste and smell	
C. Integumentary system	

D. Nervous system

E. Musculoskeletal system

F. Respiratory system

G. Cardiovascular system

H. Gastrointestinal system

I. Urinary system

J. Reproductive system

CERTIFICATION REVIEW

These questions are designed to mimic the certification examination. Select the best response.

1. When giving instructions to older adults, it is always a good idea to *(circle all that apply):*
   a. speak really loud
   b. write them in large print
   c. have patients repeat the instructions back to you if you think they did not understand completely
   d. a. and b.
   e. a., b., and c.
2. Dementia can include:
   a. memory loss
   b. confusion
   c. depression and agitation
   d. all of the above

3. The nervous system is affected by aging, resulting in all of the following *except*:
   a. insomnia
   b. problems with balance
   c. increased pain sensation
   d. problems with temperature regulation
4. The buildup of plaque in blood vessels is called:
   a. incontinence
   b. heart attack
   c. arteriosclerosis
   d. cardiopulmonary dysfunction
5. The progressive loss of hearing ability caused by the normal aging process is called:
   a. senility
   b. presbycusis
   c. deafness
   d. audio deficiency

LEARNING APPLICATION

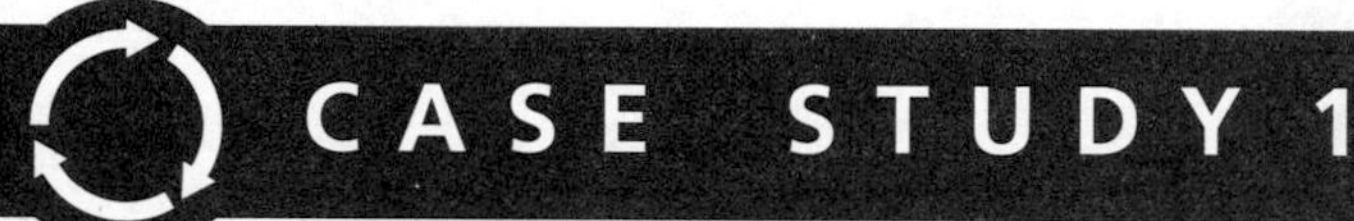

CASE STUDY REVIEW QUESTION

1. Sam Jones, 84 years old, has been examined by the provider and is ready to leave the office. Mr. Jones tells you that he is having trouble remembering to take the many medications the doctor has given him. As a medical assistant, what can you do to help him remember to take his medication?

____

____

____

____

____

CASE STUDY 2

CASE STUDY REVIEW QUESTION

1. Sandy Jones, granddaughter of Sam Jones, has come to the office with her grandfather. She tells you that she is concerned because of her grandfather's recent weight loss. She shares with you that he is not eating well. Mr. Jones is 84 and lives alone. How will you respond to Sandy? Can you think of some suggestions for them?

CHAPTER POST-TEST

Perform this test without looking at your book. If an answer is "false," rewrite the sentence to make it true.

1. True or False? Older adults are less healthy today than they were a generation ago.

2. True or False? Chronic diseases do not have to be a normal part of aging.

3. True or False? Memory loss is Alzheimer's.

4. True or False? Few changes occur as people age.

____

____

5. True or False? As people age, their senses of sight, hearing, taste, and smell diminish.

____

____

6. True or False? There is much a person can do to counteract the effects of aging.

____

____

SELF-ASSESSMENT

Without looking in the textbook, list 15 adjectives that describe older adults. Then list 15 adjectives that describe young adults. As you make your list, consider your personal biases toward older adults. Consider the differences in the two lists and think of why you chose those descriptors. When you are finished, discuss your lists with classmates. Share stories about people in your lives who are extraordinarily healthy and happy as they age. Think about the prejudices and assumptions you carry toward aging patients. Try to remember these as you work with those patients. It might be a good idea to create a list of tips to remember about geriatrics and keep it posted by your workstation.

____

____

____

____

Name ______________________ Date ____________ Score ______

CHAPTER 18

Examinations and Procedures of Body Systems

CHAPTER PRE-TEST

Perform this test without looking at your book. If an answer is "false," rewrite the sentence to make it true.

1. True or False? Urinary catheterization is performed only in hospitals during surgeries.

____

____

2. True or False? Instillation and irrigation mean the same thing.

____

____

3. An upper GI series (barium swallow) is used to examine the:
   a. entire large intestine
   b. stomach and entire small intestine
   c. esophagus, stomach and part of the small intestine
   d. esophagus, stomach, and small and large intestines
4. True or False? To test visual acuity, the patient must be able to recognize the letters of the English alphabet.

____

____

5. Medical assistants cannot remove casts.

____

____

6. True or False? Pulse oximetry is a way of counting the pulse at the wrist to determine the heart rate.

____

____

VOCABULARY BUILDER

Misspelled Words I

Find the words below that are misspelled; circle them, and correctly spell them in the spaces provided. Then fill in the blanks in the sentences below with the correct vocabulary terms listed below with their proper definitions.

alveoli	biopsy	comedome
aphasia	bronchi	demyelination
aurical	carbuncle	erythemia
____________	____________	____________

1. A ____________________________ is an inflammation of the skin and deeper tissues that terminates in slough and suppuration.
2. ____________________________ is a form of macula showing diffused redness of the skin.
3. Destruction or removal of the myelin sheath is ____________________________.
4. The ____________________________ are the two main branches leading from the trachea to the lungs.
5. The provider obtains a representative tissue sample for microscopic examination during a ____________________________.
6. ____________________________ is the absence or impairment of the ability to communicate through speech.
7. ____________________________ are air sacs in the lungs.
8. The typical small lesion of acne vulgaris is ____________________________.
9. The ____________________________ is the portion of the external ear that is not connected to the head.

Misspelled Words II

Find the words in Column A that are misspelled; circle them, and then correctly spell them in the spaces provided. Then match each of the correct vocabulary terms listed below with its proper definition.

	Column A	Correct Spelling
___	1. Akinesia	______________
___	2. Vescicle	______________
___	3. Spirometer	______________
___	4. Ossicle	______________
___	5. Opthalmoscope	______________
___	6. Ocluder	______________
___	7. Obturator	______________
___	8. Nebulizer	______________
___	9. Lesion	______________
___	10. Hydronephrosis	______________
___	11. Gate	______________

Column B

A. A device for producing a fine spray

B. A device used to close or obstruct an eye

C. A wound, an injury, or any pathologic change in body tissue

D. A device for examining the interior of the eye

E. A collection of urine in the renal pelvis caused by obstructed outflow forming a cyst by distention or atrophy

F. Small raised skin lesion containing fluid

G. A small bone such as the malleus, incus, and stapes

H. A manner of walking

I. A device used to close or block a canal, vessel, or passage of the body

J. Complete or partial loss of muscle movement

K. An instrument used to measure and record the volume of inhaled and exhaled air

LEARNING REVIEW

Multiple Choice

1. Common symptoms of urinary tract diseases and disorders are:
   a. dysuria, proteinuria, hematuria, and frequency
   b. dysuria, frequency, oliguria, and headache
   c. hematuria, pain, frequency, and headache
   d. frequency, hematuria, vaginal discharge, and dysuria
2. Cystitis is another name for what disorder?
   a. Kidney cysts
   b. Gallbladder disease
   c. Multiple cysts of the breasts or other area
   d. Bladder inflammation
3. UTI means:
   a. urinary tract infection
   b. urinary tract inflammation
   c. urinary tract involvement
   d. urinary treatment initiated

4. The medical term meaning "hidden" is:

   a. cult

   b. occult

   c. crypt

   d. retro

5. Which of the following is(are) an eating disorder(s)?

   a. Bulimia

   b. Anorexia nervosa

   c. Diverticulosis

   d. Crohn's disease

   e. a. and b.

6. The medical condition of having an increase in intraocular pressure is called:

   a. glaucoma

   b. retinal detachment

   c. cataract

   d. macular degeneration

7. Ear lavage or irrigation is performed for:

   a. impacted sebum

   b. impacted cerumen

   c. impacted lacrimal glands

   d. otitis media

8. The leading cause of blindness in the United States is:

   a. retinal detachment

   b. cataract

   c. glaucoma

   d. diabetes

9. A cholecystectogram is a test for:

   a. kidney stones

   b. diseases of the gallbladder

   c. diseases of the blood vessels

   d. gastrointestinal disorders

10. Which of the following is not determined by a chest radiograph?

    a. Bronchitis

    b. Pneumonia

    c. Pharyngitis

    d. Tuberculosis

11. Coronary artery bypass surgery might be used to help prevent which of the following cardiovascular conditions?

    a. Myocardial infarction

    b. Pericarditis

    c. Thrombophlebitis

    d. Coronary artery disease

12. Which of the following cardiovascular diseases may be treated with antibiotics?

    a. Thrombophlebitis

    b. Pericarditis

    c. Angina pectoris

    d. Valve stenosis

13. Which of the following diseases is caused by a lack of dopamine?

    a. Epilepsy

    b. Depression

    c. Reye's syndrome

    d. Parkinson's disease

14. Shingles is a type of:

    a. herpes

    b. psoriasis

    c. dermatitis

    d. acne

15. The type of disease in which the white blood cells become prolific is:

    a. anemia

    b. infectious mononucleosis

    c. leukemia

    d. lymphedema

Labeling

1. Identify the parts of the digestive system.

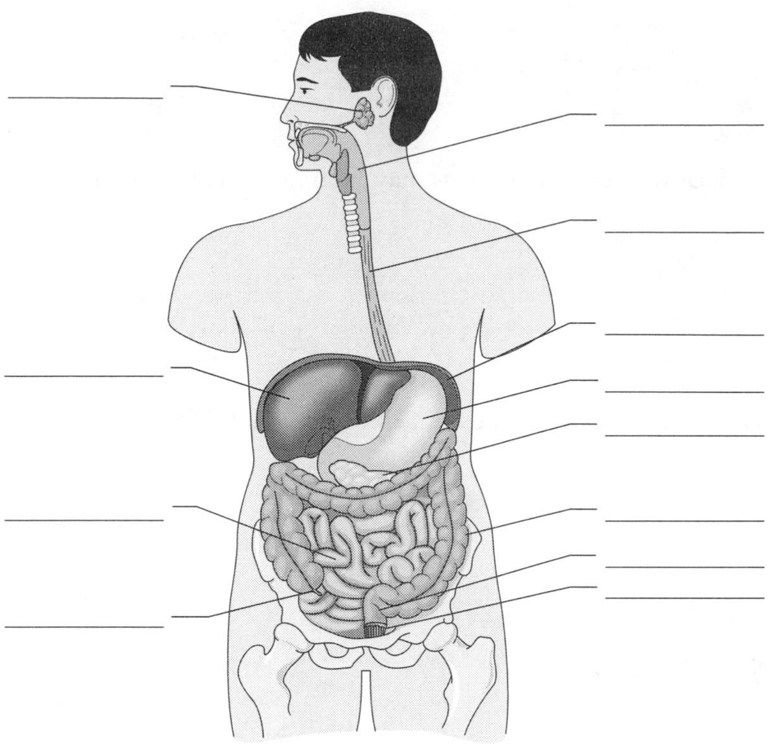

2. Identify the parts of the eye.

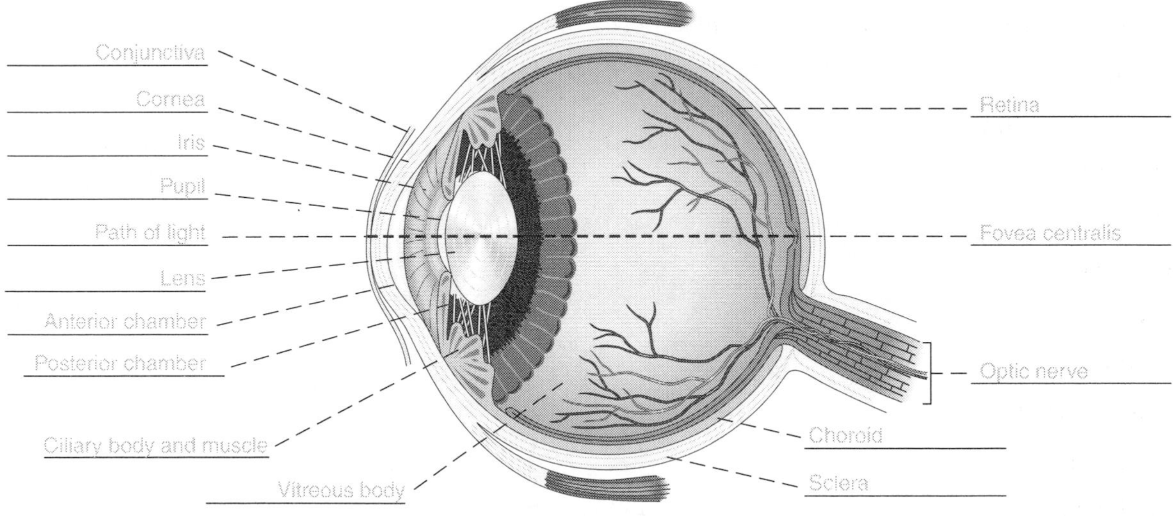

3. Identify the parts of the ear.

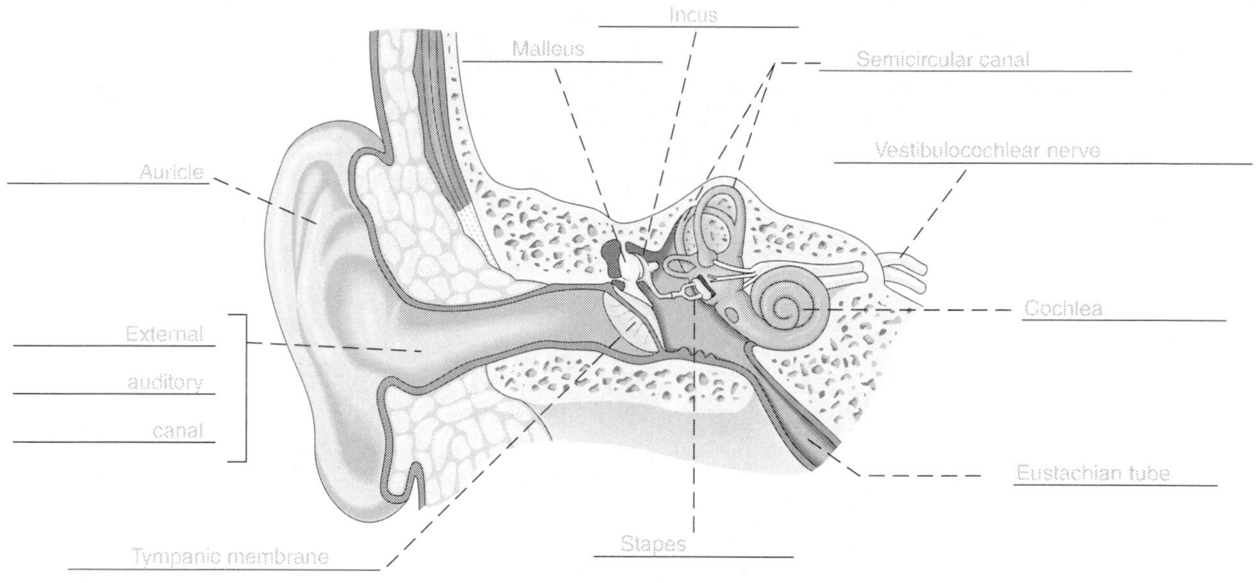

CERTIFICATION REVIEW

These questions are designed to mimic the certification examination. Select the best response.

1. Bacteria that reach the urinary tract through the blood cause ________________ infection.
   a. homogenous
   b. hematogenous
   c. ascending
   d. descending
2. High levels of nitrogenous waste in the blood may result in:
   a. polyuria
   b. oliguria
   c. uremia
   d. pyuria
3. A sigmoidoscopy is a diagnostic examination of:
   a. the inner ear
   b. the bladder
   c. a part of the colon
   d. the eye

4. Guaiac slides are used to detect:
   a. occult blood in the stool
   b. the type of bacteria found in otitis media
   c. thrush of the mucous membranes of the mouth
   d. cholelithiasis
5. A diagnostic test done to determine the presence of stones, duct obstruction, or inflammation of the gallbladder is called a:
   a. barium enema
   b. barium swallow
   c. cholecystogram
   d. gastroscopy

LEARNING APPLICATION

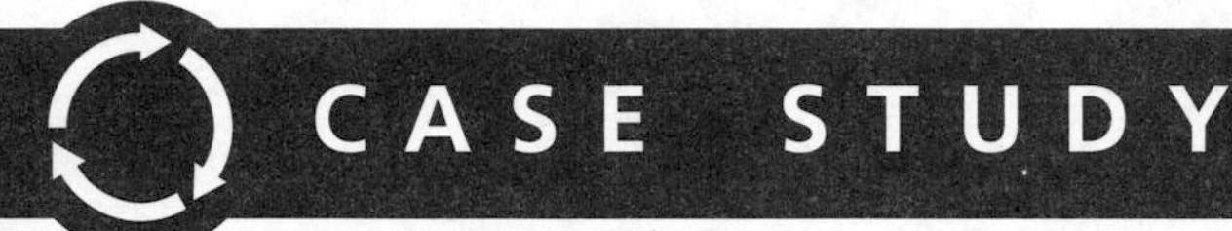

CASE STUDY REVIEW QUESTIONS

1. While visiting with family members, your elderly aunt shares with you that she has noticed that her stools are black. This has been happening off and on for several months and now she says her "belly feels swollen" and she is constipated a lot, which is not normal for her. How will you respond?

____

____

____

2. Your aunt becomes alarmed and says she is afraid of what they will do to her; maybe she will need surgery, and she cannot leave her husband alone, and what if it is cancer. She obviously has many concerns and is quite worried. How can you assist her?

____

____

____

____

____

____

____

____

CHAPTER POST-TEST

Perform this test without looking at your book. If an answer is "false," rewrite the sentence to make it true.

1. True or False? Urinary catheterization often is performed in clinics, hospitals, and surgery centers.

____

____

2. True or False? Instillation and irrigation are different procedures.

____

____

3. An upper GI series (barium swallow) is used to examine:
   a. the esophagus, the stomach, and the small and large intestines
   b. both the small and the large intestine
   c. the stomach and the entire small intestine
   d. the esophagus, stomach and part of the small intestine

4. True or False? To test visual acuity, the patient does not need to recognize the letters of the English alphabet.

____

____

5. True or False? Medical assistants often remove casts.

____

____

6. True or False? Pulse oximetry is used to determine the oxygen concentration of the blood in a noninvasive way.

____

____

SELF-ASSESSMENT

Think of a time when you or a close family member had to go to the provider's office and then go through a diagnostic procedure or test for a medical disorder or a disease. Fill in the following outline with as much information as you can remember.

1. What were the patient's symptoms? Try to list two or three.

____

____

____

____

____

2. Describe how the disease started. (Suddenly? Gradually? Over time? Related to an injury?)

3. Did the patient go to the emergency department or to the provider's office first?

4. Did the provider, or his or her staff, clearly explain the test or procedure to the patient or the patient's family?

5. What were some of the feelings that you had during the process? List two or three.

6. Could the medical assistant and doctor have reassured you better or kept you better informed, or did they do a good job of answering your questions and meeting your needs and the needs of the patient?

7. How will your experience influence your interaction with your patients when you are assisting with a diagnostic test or procedure? What will you pay special attention to that you might not have if you had not had the experience described above?

Name ______________________ Date __________ Score ______

CHAPTER 19

Assisting with Office/ Ambulatory Surgery

CHAPTER PRE-TEST

Perform this test without looking at your book. If an answer is "false," rewrite the sentence to make it true.

1. True or False? The anesthesia used in ambulatory care surgery is different from anesthesia used in major surgeries.

   ____

   ____

2. True or False? "Dressing" and "bandage" are different words that mean the same thing.

   ____

   ____

3. True or False? "Inflammation" means infection.

   ____

   ____

4. The signs of inflammation are:
   a. redness, drainage, pain, and swelling
   b. redness, pain, and swelling
   c. redness, pain, swelling, and tenderness
   d. redness, pain, swelling, and warmth

5. True or False? A sterile item is free from all microorganisms and their spores.

   ____

   ____

6. True or False? Only major surgeries require the patient to sign an informed consent form.

   ____

   ____

VOCABULARY BUILDER

Misspelled Words

Find the words in Column A that are misspelled; circle them, and correctly spell them in the spaces provided. Then match each of the vocabulary terms below with the correct definition in Column B.

	Column A	Correct Spelling
____	1. Inflamation	________________
____	2. Ephinephrine	________________
____	3. Ligature	________________
____	4. Sodium hydroxide	________________
____	5. Hibeclens®	________________
____	6. Anestesia	________________
____	7. Betadine	________________
____	8. Silver nitrate	________________
____	9. Isopryl alcohol	________________
____	10. Hydrogen proxide	________________
____	11. Strictures	________________
____	12. Tetnus	________________
____	13. Surgical asepsis	________________

Column B

A. The trade name for povidone-iodine, a topical anti-infective

B. A toxic preparation important as a germicide and local astringent

C. Partial or complete loss of sensation, with or without loss of consciousness

D. A hormone secreted by the adrenal medulla in response to stimulation of the sympathetic nervous system; used in conjunction with a local anesthetic. It constricts blood vessels to help lessen bleeding during ambulatory surgery.

E. A condition free from germs, infection, and any form of life

F. A narrowing or constriction of the lumen of a tube, duct, or hollow organ

G. Trade name for chlorhexidine gluconate, a topical antiseptic

H. A thread or wire for tying a blood vessel or other structure to constrict or fasten it

I. The nonspecific immune response that occurs in reaction to any type of bodily injury

J. NaOH, a caustic antacid used in detergents and other chemical compounds

K. An acute infectious disease of the central nervous system (CNS) caused by an exotoxin

L. A clean, flammable liquid used in medical preparations for external use

M. Used in aqueous solution as a mild antiseptic, germicide, and cleansing agent

Definitions

Match the vocabulary words below with their correct definitions.

____ 1. Allergies

____ 2. Antibacterial

____ 3. Approximate

____ 4. Bandage

____ 5. Cautery

____ 6. Contamination

____ 7. Dressings

____ 8. Infection

____ 9. Informed consent

____ 10. Liquid nitrogen

____ 11. Mayo stand/instrument tray

____ 12. Ratchets

____ 13. Surgery cards/computer

____ 14. Suture

____ 15. Swaged/atraumatic

A. To bring together the edges of a wound

B. A written reference for surgeries and procedures

C. Gauze or other material applied directly to a wound to absorb secretions and for protection

D. A surgical needle is attached to a length of suture material

E. Surgical material or thread; may describe the act of sewing with the surgical material and needle

F. Being sensitive to a normally harmless substance that causes an autoimmune reaction

G. An invasion of pathogens into living tissue

H. A voluntary agreement to have a procedure or surgery after a patient has been informed about the risks and benefits

I. A portable metal tray table used for setting up a sterile field for minor surgery and procedures

J. Capable of destroying bacteria

K. Commonly and incorrectly referred to as "dry ice"; a volatile freezing agent used to destroy unwanted tissue such as warts

L. The locking mechanisms on the handles of many surgical instruments

M. The destruction of tissue by burning

N. Gauze or other material applied over a dressing to protect and immobilize

O. To make something unclean, often used to describe a sterile area being made "unsterile" or exposing a clean area to a pathogenic substance

LEARNING REVIEW

True or False?

Identify each statement as true or false. If an answer is "false," rewrite the sentence to make it true.

___ 1. Suture material may also be called ligature.

____

____

___ 2. The word *ligature* means "to tie."

___ 3. Tissue forceps have teeth; dressing forceps do not.

___ 4. Epinephrine causes blood vessels to dilate.

___ 5. Sterile technique is a term used interchangeably for surgical asepsis.

Short Answer

1. Identify each entry below as an example that follows strict sterile principles or in which the sterile area, field, or tray is contaminated. Write "sterile" or "contaminated" in the spaces provided. If the entry is "contaminated," write what was done to render it contaminated.

   A. Bruce Goldman, CMA (AAMA), collects used instruments handed to him by Dr. Mark Woo during a minor surgical procedure to excise an infected sebaceous cyst by placing the instruments in a separate container or area out of view of the patient.

   B. Ellen Armstrong, CMA (AAMA), sets up a sterile field for a minor surgical procedure. After setting up the field, she remembers that a sterile solution is required and leaves the room to obtain the solution to be poured into a sterile cup.

   C. Wanda Slawson, CMA (AAMA), removes a dressing from a wound on a patient's arm and reaches over the sterile field to discard the used dressing in a biohazard waste container she has placed on the other side of the sterile field that she set up for the procedure.

   D. Patient Edith Leonard will not stop talking and asking questions as Liz Corbin, CMA (AAMA), removes sutures from a small wound on Edith's arm sustained during a recent fall. The medical assistant is careful to time her responses to Edith so that she is not talking when she is working directly over the sterile field.

E. Anna Preciado, CMA (AAMA), applies sterile gloves in preparation to assist Dr. Lewis with a minor surgical procedure. During the procedure, she comforts the patient and assists the physician as required. When Anna's hands are not in use, she keeps them down at her sides, careful not to touch her gloved hands to her clothing or any other nonsterile item.

2. Living tissue surfaces, such as skin, cannot be sterilized. Name two examples of ways that skin can be rid of as many pathogens as possible before the use of a sterile covering.

3. Identify and describe the most widely used method of sterilization in the ambulatory care setting.

4. List six general rules that ensure proper sterilization when using an autoclave.

5. Identify the recommended requirements for effective sterilization in an autoclave.

Temperature

Time for sterilization of unwrapped items

Time for sterilization of loosely wrapped items

Time for sterilization of tightly wrapped items

Frequency of draining of water and cleaning of autoclave

Matching I

Match the following equipment with the correct aseptic method. For each instrument or item below, identify the method used for proper asepsis: chemical disinfection (CD), chemical sterilization (CS), or steam sterilization (SS) in an autoclave.

_____ 1. Percussion hammer

_____ 2. Wrapped surgical instruments

_____ 3. Stethoscopes

_____ 4. Fiber-optic endoscopes

_____ 5. Countertops

_____ 6. Wheelchairs

_____ 7. Gynecologic instruments

_____ 8. Examination tables

Matching II

Identify each action that follows as an action appropriate to medical aseptic hand washing technique (MAH) or surgical aseptic hand washing technique (SAH).

_______ 1. Do not apply lotion.

_______ 2. Glove for sterility.

_______ 3. 1 minute duration

_______ 4. Hold hands up during washing and rinsing.

_______ 5. Apply lotion.

_______ 6. Wash hands, wrists, and forearms to the elbows.

_______ 7. Hold hands down during rinsing.

_______ 8. 3- to 6-minute duration

CERTIFICATION REVIEW

These questions are designed to mimic the certification examination. Select the best response.

1. Surgical instruments that have opposing cutting edges are classified as:
   a. hemostats
   b. probes
   c. scissors
   d. scalpels

2. Surgical instruments that have ratchets are used for:

   a. cutting

   b. clamping

   c. probing

   d. exploring

   e. opening

3. Thumb forceps may also be called:

   a. pickups

   b. towel clamps

   c. hemostats

   d. Allis forceps

4. The recommended temperature for effective sterilization in an autoclave is:

   a. 212°F

   b. 270°F

   c. 150°F

   d. 220°F

5. An acceptable border between a sterile and a nonsterile area is:

   a. 1 inch

   b. 2 inches

   c. 4 inches

   d. 5 inches

6. The preferred length for suture material because it is manageable yet long enough to complete most suture procedures is:

   a. 10 inches

   b. 8 inches

   c. 12 inches

   d. 18 inches

7. Suture material that is used when more time is needed for healing is coated with:

   a. magnesium

   b. chromium

   c. calcium

   d. iodine

8. Application of a caustic chemical or destructive heat that burns tissue is called:

   a. cryotherapy

   b. evisceration

   c. approximation

   d. cauterization

9. Mechanism located between the rings of the handles of surgical instruments that is used for locking the instrument is called the:

   a. serration

   b. box-lock

   c. ratchet

   d. probe

LEARNING APPLICATION

Preparing Surgical Packs

Pretend the areas outlined below are labels on surgical packs that you have just wrapped. Label them with the proper information.

a. Iris scissors and 4 × 4 gauze.

b. Needle driver and a #3 scalpel handle.

c. Thumb tissue forceps and a #3 scalpel handle.

CASE STUDY 1

Joyanna Evans, CMA (AAMA), is responsible for maintaining and cleaning the autoclave at Inner City Health Care. Because this equipment is used every day to sterilize instruments, Joyanna cleans the inner chamber of the autoclave daily. Once a week she gives the autoclave a thorough cleaning.

CASE STUDY REVIEW QUESTIONS

1. Describe Joyanna's daily cleaning procedure.

2. Describe Joyanna's weekly cleaning procedure.

3. Why is proper maintenance and cleaning of the autoclave important?

CASE STUDY 2

Joyanna works with a variety of instruments and supplies as she assists in ambulatory care surgery. Answer the following questions related to surgical instruments and supplies.

CASE STUDY REVIEW QUESTIONS

1. From the selection that follows, identify each instrument by name. In the spaces provided, give a brief description of each instrument's use.

Instrument	Instrument Name	Uses
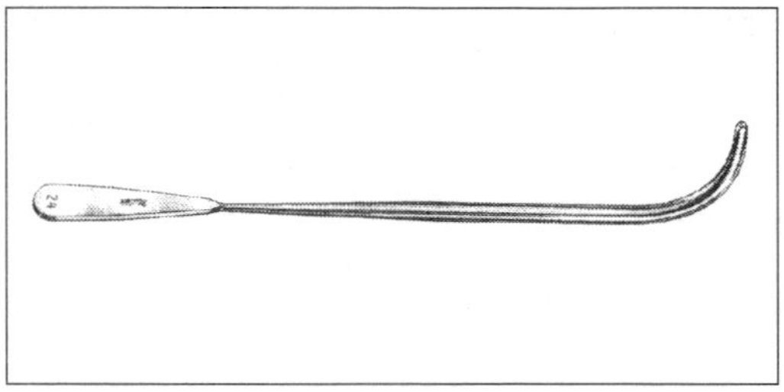	______________	______________
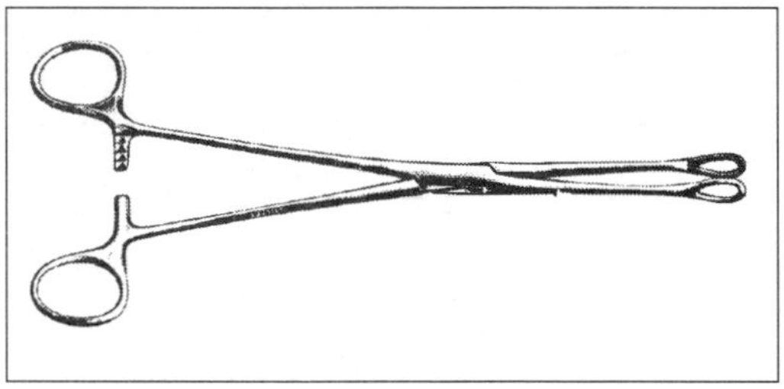	______________	______________
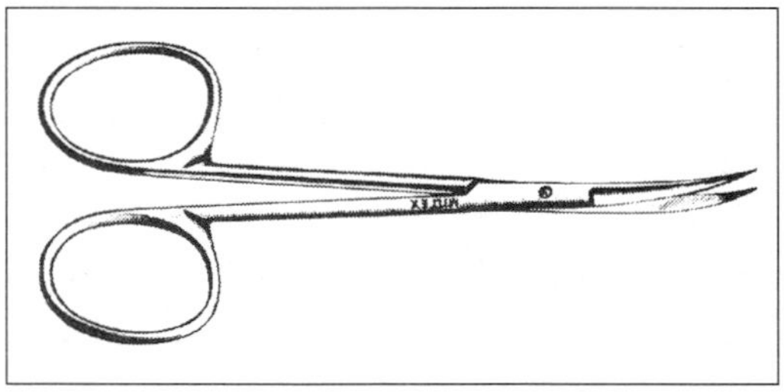	______________	______________
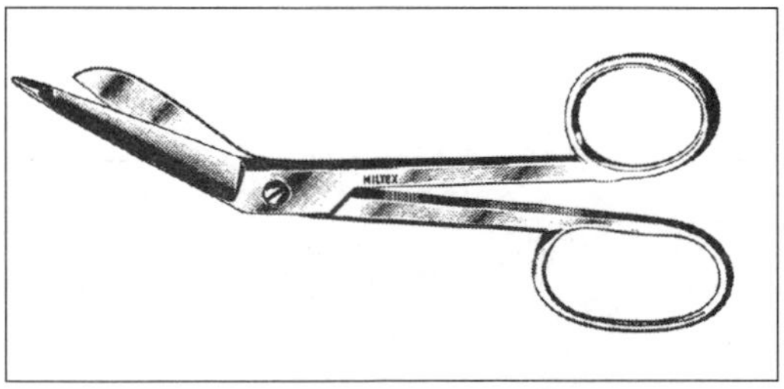	______________	______________

continues

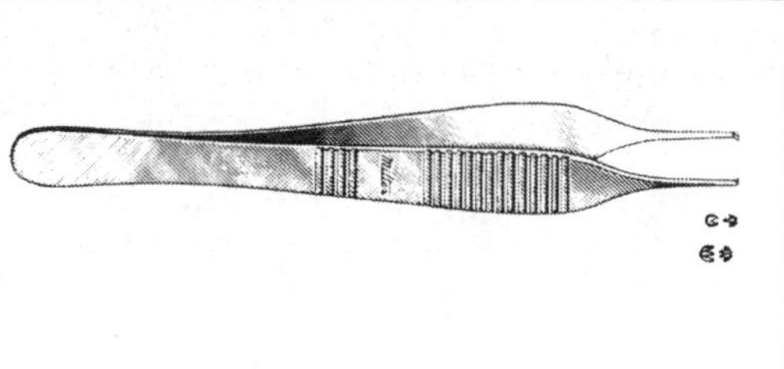

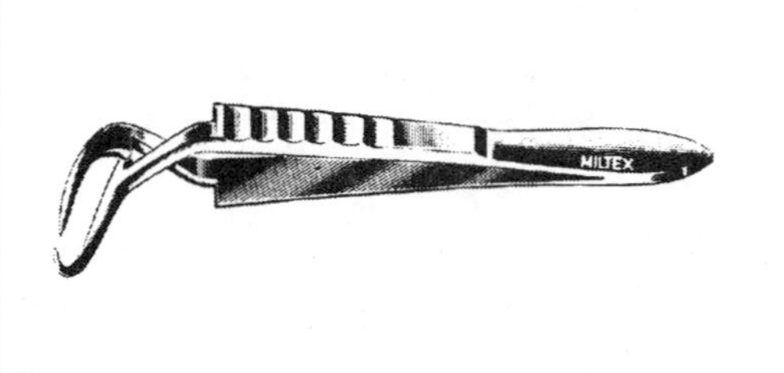

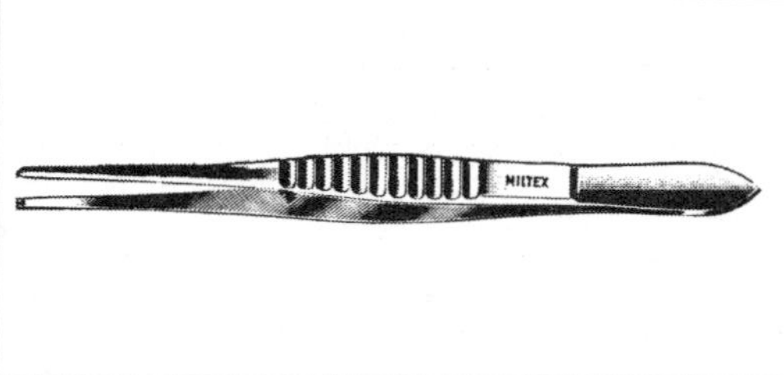

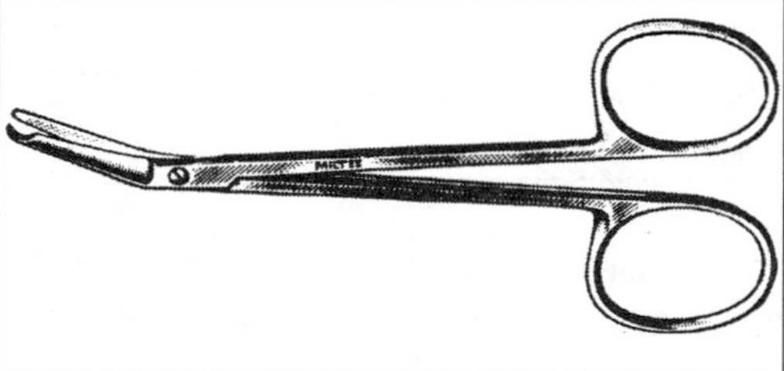

2. Joyanna will be removing stitches today. Which two instruments from above will she need for removing sutures?

CHAPTER POST-TEST

Perform this test without looking at your book. If an answer is "false," rewrite the sentence to make it true.

1. True or False? Anesthetics used in ambulatory care surgery are different from anesthetics used in major surgeries.

2. True or False? Dressings and bandages differ in that bandages are sterile and dressings are not.

3. True or False? Inflamed wounds are always infected.

4. The cardinal signs of inflammation are:
   a. redness, pain, swelling, and tenderness
   b. redness, drainage, pain, and swelling
   c. redness, pain, and swelling
   d. redness, pain, swelling, and warmth

5. True or False? A sterile item is free from all viruses and their spores.

6. True or False? Patients are required to sign an informed consent form only if they are having major surgery.

7. True or False? Patients must be told, in writing, all the things that can go wrong in a surgery and what other options they have besides surgery.

SELF-ASSESSMENT

Think of a time when you or a family member experienced a surgical event. If you have not had a personal surgical experience, interview a friend or family member and gather answers to the following questions.

1. Did the doctor or his or her staff explain the procedure clearly?

2. Were your questions answered to your satisfaction?

3. What was of greatest concern to you (financial concerns, pain, recovery, results, etc.)?

4. Did the recovery go as expected?

5. Were the results what you expected?

6. What could have made the experience better?

Name ______________________ Date __________ Score ______

CHAPTER 20

Diagnostic Imaging

CHAPTER PRE-TEST

Perform this test without looking at your book. If an answer is "false," rewrite the sentence to make it true.

1. True or False? Medical assistants may perform limited radiograph procedures in all states.

____

____

2. True or False? X-rays for fractures require no special patient preparation.

____

____

3. True or False? Radiopaque means that X-rays cannot penetrate it.

____

____

4. True or False? Ultrasound uses no X-rays and can view organs while they are in motion.

____

____

5. MRI stands for:

   a. magnetic realistic imaging

   b. magnetic resonance imaging

   c. magnetic ray imaging

   d. magnetic radiologic imagining

6. True or False? Radiation as a treatment for tumors uses X-rays to kill cancer cells.

____

____

VOCABULARY BUILDER

Misspelled Words

Find the words below that are misspelled; circle them, and correctly spell them in the spaces provided. Then write the following correct vocabulary terms next to their corresponding definitions.

computerized tomography	magnetic resonance imaging	radialpaque
dosimeter	MRA	radiolucent
flat plate	noninvasive	transducer
flouroscopy	position emission tomography	

_______________ _______________ _______________

_______________ 1. Use of fluorescent screen that shows the images of objects inserted between the tube and the screen

_______________ 2. Sound waves emitted from its head during ultrasound

_______________ 3. A noninvasive procedure where the patient lies inside a cylinder-shaped machine, or an open-bore machine, in which there is an electromagnet

_______________ 4. A noninvasive procedure that uses a small amount of radiation and beams that produce a series of cross-sectional images

_______________ 5. A radiographic procedure using a computer and radioactive substance

_______________ 6. Term a structure is called if X-rays do not penetrate it.

_______________ 7. "Plain" films

_______________ 8. Small, badgelike device worn above the waist which measures the amount of X-ray a person is exposed to

_______________ 9. Not entering the body

_______________ 10. Term a structure is called if X-rays penetrate it easily

_______________ 11. MRI for arteries and veins

LEARNING REVIEW

Short Answer

1. Describe the positions used during X-rays and include the direction of the X-rays, if applicable.

Position	Description	Direction of X-rays
Anteroposterior view (AP)	_______________	_______________
	_______________	_______________
	_______________	_______________
Posteroanterior view (PA)	_______________	_______________
	_______________	_______________
	_______________	_______________

Lateral view

Right lateral view (RL)

Left lateral view (LL)

Oblique view

Supine view

Prone view

2. For each radiologic test listed below, explain the purpose of the test.

Test	**Purpose**
Angiography	
Barium swallow (upper GI series)	
Barium enema (lower GI series)	
Cholangiography	
Cholecystography	
Cystography	
Hysterosalpingography	

Intravenous pyelography (IVP) ______________________________

Mammography ______________________________

Retrograde pyelography ______________________________

3. Describe the patient preparation needed for each test: before, during, and after. *NOTE*: instructions to the following exams may differ depending on the facility and technology involved.

Test	Patient Preparation
Angiography	
Barium swallow (upper GI series)	
Barium enema (lower GI series)	
Cholangiography	
Cholecystography	
Cystography	
Hysterosalpingography	

Intravenous pyelography (IVP) ____

Mammography ____

Retrograde pyelography ____

4. Why is exposure to radiation dangerous?

5. What test is performed to study the colon for disease?

CERTIFICATION REVIEW

These questions are designed to mimic the certification examination. Select the best response.

1. If a patient needs to be NPO before a radiologic procedure and the patient drinks a glass of water 3 hours before the appointment, what must you do?
   a. Water is allowed but nothing else.
   b. The procedure will need to be rescheduled.
   c. The patient needs a clearer explanation of what NPO means.
   d. Three hours is long enough for the water to be through the patient's system.
   e. b. and c.
2. Possible side effects of radiation include:
   a. hair loss, weight loss, nausea, and diarrhea
   b. hair loss, nausea, dizziness, and diarrhea
   c. nausea and vomiting, inflammation of the mouth, and hair loss
   d. all of the above
3. Palliative means:
   a. relieving symptoms, as well as curing
   b. curing but not offering much relief of symptoms
   c. placebo, or an agent that does nothing but the patient thinks it helps
   d. agents, such as pain relievers, used to relieve or alleviate painful or uncomfortable symptoms but do not cure the condition

4. When storing and safeguarding radiographs:
   a. they must be protected from light, heat, and moisture
   b. the environment is of little concern; they are basically plastic and can be wiped clean
   c. they must be kept in a cool, dry place
   d. a. and c.
5. What part of the X-ray machine produces X-rays?
   a. The control panel
   b. The tube
   c. The table
   d. The particle beam
6. Diagnostic imaging:
   a. is accessible to all offices and hospitals
   b. is an inexpensive form of testing
   c. results are easy to read
   d. results can be stored on computer systems

CASE STUDY

You begin working in an office where X-ray procedures are done. The provider has informed you that he will teach you the procedure for taking X-rays. In your state, special education and licensure are needed for a medical assistant to perform X-ray procedures. You also notice that no one in the office wears a dosimeter, although all are near the X-ray room during the day. Lead aprons are also not used on patients during X-ray procedures.

CASE STUDY REVIEW QUESTION

1. How will you handle this situation?

____

____

____

____

____

____

____

CHAPTER POST-TEST

Perform this test without looking at your book. If an answer is "false," rewrite the sentence to make it true.

1. True or False? Medical assistants and other health care professionals may perform limited X-ray procedures in most states.

2. True or False? X-rays for fractures require special patient preparation.

3. True or False? Radiopaque means that X-rays can penetrate a body part.

4. True or False? Ultrasound uses X-rays and can view organs while they are in motion.

5. MRI stands for:

   a. magnetic realistic imaging

   b. machine for radiologic imagining

   c. magnetic resonance imaging

   d. magnetic ray imaging

6. True or False? Radiation as a treatment for malignant tumors uses X-rays and radiopharmaceuticals to kill cancer cells.

SELF-ASSESSMENT

As a clinical medical assistant, if you are taking X-rays or assisting with X-ray procedures, what protective measures would you take? Would the patient take the same precautions? Why would you need more precautions than the patient?

Name ______________________ Date __________ Score ______

CHAPTER **21**

Rehabilitation and Therapeutic Modalities

CHAPTER PRE-TEST

Perform this test without looking at your book. If an answer is "false," rewrite the sentence to make it true.

1. True or False? To adduct is to move away from the midline.

____

____

2. True or False? Range of motion is measured in inches.

____

____

3. True or False? When lifting a heavy object, always bend from the waist and keep the object close to your body.

____

____

4. True or False? It helps to have patients put their arms around your neck when you lift them.

____

____

5. True or False? If a patient falls, you should protect his or her head, but otherwise, let the patient fall.

____

____

6. True or False? Medical assistants often perform range-of-motion exercises on patients in the office.

____

____

VOCABULARY BUILDER

Misspelled Words

Find the words below that are misspelled; circle them, and correctly spell them in the spaces provided. Then write the correct vocabulary terms next to the example below that best describes it.

activities of daily living
ambulation
assistive devices
atrophy
body mechanics
contractures
criotherapy
gait
gait belt
goniometer
goniometry
hemaplegia
modality
muscle testing
range of motion
thermaltherapy
ultrasound
vasoconstriction
vasodialation

________________ ________________ ________________

____

________________ 1. Patient Lenore McDonell, confined to a wheelchair since early childhood, receives continuing physical therapy to minimize the effects of any decrease of mobility and/or shrinkage of muscle tissue in her legs caused by inactivity.

________________ 2. When examining a new patient, a physical therapist must determine which of the physical agents, such as heat, cold, light, water, and electricity, will be most beneficial in treating the patient's condition.

________________ 3. As Margaret Thomas, diagnosed with Parkinson's disease, began to experience balance problems and difficulties in walking, her physical therapist prescribed the use of high-frequency sound waves to generate heat in the deep tissue of her right leg, producing a therapeutic effect.

________________ 4. Cold applications may be used to constrict blood vessels to slow or stop the flow of blood to an area.

________________ 5. Lenny Taylor, suffering the early stages of dementia from Alzheimer's disease, works with an occupational therapist to practice methods of making these everyday tasks easier to perform.

________________ 6. Heat is a modality that creates a therapeutic effect by causing blood vessels to dilate, thereby increasing circulation to an area and accelerating the healing process.

________________ 7. When construction worker Jaime VanBeek suffers a shoulder injury on the job, Dr. James Whitney performs this test for assessing the motion, strength, and task potential of the muscle group, tendons, and associated tissues.

________________ 8. Dr. Winston Lewis recommends this heat modality to help relieve Herb Fowler's chronic lower back pain, which is caused by strain on the back muscles created by the patient's overweight condition.

________________ 9. When patient Linda Maier comes to Inner City Health Care describing a sore back and several recent falls, Dr. Whitney asks clinical medical assistant Bruce Goldman to secure a gait belt around Linda's waist and have her walk across the room. With Bruce staying a step behind her and slightly to the side, Dr. Whitney carefully observes Linda's progress when performing this task.

________________ 10. As a muscle atrophies, shrinking and losing its strength, joints become stiff and experience development of these deformities. Without constant exercise, the musculoskeletal system deteriorates.

________________ 11. Dr. Susan Rice recommends that patient Linda Maier begin to use a walker at home to prevent further falls. Bruce Goldman, CMA (AAMA), secures this safety device around Linda's waist and positions her inside the walker as he gives her verbal instructions to begin the procedure of learning to ambulate with a walker.

________________ 12. Older adult patient Abigail Johnson is afraid that because she has diabetes mellitus she is at increased risk for stroke. "I don't want to end up a vegetable and a burden to my family," she tells Dr. Elizabeth King, "all paralyzed on one side like that."

________________ 13. Clinical medical assistant Joe Guerrero applies this practice of using certain key muscle groups together with correct body alignment to avoid injury when assisting patient Lenore McDonell in performing a transfer from her wheelchair to the examination table.

________________ 14. Margaret Thomas's neurologist uses this instrument to measure the angle of her shoulder joint's ROM during a follow-up examination for Parkinson's disease.

________________ 15. Dr. Mark Woo chooses this cold modality to treat the sprained wrist of an emergency patient, reducing inflammation.

________________ 16. Canes, walkers, and crutches are examples of walking aids.

________________ 17. When lying flat with arms at the sides, the average person should be able to move from a 20-degree hyperextension of the elbow joint to a 150-degree flexion.

________________ 18. A physical therapist uses the measurement of joint motion to help evaluate a patient's ROM.

Matching

Match each of the joint movement terminology listed below to its proper definition.

1. Extension	____	A. Moving the arm so the palm is up
2. Circumduction	____	B. Moving a body part outward
3. Plantar flexion	____	C. Straightening of a body part
4. Dorsiflexion	____	D. Motion toward the midline of the body
5. Eversion	____	E. Moving a body part inward
6. Adduction	____	F. Turning a body part around its axis
7. Hyperextension	____	G. A position of maximum extension, or extending a body part beyond its normal limits
8. Flexion	____	H. Motion away from the midline of the body
9. Inversion	____	I. Circular motion of a body part
10. Pronation	____	J. Moving the arm so the palm is down
11. Supination	____	K. Moving the foot downward at the ankle
12. Rotation	____	L. Moving the foot upward at the ankle joint
13. Abduction	____	M. Bending of a body part

LEARNING REVIEW

1. Some patients require assistive devices to ambulate. Name each assistive device shown below, then name the physical conditions each style is best suited to be used with as part of a physician's treatment plan. The first row has been completed for you as an example.

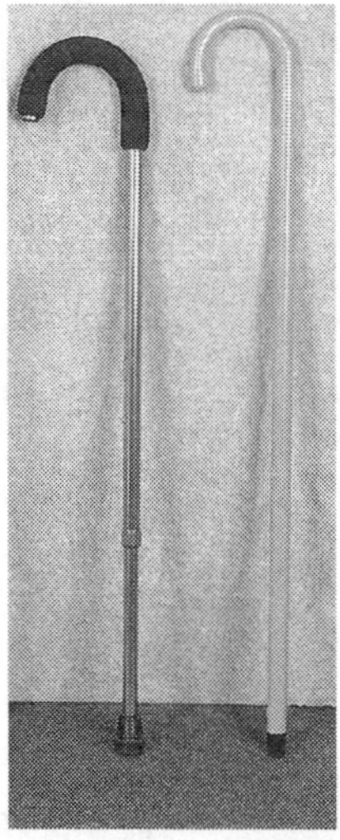

Name	Uses
Standard cane	The standard cane is good for patients with only one good arm, lateral instability, or balance conditions.

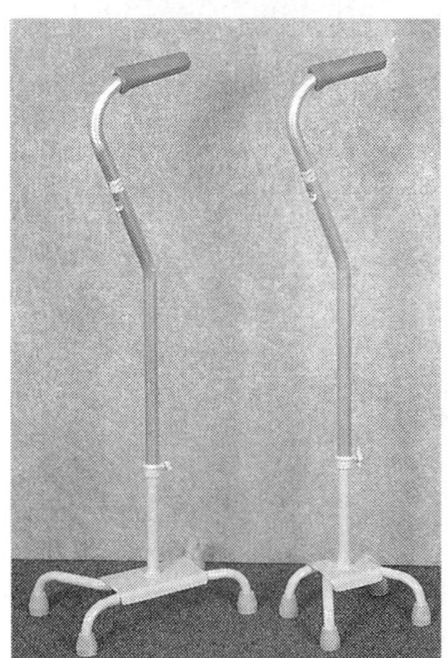

Name: ____________________

Uses: ____________________

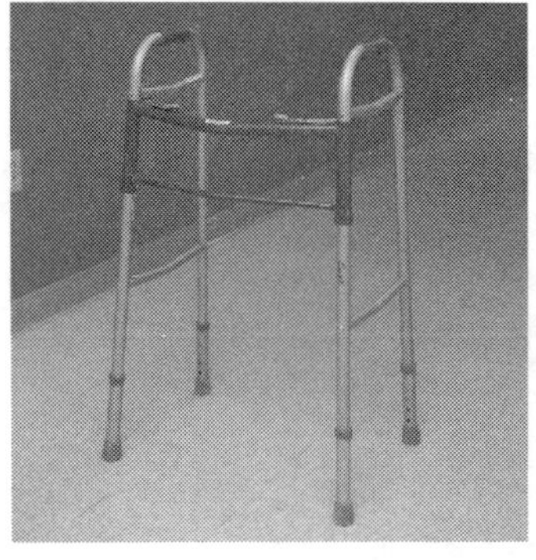

Name: ____________________

Uses: ____________________

Name	**Uses**
______________________	______________________________________
______________________	______________________________________
	______________________________________
	______________________________________
	______________________________________
	______________________________________

Name	**Uses**
______________________	______________________________________
______________________	______________________________________
	______________________________________

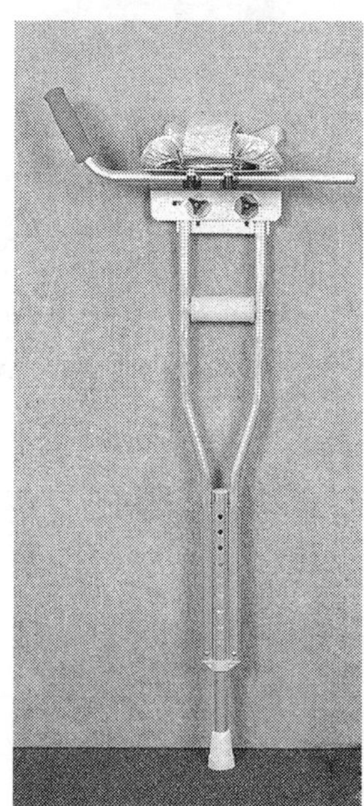

Name	**Uses**
______________________	______________________________________
______________________	______________________________________
	______________________________________
	______________________________________

2. Name four types of exercise programs that are used for therapeutic or preventative purposes.

____

____

3. Using the four types of exercise programs identified above, match each one to the example below that best describes it.

_______________ Pat Tidmarsh, who is suffering a sports injury to the muscles surrounding the knee, performs exercises with the help of a rubber exercise band.

_______________ Lourdes Austen performs self-directed exercises at home to improve the ROM and increase strength in her left arm, after lumpectomy and axillary lymph node dissection.

_______________ Lenore McDonell, who is confined to a wheelchair and unable to move her legs voluntarily, works regularly with a physical therapist to avoid atrophy and contractures in the legs and to improve overall circulation.

_______________ Luanne Moore, who is recovering from a shoulder injury, rebuilds upper body strength with a daily regimen of push-ups, first against the wall and then on the floor.

4. Therapeutic exercise is not the only way to treat painful joints or tissues. Many patients respond well to the therapeutic modalities of heat and cold, thermotherapy and cryotherapy. List six precautions that medical assistants must take when applying heat or cold modalities.

____

____

____

____

____

____

____

____

____

____

____

____

5. Identify each modality listed below as either a dry heat therapy (DHT), a moist heat therapy (MHT), a moist cold therapy (MCT), or a dry cold therapy (DCT) by placing the proper letters in the space provided. Then identify whether the modality can be performed at home by the patient, with or without caregiver assistance, or whether the modality must be performed in a clinical setting under the supervision of a health care professional.

_______ A. Ice pack _______________________________

____

_______ B. Paraffin wax bath _______________________________

____

____

_______ C. Cold compress ____

____

____

_______ D. Hot water bottle ____

____

____

____

_______ E. Warm compress ____

____

____

_______ F. Whirlpool bath ____

____

____

____

_______ G. Heating pad ____

____

____

____

____

_______ H. Warm soak of one extremity ____

____

____

_______ I. Warm pack ____

____

____

_______ J. Total body immersion in a Hubbard tank ____

____

____

____

6. For each of the following, identify the proper temperature and correct amount of time the modality should be administered to the patient. The first row has been completed for you as an example.

Modality	Temperature	Time
Aquamatic K-Pad for an older adult patient	Water temperature between 104°F and 113°F (41°C and 46°C)	Administered for no more than 30 minutes
Paraffin wax bath for a patient with rheumatoid arthritis	________________	________________
An ice pack for a patient with an ankle sprain	________________	________________
Hot water bottle for an adult patient	________________	________________
A warm compress to drain pus from a patient's skin infection	________________	________________
Warm soak of the arm and hand for a patient with osteoarthritis	________________	________________

7. How do ultrasound waves best travel? What are the special concerns of ultrasound treatment, how long can ultrasound be administered, and who is authorized to perform ultrasound procedures on patients?

____

____

____

____

____

____

____

CERTIFICATION REVIEW

These questions are designed to mimic the certification examination. Select the best response.

1. When lifting or carrying heavy objects, you should rely on the following muscle groups:

   a. abdominal

   b. thoracic

   c. legs and arms

   d. back

2. The type of assistive device that does not require much upper body strength but is not recommended for older adults is the:

   a. walker

   b. cane

   c. crutches

   d. wheelchair

3. When a patient is standing with hands on the grip of a walker, the elbow should be bent at a ______-degree angle.

   a. 90

   b. 45

   c. 15

   d. 30

4. The type of crutch that may be used temporarily while a lower extremity heals is:

   a. axillary

   b. forearm

   c. platform

   d. Lofstrand

5. A quad cane is:

   a. two-legged

   b. four-legged

   c. one-legged

   d. three-legged

LEARNING APPLICATION

CASE STUDY 1

Ellen Armstrong, CMA (AAMA), performs the annual task of assembling and moving inactive patient files into a storage filing area for safekeeping. It is the end of the day and Ellen is tired and eager to finish the job; this task has never been one of Ellen's favorites. When she gets to filling the last of three cartons of files, Ellen moves the carton to a shelf, about shoulder high, in the storage room. She returns and decides to take both of the remaining cartons in one trip. Fatigued, she bends at the waist to pick them up.

CASE STUDY REVIEW QUESTION

1. Describe the proper lifting technique that Ellen should use.

CASE STUDY 2

After explaining the procedure to the patient and her son, Wanda Slawson, CMA (AAMA), applies a gait belt and performs the transfer of Mary Craig, an older adult blind patient with diabetes mellitus who is suffering from atrophy of the legs, from a car to a wheelchair in the parking lot of Inner City Health Care. Unfortunately, because of Mary's position in the car, the patient must be transferred with her weaker side closest to the wheelchair. The patient panics during the transfer and throws her arms around Wanda's neck as she is lifting and pivoting Mary to the right to position her in the wheelchair. The patient's son, John, rushes forward to grab on to his mother.

CASE STUDY REVIEW QUESTIONS

1. What is the best action of the medical assistant?

continues

2. What is the best therapeutic response of the medical assistant?

3. Could the situation have been avoided? If so, how? If not, why not?

CASE STUDY 3

Dr. Susan Rice asks Bruce Goldman, CMA (AAMA), to instruct patient Dottie Tate in the use of a walker to prevent further falls at home. Dottie is silent as Dr. Rice leaves the examination room and Bruce proceeds to set the walker correctly. However, when Dottie sees that Bruce must once again put Dottie in a gait belt for her protection—the belt was used earlier in the examination to assess Dottie's ability to ambulate—the patient gets feisty. She is visibly tired and ready to go home. "I'll learn to use the walker if I have to, but I won't wear that infernal contraption. It makes me feel like a baby. And it's such a bother. Who wants to go through all that? We just don't need it."

CASE STUDY REVIEW QUESTIONS

1. What is the best action of the medical assistant?

2. What is the best therapeutic response of the medical assistant?

3. Could the situation have been avoided? If so, how? If not, why not?

CHAPTER POST-TEST

Perform this test without looking at your book. If an answer is "false," rewrite the sentence to make it true.

1. True or False? To abduct is to move away from the midline.

2. True or False? ROM is measured in degrees.

3. True or False? When lifting heavy objects, always bend from the waist and keep the object close to your body.

4. True or False? It helps to have patients put their arms on your shoulders when you help them to ambulate.

5. True or False? If a patient falls, you should gently ease him or her to the floor.

6. True or False? Medical assistants must be familiar with ROM exercises that will be performed on patients by other members of the health care team.

SELF-ASSESSMENT

1. Have you ever considered the field of physical or occupational therapy as a career?

2. What makes you think you would do well or not do well in those fields?

3. What do you think you would not care for in working with rehabilitative medicine? What would you like the most?

____

____

____

____

4. What are some of the skills, talents, interests, and abilities a person would need to have to do well in rehabilitative medicine? List a dozen or more, and then consider and circle all of those that you possess. Which on the list could you learn in a rehabilitative medicine program (insert an S for school), and which would be a natural part of your makeup (insert an N for natural)? Is there a direct relation between the skills, talents, interests, and abilities you possess and those that you marked with an N? Discuss your results with a small group of fellow students. What conclusion(s) did you reach?

____

____

____

____

Name ______________________ Date ____________ Score ______

CHAPTER 22

Nutrition in Health and Disease

CHAPTER PRE-TEST

Perform this test without looking at your book. If an answer is "false," rewrite the sentence to make it true.

1. True or False? Homeostasis depends on proper nutrients being made available for the body to use.

2. True or False? Some nutrients provide energy, whereas others help with bodily processes.

3. True or False? Fats, carbohydrates, and proteins provide energy.

4. True or False? Fat-soluble vitamins are those vitamins that need oil to be used and stored.

5. True or False? Water-soluble vitamins are readily depleted, and therefore must be taken in daily.

6. True or False? Antioxidants are those substances that help the body cells recover from the damaging effects of day-to-day living.

7. True or False? Fiber is primarily a carbohydrate and comes only from plant sources.

VOCABULARY BUILDER

Misspelled Words

Find the words below that are misspelled; circle them, and then correctly spell them in the spaces provided. Then fill in the blanks below with the correct vocabulary term from the following list.

absorbtion	digestion	metabolism
amino acids	electrolytes	nutrients
antioxident	elimination	nutrition
basal metabolic rate	extracellular	oxidation
calories	fat-soluble	preservatives
catalist	glycogen	processed foods
cellulose	homostasis	saturated fats
coenzyme	ingestion	trace minerals
diaretics	major minerals	water soluable

_______________ _______________ _______________

_______________ _______________ _______________

1. Artificial flavors, colors, and _______________, chemicals that keep food fresh longer, are non-nutritive substances commonly added to processed foods.
2. _______________ is the study of the intake of nutrients into the body and how the body processes and uses these nutrients.
3. Toxicity is most likely to occur with _______________ vitamins because they are stored in tissues composed of lipids and in the liver and are not carried easily into the bloodstream.
4. The best source of complete proteins are meats and animal products such as milk and eggs; complete proteins contain all eight of the essential _______________.
5. Beverages that contain caffeine and alcohol, which are _______________, will cause the body to increase urinary output and lose water. These substances should be avoided when performing activities, such as a good physical workout, and entering environments, such as an airplane passenger cabin, that promote dehydration.
6. A _______________ is a nonprotein substance that acts with a catalyst to facilitate chemical reactions in the body.
7. _______________ is the process of the digestive system involving the transfer of nutrients from the gastrointestinal tract into the bloodstream.
8. Chlorine (Cl) is a mineral with an important _______________ function, one that takes place outside the cells of body tissues in the spaces between layers or groups of cells.
9. The total of all changes, or energy, chemical and physical, that takes place in the body is called _______________.
10. Some minerals are considered _______________ in that they become ionized and carry a positive or negative charge; these minerals must be carefully balanced in the body.
11. _______________ begins at the mouth with chewing and progresses through the gastrointestinal tract to the small intestine.
12. _______________ are ingested substances that help the body maintain a state of homeostasis.
13. The process of _______________ maintains a constant internal environment of the human body, including such functions as heartbeat, blood pressure, respiration, and body temperature.

14. A ______________________________ facilitates chemical reactions by speeding up the reaction time without the need for a high-energy output.

15. It is always important to analyze the nutritional labels on ______________________________ purchased in the supermarket.

16. Lard is one example of ______________________________, which have been found to increase the level of fats and cholesterol in the blood and are hydrogenated, or contain hydrogen.

17. The ability to reduce ______________________________ is a characteristic of vitamin E that has led some researchers to suggest that vitamin E may slow the aging process, although its true effectiveness has not yet been demonstrated.

18. The excretion of waste through the anus is called ______________________________, the final step of the digestive process.

19. The amount of energy a substance is able to supply is measured in large ______________________________.

20. Potassium is one of the seven ______________________________ found in the body.

21. Vitamins that are ______________________________ must be constantly ingested to maintain proper blood levels, because these vitamins are not easily stored in the body.

22. Vitamin E is a fat-soluble vitamin that belongs to a group of compounds called ______________________, which counteract the damaging effects of oxidation. Beta-carotene is another substance in this group.

23. Despite their name, ______________________________ are vital to body functioning and include molybdenum and fluorine.

24. ______________________________ begins the digestive process when we put food in our mouths to eat.

25. Children, pregnant women, and people with a lean body mass will have a higher ______________________ because it takes more energy to fuel the muscles than it does to store fat.

26. A type of carbohydrate, ______________________________, is derived from a plant source and supplies fiber in the human diet.

27. Ingested only in small quantities, ______________________________ is an important carbohydrate form for storage of glucose in the body.

LEARNING REVIEW

1. Vitamins are a class of nutrients in which each specific vitamin has a function entirely of its own. These complex molecules are required by the body in minute quantities. What are the two functions of vitamins in the body?

____

____

____

2. Identify the correct chemical name for each vitamin listed. Then describe what each vitamin does in the body to promote good health.

   A. One of the B-complex vitamins, also called nicotinic acid:

   ____

   ____

   B. Vitamin B_1:

   ____

   ____

C. Vitamin E:

D. Vitamin D:

E. One of the B-complex vitamins, also called folacin:

F. Vitamin A:

G. Vitamin B_{12}:

H. Vitamin C:

I. Vitamin B_2:

J. Vitamin B_6:

3. Nutrients are divided into two groups: those that provide energy and those that do not. Identify the nutrients listed below as providing energy or not providing energy by placing an X in the appropriate column.

	Energy	**No Energy**
Vitamins		
Carbohydrates		
Fiber		
Minerals		
Lipids (fats)		
Proteins		
Water		

4. What three chemical elements do carbohydrates, fats, and proteins all contain?

____

____

5. Name the most important dietary complex carbohydrate. ____________________

6. Name the only true essential fatty acid in the human diet. ____________________

7. What additional chemical element does protein alone contain? ____________________

8. What happens when the body does not have enough carbohydrates or fats in supply as an energy source? What effect does this have on the body?

____

____

____

9. Name two conditions associated with deficiencies in protein.

____

____

____

10. List two distinct ways in which minerals differ from vitamins.

____

____

____

____

11. For each food source, list the mineral or minerals that each provides.
    (1) Eggs: ____
    (2) Milk: ____
    (3) Cheese: ____
    (4) Salmon: ____
    (5) Bananas: ____
    (6) Green vegetables: ____

12. List six types of fiber that are carbohydrates.

13. What important fiber is *not* a carbohydrate?

14. Americans generally do not consume enough fiber. How much fiber should be consumed each day?

15. Why does brown rice contain more fiber than white rice?

16. What happens when the body takes in more calories than will be expended by the body as energy?

17. What happens when the body uses more energy than the calories it takes in will produce?

18. What is the ideal percentage of total calories for adults that should be consumed as carbohydrates, fats, and proteins?

19. Compare the advantages and disadvantages of the following diets: U.S. southern, Jewish, and Japanese.

20. Obesity is a major health concern in the United States and often begins in childhood. What can you do as a medical assistant to assist parents to help their children avoid obesity?

____

____

____

____

Matching

For each of the following in Column A, identify the substance as a water-soluble vitamin (WSV), fat-soluble vitamin (FSV), a major mineral (MM), or a trace mineral (TM) in Column B. Then match the substance to the response in Column C that best fits its character or properties. The first one has been completed for you as an example.

	Column A	Column B
H	1. Sulfur	MM
____	2. Vitamin B_{12}	________
____	3. Iron	________
____	4. Vitamin K	________
____	5. Sodium	________
____	6. Pyridoxine	________
____	7. Iodine	________
____	8. Biotin	________
____	9. Retinol	________
____	10. Vitamin D	________

Column C

A. This substance works with potassium to maintain proper water balance and proper pH balance; the two also are involved in nervous muscular conduction and excitability.

B. This substance is part of the pigment rhodopsin found in the eye and is responsible in part for vision, especially night vision.

C. This substance is vital to life because of its role in the heme molecule, which carries oxygen to every cell in the body.

D. Rickets and osteomalacia are diseases caused by deficiencies in this substance; when deficiencies occur, usually in childhood, malformation of the skeleton is seen.

E. This member of the B-complex, together with pantothenic acid, is generally responsible for energy metabolism.

F. Because this substance is found only in foods from animal sources, such as liver, kidney, and dairy products, pernicious anemia, the result of deficiencies, may be a problem for some vegetarians.

G. This substance, found in rice, beans, and yeast, is important to protein metabolism.

H. This substance is a component of one of the amino acids and is found in protein; it is also involved in energy metabolism.

I. About half of the body's requirement for this substance is fulfilled through synthesis by intestinal bacteria; bile is required for its absorption into the bloodstream.

J. This substance is found only in the thyroid hormones; without it, the thyroid gland would be unable to regulate the overall metabolism of the body.

CERTIFICATION REVIEW

These questions are designed to mimic the certification examination. Select the best response.

1. Carbohydrates, fats, and proteins have one thing in common. What is it?
   a. High calcium content
   b. Their ability to convert into energy
   c. Low sodium content
   d. All of the above
2. Examples of monosaccharides are:
   a. fructose
   b. sucrose
   c. a. and d.
   d. glucose
3. The compounds composed of carbon, hydrogen, and oxygen that exist as triglycerides in the body are:
   a. fats
   b. fiber
   c. vitamins
   d. minerals
4. The basic structural unit of a protein is:
   a. simple sugar
   b. complex sugar
   c. lipids
   d. amino acids
5. Herbal supplements are also known as:
   a. phytomedicines
   b. antioxidants
   c. amino acids
   d. trans acids

LEARNING APPLICATION

Research Activities

1. Identify each organ of the digestive system below. Describe the healthy functioning of each organ in the space provided. Then, using a medical dictionary or encyclopedia, look up each organ and list one common disorder that would adversely affect the digestive process.

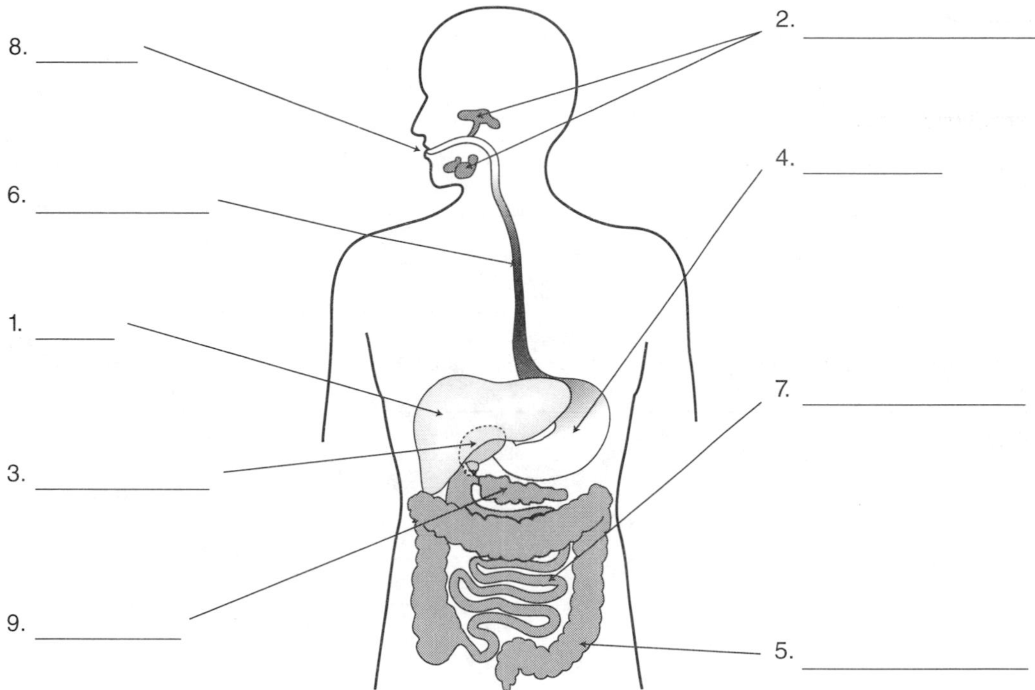

Healthy Function	Common Disorders
1. ______	______
______	______
______	______
______	______
______	______
2. ______	______
______	______
______	______
______	______
3. ______	______
______	______
______	______

4. __________

5. __________

6. __________

7. __________

8. __________

9. __________

2. When helping patients modify their diets, medical assistants need to be knowledgeable about the nutrients in the food we eat. The nutritional analysis label on the back or side of a food package is helpful when figuring out the levels of fat, cholesterol, sodium, carbohydrates, protein, and vitamins contained in a particular food. Obtain a food label and answer the following questions.

   A. The percentage of daily values listed on a food label report the amount of a nutrient obtained by eating how many servings of a product? ________

   B. The percentages are based on a ________-calorie diet.

   C. The listing for total carbohydrates is broken down into what two additional listings? Which type of carbohydrate is more beneficial and why?

D. A patient should look for a food product in which the sodium content is relatively low. What is the greatest number of milligrams of sodium a person should eat each day?

____

____

E. Why is a high-fiber diet important?

____

____

____

____

3. Compare the nutrition label from a box of muesli with fruit, nuts, and seeds with the label from a package of pretzel snacks. Which is more nutritious and why? Note that one serving of the muesli, a half cup or 55 grams, is roughly equivalent to 2 servings of pretzels, 14 pretzels or 60 grams.

Muesli

Nutrition Facts

Serving Size: 1/2 cup (55g)
Servings Per Container: about 8

Amount Per Serving	Cereal	Cereal + 125 mL Vitamin A & D fortified skim milk
Calories	210	250
Calories from Fat	30	35
	% Daily Value**	
Total Fat 3g*	5%	5%
Saturated Fat 0.5g	3%	3%
Cholesterol 0mg	0%	0%
Sodium 30mg	1%	4%
Total Carbohydrate 40g	13%	15%
Dietary Fiber 5g	21%	21%
Sugars 13g		
Protein 6g		
Vitamin A	0%	8%
Vitamin C	8%	8%
Calcium	4%	20%
Iron	35%	35%
Vitamin D	0%	10%
Thiamine	35%	40%
Riboflavin	25%	35%
Niacin	2%	2%
Vitamin B_6	15%	20%
Folate	10%	10%
Pantothenic Acid	4%	10%

*Amount in Cereal. One half cup skim milk contributes an additional 40 calories. 65 mg sodium. 6g total carbohydrate (6g sugars). and 4g protein

**Percent Daily Values are based on a 2.000 calorie diet. Your daily values may be higher or lower depending on your calorie needs.

	Calories	2.000	2.500
Total Fat	Less than	65g	80g
Sat Fat	Less than	20g	25g
Cholesterol	Less than	300mg	300mg
Sodium	Less than	2.400mg	2.400mg
Total Carbohydrate		300g	375g
Dietary Fiber		25g	30g

Calories per gram:
Fat 9 • Carbohydrate 4 • Protein 4

Pretzels

Nutrition Facts

Serving Size: 7 Pretzels (30g)
Servings Per Container: 9.4

Amount Per Serving	
Calories 120	
Calories from Fat 10	
	% Daily Value*
Total Fat 1g	2%
Saturated Fat 0g	0%
Cholesterol 0g	0%
Sodium 360mg	15%
Total Carbohydrate 24g	8%
Dietary Fiber 1g	4%
Sugars 1g	
Protein 3g	

Vitamin A 0% Σ Vitamin C 0%
Calcium 0% Σ Iron 2%

*Percent Daily Values are based on a 2,000 calorie diet. Your daily values may be higher or lower depending on your calorie needs:

	Calories	2,000	2,500
Total Fat	Less than	65g	80g
Sat Fat	Less than	20g	25g
Cholesterol	Less than	300mg	300mg
Sodium	Less than	2,400mg	2,400mg
Total Carbohydrate		300g	375g
Dietary Fiber		25g	30g

Calories per gram:
Fat 9 Σ Carbohydrate 4 Σ Protein 4

Ingredients: Unbleached Wheat Flour, Water, Corn Syrup, Partially Hydrogenated Vegetable Oil (Soybean), Yeast Salt, Bicarbonates and Carbonates of Sodium.

Calorie Calculating Activity

1. An 8-fluid-ounce serving of 1% fat soy milk contains 110 calories with 2 grams of total fat, 20 grams of total carbohydrates, and 4 grams of total protein. Calculate the total number of calories from each energy nutrient; show your calculations in the space provided below.

   Number of calories from fat: ____

   Number of calories from carbohydrates: ____

   Number of calories from protein: ____

2. Now calculate the percentage of total calories due to each energy nutrient.

   Percentage of calories from fat: ____

   Percentage of calories from carbohydrates: ____

   Percentage of calories from protein: ______

3. Compare the percentages of total calories due to fat, carbohydrates, and protein found in soy milk with the percentages you calculated for one serving of peanut butter in the textbook's Critical Thinking box on page 655. How do the percentages relate to the ideal percentages for optimum energy balance in the body?

Case Studies

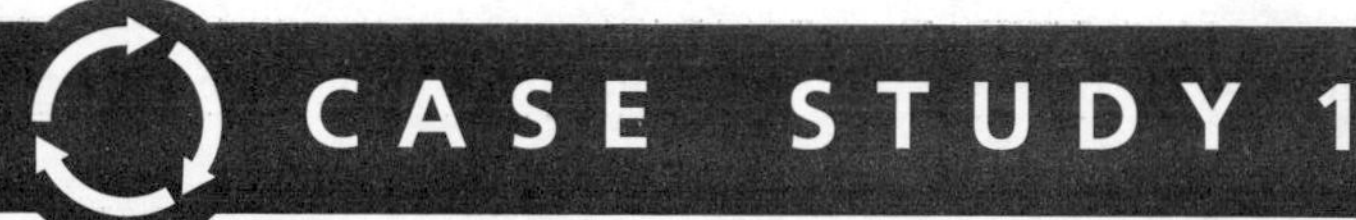

Dr. Elizabeth King has confirmed that patient Mary O'Keefe is pregnant with her third child.

CASE STUDY REVIEW QUESTIONS

1. Name two minerals that Mary must increase the intake of in her diet.

____

____

2. Name three reasons why a woman needs to increase her intake of nutrients and calories when she is pregnant.

____

____

____

____

____

3. What dietary supplement usually needs to be added to a baby's diet?

____

____

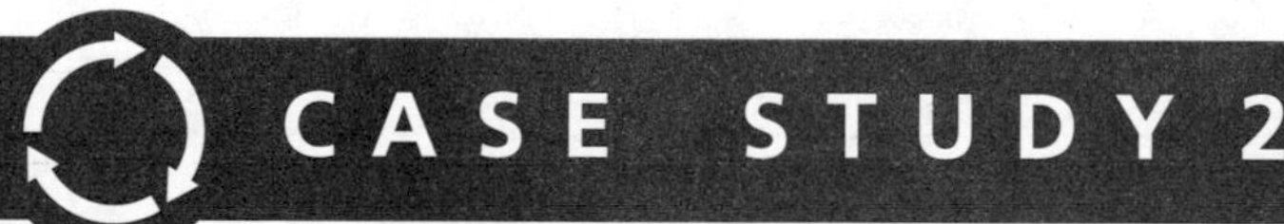

Lourdes Austen, a breast cancer survivor, regularly attends a support group for breast cancer patients and survivors held once a month. Lourdes finds the group a great source of encouragement, information, and support—a safe place to discuss her feelings and concerns about breast cancer. The group is planning a session to talk about nutrition issues, and Lourdes asks clinical medical assistant, Audrey Jones, if she would like to attend the meeting with her to contribute to the group's discussion. With permission from office manager Marilyn Johnson and Lourdes's physician, Dr. Elizabeth King, Audrey attends the meeting. The group members are enthusiastic and ask Audrey many questions, including the following: "Why is good nutrition important for cancer patients?" "I don't have much appetite anymore and get nauseous all the time. What can I do?" "I keep hearing about those macrobiotic diets. Are they any good? Should I try them?"

continues

CASE STUDY REVIEW QUESTIONS

1. What information can Audrey give in answer to the question regarding the importance of good nutrition for cancer patients?

2. What suggestion can Audrey offer to patients who have no appetite and have nausea or vomiting?

3. What can Audrey tell the group about macrobiotic diets?

4. What is the role of the medical assistant in attending the breast cancer support group meeting?

CHAPTER POST-TEST

Perform this test without looking at your book. If an answer is "false," rewrite the sentence to make it true.

1. True or False? Homeostasis occurs properly and does not depend on proper nutrients being made available for the body to use.

2. True or False? Nutrients provide energy.

3. True or False? Fats and carbohydrates provide energy, whereas proteins do not.

4. True or False? Fat-soluble vitamins are those vitamins that are stored in the fat of the body.

5. True or False? Water-soluble vitamins are not easily depleted, and therefore can build up to dangerous levels.

6. True or False? Antioxidants are those substances that help the body's cells overcome the damages of free radicals.

7. True or False? Fiber is primarily a carbohydrate and comes only from plant sources.

SELF-ASSESSMENT

1. Keep track of your diet for a couple of days. Track everything you eat and drink and the amounts of each item.

2. Either use the Internet to research the nutritional value of each item or look in a good dietary resource for the information. Figure the number of calories you ate each day, the amount of fiber, the amount and types of fats, how much protein, how many carbohydrates and sugars, and which vitamins and minerals you consumed. Hint: There are specific Web sites that can help you with this project. One example is: http://www.calorie-count.com. This Web site allows you to search through hundreds of different foods and drinks to find the "labels" for them. It is free! You can even create your own personal profile.

   A. Now figure in any vitamins and supplements you ingested.

   B. Is there any particular part of a nutritious diet that you are lacking?

   C. Are there any components that you ate too much of?

Name ______________________ Date ____________ Score ______

CHAPTER **23**

Basic Pharmacology

CHAPTER PRE-TEST

Perform this test without looking at your book. If an answer is "false," rewrite the sentence to make it true.

1. True or False? Only licensed physicians may dispense drugs.

2. True or False? All prescription drugs are considered to be controlled substances.

3. True or False? Most drugs are called by their chemical names now.

4. True or False? The *Physician's Desk Reference* (PDR) is a small, handy, easy-to-use reference for drug information.

5. True or False? An allergic reaction to a drug is considered a side effect.

6. True or False? Controlled substances should be flushed down the toilet when they become out of date.

7. True or False? "Parenteral" means to administer a drug by injection.

VOCABULARY BUILDER

Misspelled Words I

Find the words in Column A that are misspelled; circle them, and then correctly spell them in the spaces provided. Then match each of the vocabulary terms below with the correct definition in Column B.

	Column A	Correct Spelling
____	1. Abuse	________________
____	2. Administer	________________
____	3. Anaphalaxis	________________
____	4. Contradication	________________
____	5. Dispense	________________
____	6. Perscribe	________________
____	7. Pharmacology	________________

Column B

A. Term used to describe when a licensed practitioner gives a written order to be taken to a pharmacist to be filled

B. An allergic hypersensitivity reaction of the body to a foreign protein or drug

C. To give the medication to the patient to be used at another time

D. The study of drugs; the science dealing with the history, origin, sources, physical and chemical properties, uses, and effects on living organisms

E. To give a medication to a patient by mouth, injection, or any other method of delivery

F. Any symptom or circumstance for which an otherwise approved form of treatment is inadvisable

G. The misuse of legal and illegal drugs

Misspelled Words II

Find the words in the list below that are misspelled; circle them, and correctly spell them in the spaces provided. Then insert the proper terms into the spaces provided in the following text, which discusses medical uses of drugs, name of drugs, and sources of drugs.

animal	generic	replacement
chemical	genetic engineering	sinthetic
curative	mineral	therapeutic
diagnostic	plant	trade name
gene splicing	prophalactic	

________________ ________________ ________________

A drug is a medicinal substance that may be used to vary or modify the functions of a living being. Of the five basic medical uses for drugs, antibiotics are an example of ________________ drugs (agents used for the killing or removal of the causative agent of a disease). An immunizing agent is an example of a preventive or ________________ drug, which is one used to stave off or abate the severity of a disease. Another medical use for drugs is in the treatment of a condition to provide symptomatic relief; this is known as ________________. Insulin and hormones are examples of this medical use of drugs, known as ________________. A fifth basic medical use of drugs is in conjunction with radiology and allows providers to pinpoint the location of diseases' manifestations. This usage is known as ________________.

As essential to the medical assistant as the knowledge of basic uses for drugs is the knowledge of the names of drugs. The majority of drugs have three types of names. The ________________ name is the drug's official name assigned by the U.S. Adopted Names Council. Aspirin is an example of this type of name. The drug's ________________ name describes its molecular structure and identification of its chemical structure. Acetylsalicylic acid is an example of this type of name. Ecotrin is an example of a ____________________________ or brand name, which is registered by the U.S. Patent Office and approved for usage by the U.S. Food and Drug Administration.

Medical assistants must also have a comprehensive understanding of the five basic sources of drugs. The source of digitalis, the dried leaf of a foxglove plant, is an example of a ____________________________ source. Insulin, a hormone derived from the pancreas of cows and hogs, is an example of a drug derived from an ____________________________ source. Drugs that are artificially prepared in pharmaceutical laboratories are known as ____________________________ drugs. Synthetically prepared sulfur, used in pharmaceutical products (such as certain bacteriostatic drugs), is an example of a drug derived from a ____________________ source. One of the latest sources for drugs has been provided by ____________________________. Using a technique called ____________________________, scientists are able to create hybrid forms of life that can treat certain diseases; interferon for cancer treatment is an example of this process.

LEARNING REVIEW

Multiple Choice

1. All drugs available for legal use are controlled by the:
   a. Federal Food, Drug, and Cosmetic Act
   b. the Council on Pharmacy of the American Medical Association
   c. Controlled Substance Act of 1970
2. Federal law requires that at the end of the workday, controlled substances that are used on the premises must be:
   a. locked in a provider's office by a provider
   b. removed from the building and stored in a government-appointed storage space
   c. counted, verified by two individuals, and recorded on an audit sheet
3. An inventory record of Schedule II drugs must be submitted to the Drug Enforcement Administration (DEA) every:
   a. week
   b. year
   c. 2 years
4. An example of a drug requiring a prescription is the:
   a. antibiotic penicillin
   b. antihistamine Benadryl®
   c. analgesic acetaminophen
5. An example of an OTC drug is the:
   a. analgesic ibuprofen
   b. vasodilator nitroglycerin
   c. antitussive codeine
6. When a drug acts on the area to which it is administered, it has what is known as a:
   a. systemic action
   b. remote action
   c. local action

7. The four principal factors that affect drug action are absorption, distribution, biotransformation, and:
   a. elimination
   b. interaction
   c. contraindication
8. By law, outdated and expired controlled substances must be:
   a. handed over to your local law enforcement agency
   b. thrown away
   c. returned to the pharmacy
9. Patients need to realize that OTC drugs can:
   a. interact with other drugs and cause undesirable or adverse reactions or complications
   b. mask symptoms and exacerbate an existing condition
   c. a. and b.
10. The most frequently used routes of administering medication are:
   a. inhalation and sublingual
   b. parenteral and inhalation
   c. oral and parenteral

Short Answer

1. Under federal law, providers who prescribe, administer, or dispense controlled substances must register with the DEA and renew their registration as required by state law. Describe the five schedules of classification for controlled substances and give an example for each.

____

____

____

____

____

____

____

____

____

2. For each of the following, identify whether the drug involved is an OTC medication or a prescribed medication (PM). What patient guidelines for proper use are illustrated in each example?

_____ A. Nora Fowler insists that Dr. Winston Lewis cannot help her rheumatoid arthritis and that simple ibuprofen is all she needs. Nora buys bulk generic bottles of ibuprofen at the drugstore for her rheumatoid arthritis and takes as many as she needs to help ease the painful inflammation in her joints and tissues.

_____ B. When Jim Marshall experiences extreme stress while finishing the architectural designs for a new office building in the community, his girlfriend offers him a tablet or two of lorazepam, a benzodiazepine drug used to treat anxiety and insomnia. "Here, Dr. King gave me these, and they work great," she says. "You can't drive when you take this stuff, though. Oh, and these pills are about 2 years old, but I'm sure they'll still work fine."

_____ C. At the slightest sniffle or sneeze, Lenore McDonell takes the strongest multisymptom cold medication she can find. Her philosophy is: "I might as well knock it out of my system."

_____ D. Abigail Johnson hates taking so many medications. So every now and then, when she feels especially good, Abigail just decides to stop taking the antihypertensive drug that is part of Dr. Elizabeth King's treatment plan to control Abigail's high blood pressure. On a bad day, she'll take an extra pill.

_____ E. Patty McLean is susceptible to recurrent colds and ear infections. Patty's symptoms are hard to control because she will almost always stop taking the antibiotics when she starts to feel better and she does not finish the entire regimen recommended by Dr. Lewis.

3. Proper disposal of drugs has become increasingly important. How should outdated medications be disposed of?

4. The most frequently used routes of administering medication are oral and parenteral. List seven additional routes of administration.

5. Name three recently developed systems of drug delivery. Describe each and note their specific advantages.

6. List four examples of the ways in which drugs may be classified, or arranged, in groups.

7. For each drug action, identify the correct drug classification. Then list one example of a drug contained in each class. The first row has been completed as an example for you.

Action	Classification	Drug Example
Controls or stops bleeding	Hemostatic	Humafac®, Amitar®, vitamin K
Prevents or relieves nausea and vomiting		
Neutralizes acid		
Decreases blood pressure		
Reduces fever		
Loosens and promotes normal bowel elimination		
Prevents conception		

Kills or destroys malignant cells	____________	________________________
		________________________
		________________________
Prevents or relieves diarrhea	____________	________________________
		________________________
		________________________
Produces a calming effect without causing sleep	____________	________________________
		________________________
		________________________

CERTIFICATION REVIEW

These questions are designed to mimic the certification examination. Select the best response.

1. Hybrid forms of life have been created that benefit human beings by providing an alternative source of drugs; an example is:
   a. ibuprofen
   b. interferon
   c. digitalis
   d. epinephrine
2. If the symbol ® follows a drug name, no other manufacturer can make or sell the drug for:
   a. 7 years
   b. 10 years
   c. 20 years
   d. 17 years
3. One compound extracted from the adrenal gland of animals and used therapeutically is:
   a. cortisone
   b. acetaminophen
   c. insulin
   d. piroxician
4. Those drugs with a potential for abuse and dependency are monitored by the:
   a. FDA
   b. AAMA
   c. DEA
   d. CDC

5. An inventory record of Schedule II drugs must be submitted to appropriate authorities every:
   a. 2 years
   b. year
   c. 5 years
   d. 7 years

LEARNING APPLICATION

Critical Thinking Activity

1. What factor in determining the route selection for administering a medication is illustrated by each example below and why?
   A. A patient diagnosed with insulin-dependent diabetes mellitus performs three self-injections of insulin daily, according to the provider's treatment plan.

   ____

   ____

   ____

   B. Chemotherapeutic drugs are used to attack cancer cells that may be traveling throughout a patient's body, and usually they are administered intravenously.

   ____

   ____

   ____

   ____

   C. A patient in a nursing home who is in the end stages of Parkinson's disease is bedridden, has trouble swallowing, and suffers from dementia. The patient, who is also suffering from angina as a result of poor blood circulation, is prescribed a nitroglycerin transdermal system instead of a sublingual dosage, to be held under the tongue, or a time-released capsule to swallow.

   ____

   ____

   ____

   ____

   ____

Research Activities

The PDR is an invaluable resource and one of the most widely used publications in the medical industry. The annually updated publication is usually available in most clinics and medical offices. It provides medical professionals with practical information about thousands of medications and includes other useful data, such as lists of drugs new to the market and those that have been discontinued. It is essential that medical assistants become familiar with the publication and learn how to access the wealth of information stored within.

1. Use the PDR to locate the pertinent information for each of the following scenarios. Then identify the drug's source or method of production.

   A. Herb Fowler, Dr. Winston Lewis's patient, calls to report he is experiencing nausea, a symptom he believes may be a negative reaction to the Chronulac Syrup® Dr. Lewis recently prescribed for Herb's chronic constipation. Using the PDR, locate the following information:

   Chronulac Syrup's generic name: ______________________________

   The sugar Chronulac Syrup contains is ______________________________

   Identify the drug's source or method of production: ______________________________

   B. Another patient of Dr. Lewis's, Michael Zamboni, has recently been diagnosed with insulin-dependent type II diabetes. Dr. Lewis prescribes Humulin®. Using the PDR, find the following information:

   Humulin's® generic name: ______________________________

   ____

   The source from which Humulin® is derived: ______________________________

   ____

   ____

   Identify the drug's source or method of production: ______________________________

   ____

   C. Susan Marshall, a new patient of Dr. Elizabeth King's, acquired a high-pressure job about 1 month ago. Recently, she has been reporting an upset stomach, which has been attributed to her stressful job and poor eating habits. Dr. King orders prescription-strength Pepcid® for Susan. Using the PDR, locate the following information:

   Pepcid's® generic name: ______________________________

   Pepcid's® active ingredient: ______________________________

   Identify the drug's source or method of production: ______________________________

2. Camille Saunders, another patient of Dr. King's, has been taking Ortho-Tri-Cyclen®, an oral contraceptive, for 6 months. It has just been discovered that Camille has epilepsy. Using the PDR, locate the following information:

   A. Does Ortho-Tri-Cyclen® have any known contraindications to any drugs used in the treatment of epilepsy, and if so, which drugs?

   ____

   ____

   ____

   B. Identify the drug's source or method of production.

   ____

   ____

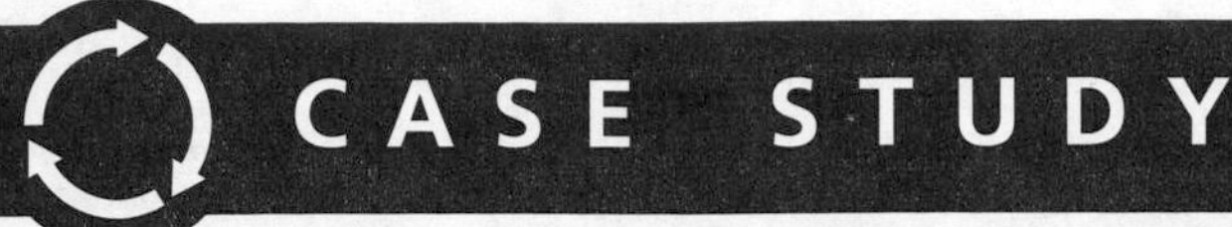

CASE STUDY

While Anna Preciado, a clinical medical assistant newly hired at the offices of Drs. Lewis and King, is performing her shift duties, she notices a fellow employee exhibiting strange behavior. Audrey Jones, CMA (AAMA), is usually the model of efficiency. Since Anna began working at the Northborough Family Medical Group, she has always known Audrey to be alert, friendly, and able to handle difficult clinical situations with grace under pressure. Lately, however, when Anna asks Audrey questions, Audrey seems irritable and easily confused. Anna also notices Audrey exhibiting a sloppy technique during routine clinical procedures. Anna is disturbed by Audrey's erratic behavior but does not mention anything to anyone. After all, Anna is new to the job. But while counting the contents of the controlled substance cabinet in preparation for the end of her shift, Anna notices that a bottle of phenobarbital is missing. Anna knows that office manager Marilyn Johnson will arrive shortly to verify and record the inventory count. Anna is now worried that perhaps Audrey is to blame for the missing drugs but is afraid of jumping to conclusions and of angering Audrey. Anna knows Audrey is in the staff lounge preparing to leave for a dinner break.

CASE STUDY REVIEW QUESTIONS

1. What is Anna's first action under the circumstances? Should she confront Audrey?

____
____
____
____
____
____
____

2. What special responsibilities do health care professionals, including medical assistants, have regarding the misuse or abuse of legal or illegal drugs?

____
____
____
____
____
____
____
____
____

CHAPTER POST-TEST

Perform this test without looking at your book. If an answer is "false," rewrite the sentence to make it true.

1. True or False? Only licensed physicians may prescribe drugs.

____

____

2. True or False? The possibility exists for any drug to be abused if a patient deliberately misuses the medication or uses it excessively.

____

____

3. True or False? Most drugs are now called by their generic names.

____

____

4. True or False? PDR stands for the *Physician's Drug Reference.*

____

____

5. True or False? An allergic reaction to a drug is considered a contraindication.

____

____

6. True or False? Outdated drugs that are not controlled substances should be flushed down the toilet.

____

____

7. True or False? Parenteral usually means to administer a drug by injection.

____

____

SELF-ASSESSMENT

Organize your medicine cabinet. Or, with permission, organize the medicine cabinet of a close family member.

1. First, determine which drugs are out of date and destroy them properly.

____

____

____

____

2. Next, determine which drugs are no longer being prescribed, but rather are basically "left over" from a previous illness.

3. Make a decision. Should those leftover drugs be disposed of, or was it the intention of the provider for those medications to be available to you (or your family member) in the future? If they are not to be used in the future, dispose of them properly.

4. Separate the OTC drugs from the prescription drugs. Organize the OTC medications into categories of actions (the analgesics together, cough and cold medicines together, etc.).

5. If you (or your family member) are on a long-term drug therapy, make up a medicine card to be carried with you (or your family member) at all times. On the card, list the drug, strength, and dosage. Place this card in your wallet or purse (or that of your family member), so the medicine list is available at all times. Keep the list updated as prescriptions change.

Name ______________________ Date ____________ Score ________

CHAPTER 24

Calculation of Medication Dosage and Medication Administration

CHAPTER PRE-TEST

Perform this test without looking at your book. If an answer is "false," rewrite the sentence to make it true.

1. True or False? A prescription is a written legal document.

____

____

2. True or False? Prescriptions for controlled substances have different requirements than prescriptions for other drugs.

____

____

3. True or False? Dosage and dose mean the same thing.

____

____

4. True or False? Dosages are determined by considering patient age, weight, sex, and other factors.

____

____

5. True or False? We are required by the "Needlestick Safety Act" to use the safest needles available.

____

____

6. True or False? The dorsogluteal site is the traditional location for a deep intramuscular (IM) injection.

____

____

7. True or False? The deltoid muscle is the easiest and most accessible IM site.

____

____

8. True or False? The ventrogluteal muscle is the muscle of choice for an infant IM injection.

____

____

VOCABULARY BUILDER

Misspelled Words

Find the words below that are misspelled; circle them, and correctly spell them in the spaces provided. Then fill in the blanks in the sentences below with the correct vocabulary term.

administer	hypoxemia	precipitate
apnea	meniskis	taut
body surface area	namogram	unit dose
dispense	parentral	weal

_______________ _______________ _______________

____

1. The absence of breathing is termed _______________.
2. _______________ is a highly accurate method for calculating medication dosages for infants and children up to 12 years of age.
3. A lack of oxygen in the blood is _______________.
4. The convex or concave upper surface of a column of liquid in a container is known as _______________.
5. A _______________ is a graph that shows the relationship among numerical values; an estimate of body surface area (BSA) of a patient can be determined by its use.
6. The term _______________ describes the injection of a liquid substance into the body via a route other than the alimentary canal.
7. _______________ is a substance in the form of fine particles that separates from a solution if allowed to stand for a period of time.
8. Stretch the skin _______________, pulling it tight, when giving an intramuscular injection.
9. A _______________ is a premeasured amount of medication, individually packaged on a per-dose basis.
10. A slight elevation of skin that can be produced as a reaction to an intradermal injection, such as allergy testing and PPDs, is a _______________.

LEARNING REVIEW

Short Answer

1. Identify the following measures as weight (W) or volume (V). Then name the measure each abbreviation stands for and what system of measurement it belongs to. The first row has been completed as an example for you.

Weight	Volume	Abbreviation	Measure	System
X		g	Gram	Metric
		tbsp	__________	__________
		mL	__________	__________
		qt	__________	__________
		gtt	__________	__________
		mcg	__________	__________

2. Perform the following conversions:

   (A) 4 tsp = ____ mL

   (B) 7 kg = ______ lbs

   (C) 3.5 in. = ______ cm

   (D) 1,200 mg = _____ gm

   (E) 8 mL = _____ gtt

3. What are proportions? How are proportions useful in calculating dosages of medication?

   ____
   ____
   ____
   ____
   ____
   ____

4. Identify the type of syringe typically used for each of the following; list the size and calibration as well.

	Type	Size	Calibration
Venipuncture	__________	______	__________
Insulin administration	__________	______	__________
Allergy testing	__________	______	__________

5. For each syringe-needle combination below, identify the most likely parenteral route: subcutaneous injection (SC), intramuscular injection (IM), or intradermal injection (ID). Also identify the proper angle of injection.

	Route	Angle of Injection
3-mL syringe/22G, 1½-inch needle	____	__________
1-mL syringe/25G, ⅝-inch needle	____	__________
U-100 (1 mL)/26G, ½-inch needle	____	__________
3-mL syringe/25G, ⅝-inch needle	____	__________

CERTIFICATION REVIEW

These questions are designed to mimic the certification examination. Select the best response.

1. The hard copy of a prescription is filed and kept for a minimum of:

   a. 10 years

   b. 7 years

   c. 5 years

   d. indefinitely

2. The portion of the prescription that gives directions to the patient is called the:

   a. superscription

   b. inscription

   c. subscription

   d. signature

3. The metric prefix that refers to 1,000 units is:

   a. kilo-

   b. milli-

   c. micro-

   d. deca-

4. Dosage of insulin is always measured in:

   a. cubic centimeters

   b. milliliters

   c. units

   d. milliequivalents

5. The hollow core of a needle is called the:

   a. bevel

   b. gauge

   c. lumen

   d. hilt

LEARNING APPLICATION

Reading Prescriptions

1. A prescription is a written legal document that gives directions for compounding, dispensing, and administering to a patient. Refer to the prescriptions shown below, and in the spaces below, "decode" the prescriptions into layperson's terms and answer the questions that follow.

____

____

____

____

Dr. King prescribes an adult dosage for epilepsy.

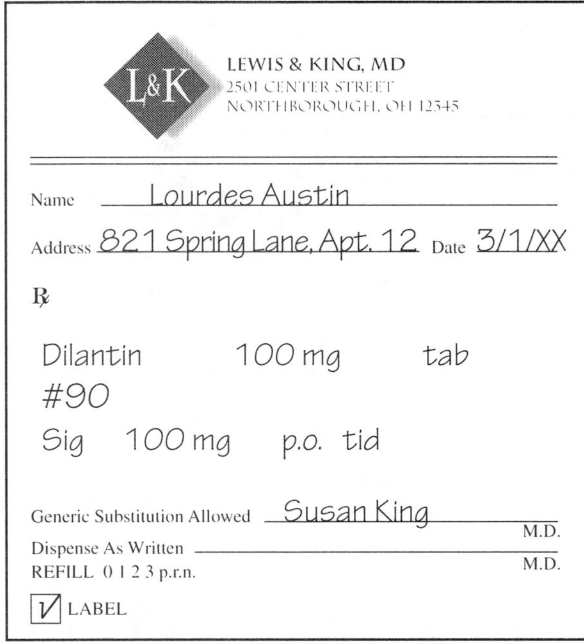

LEWIS & KING, MD
2501 CENTER STREET
NORTHBOROUGH, OH 12345

Name Lourdes Austin

Address 821 Spring Lane, Apt. 12 Date 3/1/XX

℞

Dilantin 100 mg tab
#90
Sig 100 mg p.o. tid

Generic Substitution Allowed Susan King M.D.
Dispense As Written ______ M.D.
REFILL 0 1 2 3 p.r.n.

☑ LABEL

Dr. Lewis prescribes a child's dosage for an ear infection.

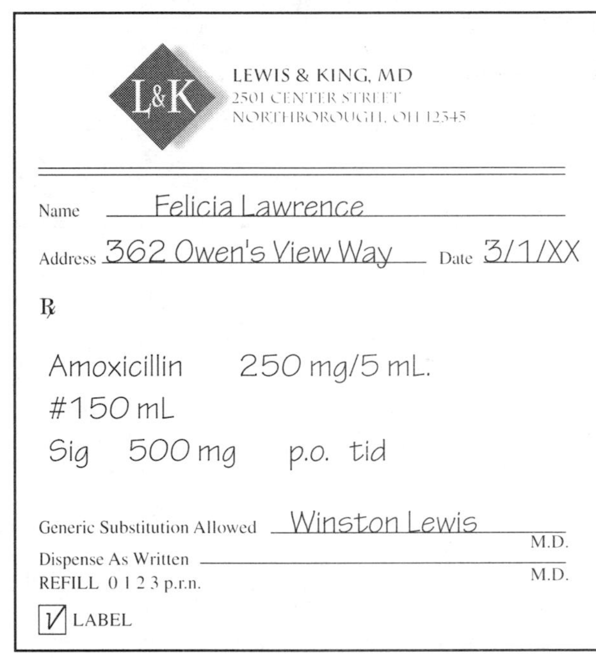

LEWIS & KING, MD
2501 CENTER STREET
NORTHBOROUGH, OH 12345

Name Felicia Lawrence

Address 362 Owen's View Way Date 3/1/XX

℞

Amoxicillin 250 mg/5 mL.
#150 mL
Sig 500 mg p.o. tid

Generic Substitution Allowed Winston Lewis M.D.
Dispense As Written ______ M.D.
REFILL 0 1 2 3 p.r.n.

☑ LABEL

1. How many grams are in each dose of Dilantin? ____________________
2. How many days of Dilantin are dispensed? ________________
3. How many teaspoons are in 5 mL? ____________________________________
4. How many doses of amoxicillin are included in the amount dispensed? ___________________________________ ________________

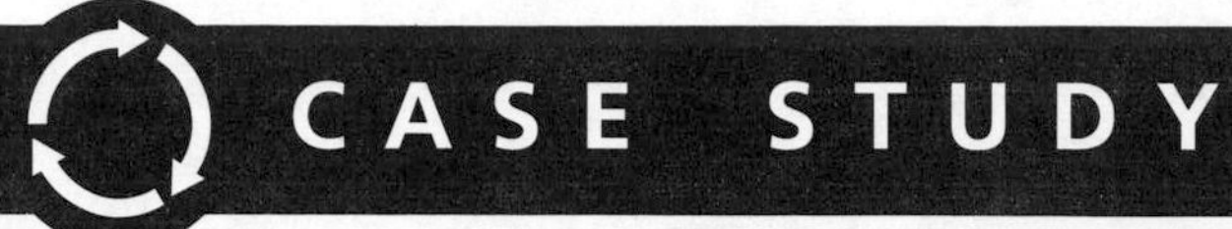

Louise Kipperley comes to the urgent care center at Inner City Health Care when she experiences the third severe migraine headache in only one month. The headache has lasted two days, and Louise has experienced symptoms of nausea and vomiting. Dr. Rice gives written orders to administer Imitrex 25 mg IM stat, together with a prescription for the patient to fill and use at home. Liz Corbin, CMA (AAMA), makes a medicine card from the provider's order sheet of Louise's medical record and prepares the STAT dosage for Louise according to the correct procedure for administering oral medications. Liz is about to transport the medication to Louise in examination room 3 when she reads the provider's order for Louise, which calls for 25 mg IM STAT. The written prescription is for Imitrex every four hours as needed. Liz discards the dosage she has prepared for the patient and instead gives Louise Dr. Rice's prescription and tells her to have it filled immediately.

CASE STUDY REVIEW QUESTIONS

1. What medication error has Liz made? What effect will the error likely have on the patient?

____

____

____

____

____

2. What should Liz have done? What standard procedures should be followed when a medication error occurs?

____

____

____

____

____

____

____

____

CHAPTER POST-TEST

Perform this test without looking at your book. If an answer is "false," rewrite the sentence to make it true.

1. True or False? A prescription is a legal document only if it is written.

____

____

2. True or False? Prescriptions for controlled substances have the same requirements as prescriptions for other drugs.

____

____

3. True or False? Dosage and dose have different meanings.

4. True or False? Doses are determined by considering patient age, weight, sex, and other factors.

5. True or False? We are required by OSHA to use the safest needles available.

6. True or False? The gluteus maximus is the traditional location for a deep IM injection.

7. True or False? The bicep muscle is the easiest and most accessible IM site.

8. True or False? The vastus lateralis muscle is the muscle of choice for an infant IM injection.

SELF-ASSESSMENT

1. Have you ever been given a shot? Do you remember how you felt just before the injection? Most people are more afraid of the pain of the injection than anything having to do with the medication. Do you think there are ways you can behave that will help your fearful patients feel less afraid? What could you do or say to alleviate their fears? Do you think it is just children who are afraid of needles? Write down a couple of things you will do and say to help your patients. Discuss your ideas with a few classmates and listen to their ideas.

Name ______________________ Date __________ Score ______

CHAPTER 25

Electrocardiography

CHAPTER PRE-TEST

Perform this test without looking at your book. If an answer is "false," rewrite the sentence to make it true.

1. True or False? The skin is a great conductor of electricity.

____

____

2. True or False? Electrolytes provide moisture, and aid in conduction.

____

____

3. True or False? The heart is a two-sided pump that routes blood where it needs to go.

____

____

4. True or False? Only certain cells in the heart are able to initiate electricity.

____

____

5. True or False? One type of artifact is an electrical interference.

____

____

6. True or False? The heart beats approximately 60 times a minute, only resting in-between beats.

____

____

VOCABULARY BUILDER

From the following terms, find the misspelled words, circle them, and spell them correctly in the spaces provided. Then, fill in the blanks in sentences below.

atria	electrocardigraph	sinoatrial node
atrioventrical node	electrocardiography	ventricles
cardiac cycle	oxygenated	
deoxygenated	Purkingi fibers	

_______________ _______________

____

1. The lower chambers of the heart are called _______________.
2. The upper chambers of the heart are called _______________.
3. _______________ blood enters the right side of the heart.
4. _______________ blood enters the left side of the heart.
5. The _______________ is the body's natural pacemaker.
6. From the sinoatrial node, the _______________ receives the current of electricity.
7. The fibers that spread the electrical impulses from the bundle branches throughout the ventricles are called the _______________.
8. The entire route of the electrical impulses through the heart is referred to as the _______________.
9. The _______________ is a machine used to perform the ECG procedure.
10. Ultrasonography and _______________ are noninvasive diagnostic procedures commonly used in the clinical setting.

LEARNING REVIEW

1. List five reasons why electrocardiography is performed.

____

____

____

____

____

____

2. The first three leads recorded on a standard ECG are Lead I, Lead II, and Lead III. These are called ____________________ leads because each of them uses two-limb electrodes that record simultaneously. For each lead, what electrical activity of the heart is recorded? Draw it on each figure.

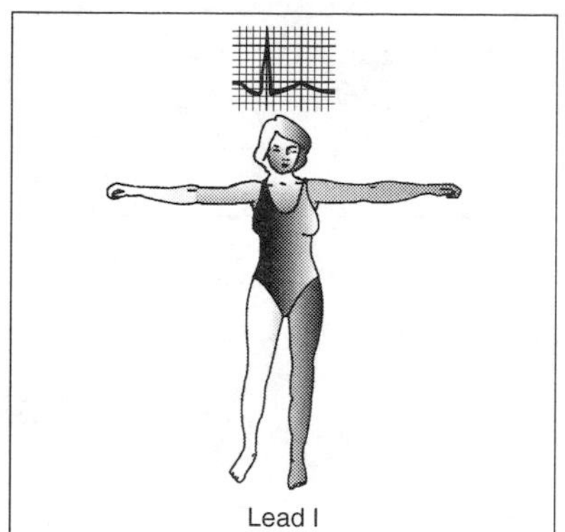

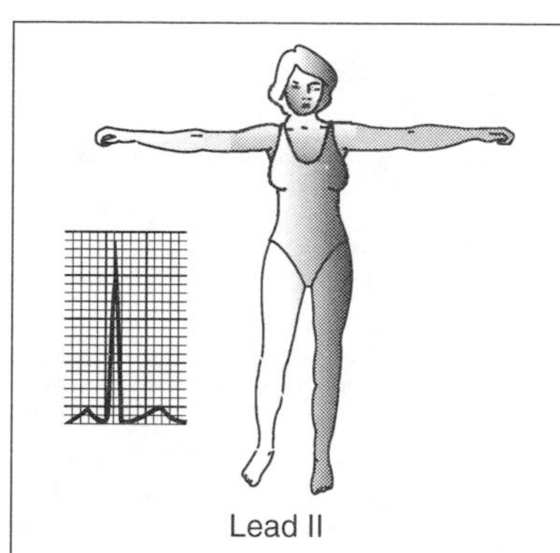

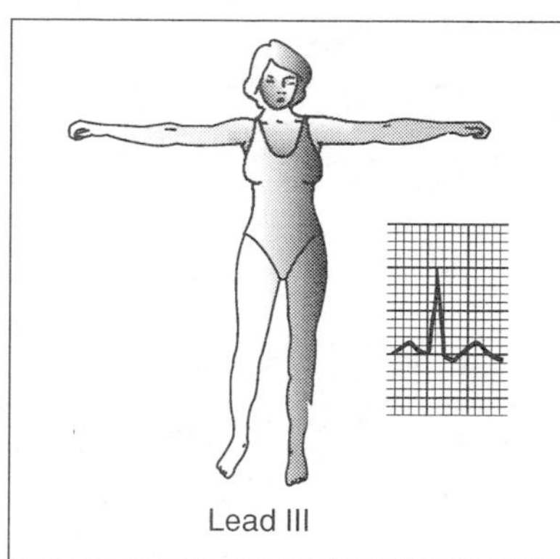

3. Fill in the blanks:

   (A) Lead I records electrical activity between the ________________ and the ________________.

   (B) Lead II records electrical activity between the ________________ and the ________________.

   (C) Lead III records electrical activity between the ________________ and the ________________.

4. The next group of leads recorded on a standard ECG are augmented leads, designated aV_R, aV_L, and aV_F. These are called ________________ leads. For each lead, what electrical activity of the heart is recorded? Draw it on each figure.

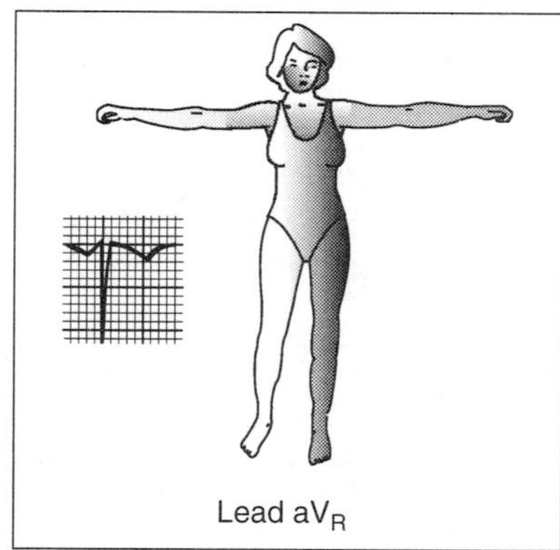

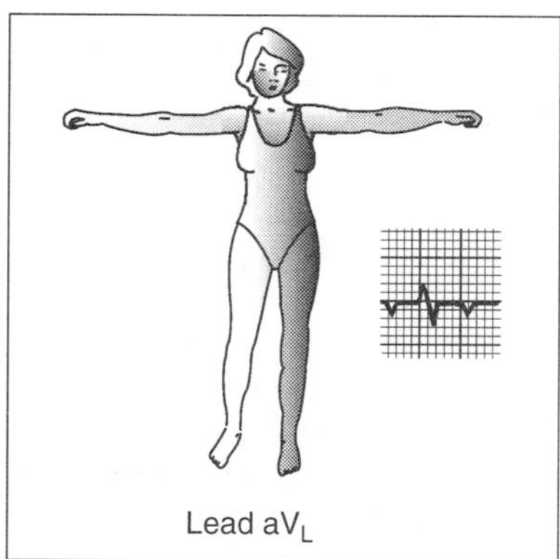

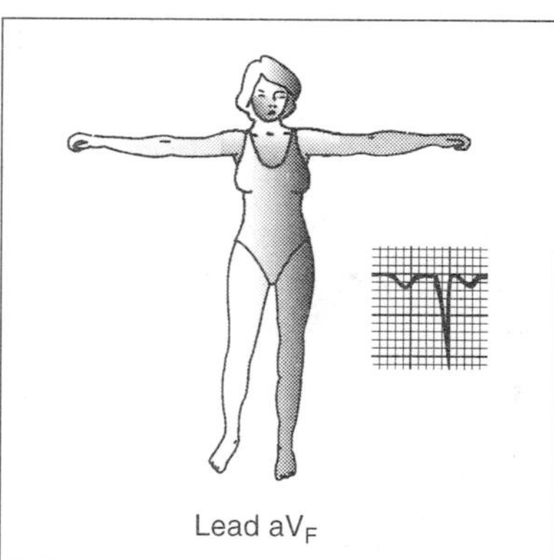

5. Fill in the blanks:

   (A) Lead aV_R records electrical activity from the ________________________________ and the ________________________________.

   (B) Lead aV_L records electrical activity from the ________________________________ and the ________________________________.

   (C) Lead aV_F records electrical activity from the ________________________________ and the ________________________________.

6. The remaining 6 leads of the standard 12-lead ECG are called the chest leads, or ____________________ leads. These leads are (*circle the correct one*) unipolar/bipolar. Where are the leads placed on the body?

   V1: ____________________

   V2: ____________________

   V3: ____________________

   V4: ____________________

   V5: ____________________

   V6: ____________________

CERTIFICATION REVIEW

These questions are designed to mimic the certification examination. Select the best response.

1. Repolarization takes place while the heart muscle:
   a. contracts
   b. stops
   c. skips a beat
   d. relaxes
2. Chest leads are also called ____________________ leads
   a. precordial
   b. limb
   c. augmented
   d. bipolar
3. Augmented leads are also called:
   a. unipolar
   b. bipolar
   c. precordial
   d. standard
4. One millivolt of cardiac electrical activity will deflect the stylus exactly:
   a. 5 mm high
   b. 10 mm high
   c. 25 mm high
   d. 40 mm high
5. A wandering baseline may be caused by:
   a. lotions, creams, or oils on the patient's skin
   b. electrical interference
   c. crossed lead wires
   d. improper grounding

LEARNING APPLICATION

Identifying Artifact Activity

Artifacts are unusual and unwanted activity in the ECG tracing not caused by the electrical activity of the heart. Match each circumstance below to the artifact ECG tracing it would produce and identify the type of artifact in the space provided.

A. A broken patient cable or lead wire has become detached from an electrode.

B. The patient sings to himself during the ECG procedure.

C. The patient uses body lotion.

D. The lead wires are crossed and do not follow the patient's body contour.

Type of Artifact **Circumstance**

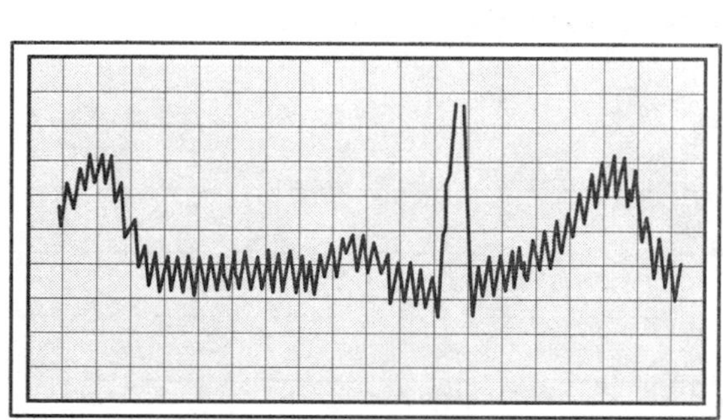

______________________________ ___

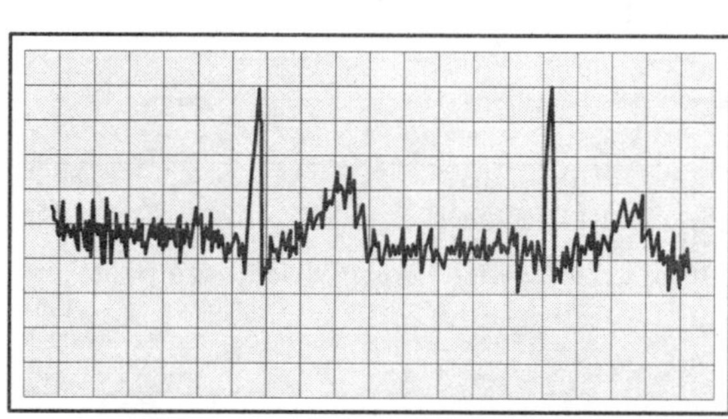

______________________________ ___

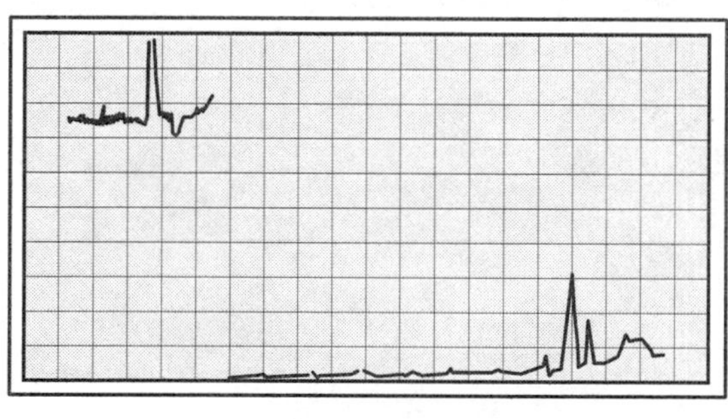

______________________________ ___

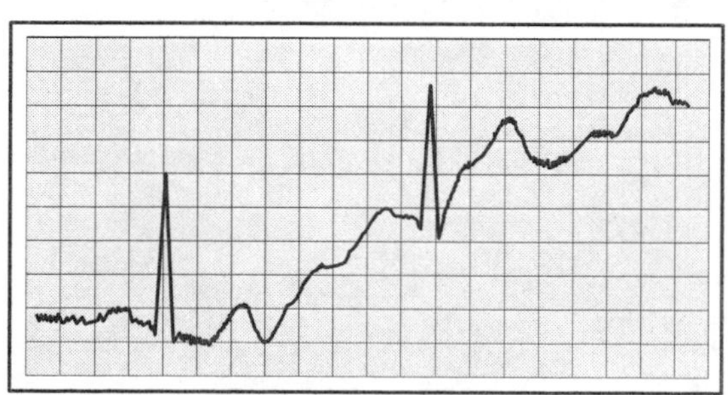

______________________________ ___

CASE STUDY

Jim Marshall, a prominent local architect in his late 30s, stays in good physical condition, works out regularly at the gym, and maintains a low-fat, low-cholesterol, low-sodium diet. Aggressive and ambitious, Jim enjoys pushing his mind and body to the limit. His favorite sports are skiing and sailing. At work, Jim is a perfectionist who puts in long hours and demands the same of his employees. Lately, though, Jim is more aware of the high-stress lifestyle he is leading and is worried about his family history of heart failure and diabetes. During periods of high physical exertion, Jim experiences mild chest pain and palpitations. Dr. Lewis prescribes an exercise tolerance test for Jim.

CASE STUDY REVIEW QUESTIONS

1. What is an exercise tolerance test? How is it performed?

____

____

____

____

____

____

____

2. Under what conditions would the test be discontinued?

____

____

____

3. At the conclusion of the test, what patient care is given? What special instructions for home care should the patient observe?

____

____

____

____

____

CHAPTER POST-TEST

Perform this test without looking at your book. If an answer is "false," rewrite the sentence to make it true.

1. True or False? The skin is a poor conductor of electricity.

2. True or False? Electrodes provide moisture and aid in conduction.

3. True or False? The heart is a four-sided pump that routes blood where it needs to go.

4. True or False? All cardiac cells are able to initiate electricity.

5. True or False? Alternating current artifacts are part of the heart's electrical circuitry.

6. True or False? The heart beats approximately 24 times a minute, resting only in-between beats.

SELF-ASSESSMENT

Keep a strict diary of everything you eat and drink for the next three days (a week is better).

1. Count up the total fats you have eaten each day.

2. Separate the types of fats and total each type for each day.

3. Go online and use search words such as "saturated fats" or "trans fats" to learn more about the different fats.

____

____

____

____

4. Find out about omega-3 fatty acids. Are you eating enough? How could you take in more?

____

____

____

____

5. What else should you be doing to stay "heart healthy"?

____

____

____

____

Name ______________________ Date ____________ Score ______

CHAPTER 26

Safety and Regulatory Guidelines in the Medical Laboratory

CHAPTER PRE-TEST

Perform this test without looking at your book. If an answer is "false," rewrite the sentence to make it true.

1. True or False? The Clinical Laboratory Improvement Act (CLIA) is a federal mandate that protects the laboratory worker.

____

____

2. "Aegis" means:

   a. sponsorship or protection

   b. the part of the laboratory sample that is discarded

   c. a reagent or chemical used in laboratory tests

   d. a region or area of concern

3. Quality control is a way of:

   a. ensuring that the chemicals or reagents used are of good quality

   b. ensuring the test is run correctly

   c. ensuring that the patient sample is stored correctly

   d. All of the above

4. MSDS stands for:

   a. Material Safety Data Sheet

   b. Manual for Safety Documents/Sheets

   c. Mandated Standards for Documentation and Safety

   d. Manual of Supplies and Data for Safety

5. MSDS information must be:
   a. read by all employees
   b. indexed and alphabetized in a notebook or manual
   c. made readily available to all employees
   d. All of the above

VOCABULARY BUILDER

Misspelled Words

Find the words in Column A that are misspelled; circle them, and correctly spell them in the spaces provided. Then match each of the vocabulary terms below with the correct definition in Column B.

	Column A	Correct Spelling
____	1. Spill kit	______________
____	2. Standard	______________
____	3. Proficiency testing	______________
____	4. Waved	______________
____	5. Fume hood	______________
____	6. *Federal Register*	______________
____	7. Calabration	______________
____	8. Requisition	______________
____	9. Mandate	______________
____	10. Quality control	______________

Column B

A. Rules set up and established to measure quality, weight, extent, or value

B. The determination of the accuracy of an instrument by comparing the information provided with an accepted standard known to be accurate

C. Used to describe a category of clinical laboratory tests that are simple and unvarying and require a minimum of judgment and interpretation

D. Measures used to monitor the processing of laboratory specimens

E. Commercially packaged materials containing supplies and equipment needed to clean a biohazardous spill

F. Formal order to obey certain rules and regulations

G. A written request for laboratory analysis to be performed on a specimen

H. A barrier used in the laboratory to capture chemical vapors

I. Federal agency from which written CLIA '88 documents may be obtained

J. Sample tests performed in a clinical laboratory to determine that a specific degree of accuracy is achieved

Unscramble

To test your spelling skills, unscramble the vocabulary terms that follow, then define each term in the space provided.

1. TANOECE ______________ ______________________________
2. PATMIRHEEHCUTEOC TANGES ______________ ______________________________
3. TELHY LOCOLAH ______________ ______________________________
4. DOYEFAMEDLRH ______________ ______________________________
5. RENCISOF ______________ ______________________________

LEARNING REVIEW

1. CLIA '88 requires that every facility that tests human specimens for diagnosis, treatment, and prevention of disease meet specific federal requirements. Name five specific duties a medical assistant may perform that will make an impact on the medical facility's compliance with CLIA '88 regulations.

____

____

____

____

____

2. A written chemical hygiene plan (CHP) is required of all medical facilities to comply with safety standards outlined by the Occupational Safety and Health Administration (OSHA). To comply with OSHA regulations, chemicals must be labeled using the color and number methods of the National Fire Protection Association (NFPA). Match the colors below to the type of hazard each signifies.

___	Blue	1. Fire
___	White	2. Reactivity
___	Yellow	3. Use of personal protective equipment (PPE)
___	Red	4. Health

3. For each configuration listed, use the NFPA color and number method to describe the hazardous properties of each chemical.

   (A) CHEMICAL X: Red/2; Blue/3; Yellow/3; White/F

   ____

   ____

   ____

(B) CHEMICAL Y: Red/0; Blue/1; Yellow/0; White/X

___

___

___

(C) CHEMICAL Z: Red/1; Blue/2; Yellow/1; White/E

___

___

___

CERTIFICATION REVIEW

These questions are designed to mimic the certification examination. Select the best response.

1. CLIA was passed in an effort to:
   a. teach staff how to read test results accurately
   b. establish standards to ensure the confidentiality of test results
   c. establish standards to ensure accurate test results
   d. All of the above
2. CLIA was passed in what year?
   a. 1902
   b. 1975
   c. 1988
   d. 1999
3. Which of the following procedures is a requirement of qualifying protocol for automated hematology instruments?
   a. Control samples
   b. Proficiency testing
   c. Calibration
   d. All of the above
4. Material Safety Data Sheets (MSDSs) do *not* contain:
   a. product/chemical information
   b. emergency response procedures
   c. manufacturer information
   d. training information for using the product/chemical
5. When skin comes into contact with chemicals, it is best to:
   a. wash the area with water immediately
   b. apply a neutralizing agent to the site
   c. consult the MSDS before treatment
   d. rinse area with vinegar

LEARNING APPLICATION

Research Activity

The three categories of laboratory testing are "waived," "moderate complexity" (which includes provider-performed microscopy), and "high complexity." All laboratories are required to register with CLIA '88 and receive certification to perform specific categories of tests within strict boundaries of compliance. Waived tests deliver simple unvarying results and require a minimum of judgment and interpretation. Name 10 waived tests. Use online resources such as the CLIA '88 official Web site.

____

____

CHAPTER POST-TEST

Perform this test without looking at your book. If an answer is "false," rewrite the sentence to make it true.

1. True or False? CLIA is a federal mandate that protects the patient.

   ____

   ____

2. "Aegis" means:

   a. a reagent or chemical used in laboratory tests

   b. the part of the laboratory sample that is discarded

   c. sponsorship or protection

   d. a region or area of concern

3. Quality control is a way of:

   a. ensuring that the test is run correctly

   b. ensuring that the chemicals or reagents used are of good quality

   c. ensuring that the patient sample is stored correctly

   d. All of the above

4. MSDS stands for:

   a. Material Safety Data Sheet

   b. Mandated Standards for Documentation and Safety

   c. Manual for Safety Documents/Sheets

   d. Manual of Supplies and Data for Safety

5. MSDS information must be:

   a. readily available to all employees

   b. organized in a notebook or manual

   c. indexed and alphabetized

   d. All of the above

SELF-ASSESSMENT

1. Choose a chemical you have at home or in the basement, garage, or storage area.

2. Look at the label.
   a. Does it have any precautionary statements or warnings?

   b. Does it have any fire hazard information?

3. Complete the following:

   Name of chemical (brand name) __________

   What chemicals are included in the active ingredients? __________

   What precautions are listed? __________

   What instructions are listed for contamination of eyes or skin, ingestion, and so forth? __________

   What is the number in your area for Poison Control? __________

Name ______________________ Date __________ Score ______

CHAPTER 27

Introduction to the Medical Laboratory

CHAPTER PRE-TEST

Perform this test without looking at your book. If an answer is "false," rewrite the sentence to make it true.

1. True or False? Cytology is the study of cells.

____

____

2. A urine culture would be performed in which department of a regional laboratory?
   a. Bacteriology department
   b. Urinalysis department
   c. Culture department
   d. Cytology department
3. Which of the following is a description of a profile?
   a. many tests all billed together at one time
   b. all the tests for one patient during one calendar year
   c. all the tests a doctor orders consistently throughout her or his practice
   d. a related set of tests about an organ, system, or function
4. True or False? Proficiency tests are required by the Occupational Safety and Health Administration (OSHA).

____

____

5. True or False? Fasting means that the patient may have water but nothing else by mouth for 12 hours.

____

____

VOCABULARY BUILDER

Misspelled Words

Find the words below that are misspelled; circle them, and correctly spell them in the spaces provided. Then insert the proper correct vocabulary terms into the sentences below. Each sentence describes a situation you might find in a POL or in a reference laboratory.

assay	diagnosis	objective
asymptomatic	diaphram	profile
baseline	differential diagnosis	qualitative tests
biopsy	electrolytes	quantative tests
clinical diagnosis	glucose	reagents
condensor	invasive	requisition
control test	normal flora	serum

________________ ________________ ________________

1. Wanda Slawson, CMA (AAMA), is examining a specimen in the laboratory using a compound microscope. The ________________ is the lens system closest to the specimen she is viewing.
2. Dr. Mark Woo orders laboratory tests for a female emergency patient experiencing severe abdominal cramps to make a ________________ that will distinguish between a diagnosis of appendicitis and a diagnosis of an ovarian cyst.
3. Richard Butts receives a job offer from a construction company that requires all employees to be tested for misuse or abuse of legal or illegal drugs before they can work on the site. Bruce Goldman, CMA (AAMA), performs Richard's blood test under the direction of Dr. Whitney; his test comes back clean. The results of Richard's test can be used in the future as a ________________ measurement, a record of healthy normal results.
4. Dr. King needs a red blood cell (RBC) count, a white blood cell (WBC) count, and a platelet count for Melinda Cool. Joe Guerrero, CMA (AAMA), performs a venipuncture on Melinda and sends a tube of her blood to the laboratory, together with a written ________________ containing specific information and instructions about what tests to perform on the specimens.
5. Bruce Goldman, CMA (AAMA), is examining a specimen under a compound microscope. Because he is having difficulty seeing clearly, Bruce opens the microscope's ________________ to increase the amount of light on the specimen.
6. Dr. Lewis asks Audrey Jones, CMA (AAMA), to send a tube of Herb Fowler's blood to the laboratory for analysis. Dr. Lewis wants to determine the constituents and relative proportion of each of the enzymes in Herb's serum; this type of analysis is called an ________________.
7. Jacquie Cavanaugh comes to see Dr. Lewis and reports that she has been constantly tired for the past two or three months. Because Jacquie's symptoms are so vague, Dr. Lewis orders a blood ________________ to help narrow the diagnosis possibilities.
8. Bruce Goldman, CMA (AAMA), always follows Standard Precautions and washes his hands before touching a patient. Although everyone's body contains many natural microorganisms, called ________________, aseptic hand washing reduces the potential for exposure to or transmission of pathogens.
9. Hematology laboratories count the WBCs or RBCs in a sample of a patient's blood. In general, these type of counting tests are known as ________________.
10. As a method of quality control, a ________________ sample is tested together with a patient's sample as a method of ensuring the accuracy of test results.
11. Joe Guerrero, CMA (AAMA), asks Abigail Johnson, who he knows is diagnosed with diabetes mellitus, whether she regularly tests her blood at home to measure her ________________ level.

12. The hematology laboratory performs tests that measure characteristics of blood such as size, shape, and maturity of cells. These types of tests are known in general as ______________________.

13. Histology is the study of tissue samples to determine disease. In most cases, a frozen tissue sample or ______________________ is sliced, stained, and microscopically examined for anomalies.

14. Urinalysis performed on a urine specimen from patient Irina Panasenko shows that she has a mild bladder infection. Irina is surprised at this diagnosis; she does not feel sick. Dr. Esposito explains that it is possible to be ______________________ and still have an infection.

15. Most of the patient samples that Audrey Jones, CMA (AAMA), prepares to send to the laboratory are samples of ______________________, the liquid portion of blood obtained after blood has been allowed to clot or has been separated.

16. If a control sample shows inaccurate results after testing, one possible explanation is that the __________ are faulty or have expired.

17. In microscopic analysis of specimens, the light, or image, is reflected by the ______________________ onto the specimen to the ocular lenses for visualization.

18. Fine-needle aspiration is an ______________________ procedure used in a preliminary diagnosis of breast cancer; the test involves inserting a needle into the suspicious breast lump and extracting cells for analysis under a microscope. Because this test is not always reliable, often a mammogram is also performed.

19. A ______________________ of Lyme disease can be confirmed by performing laboratory tests on patient blood specimens.

20. Dr. Rice makes a ______________________ of asthma for patient Yuping Chen, based on subjective and objective information gathered after obtaining an in-depth patient history and performing a complete physical examination.

21. ______________________ are substances that split into electrically charged particles, or ions, when dissolved or melted. These electricity conductors are important in maintaining fluid and acid-base homeostasis in the body.

LEARNING REVIEW

Matching

Match each laboratory facility or department to the statement below that best describes it.

A. Reference laboratories
B. Clinical chemistry
C. Cytology
D. Hematology
E. Histology
F. Immunology/immunohematology
G. Hospital-based laboratories
H. Parasitology
I. Microbiology
J. Mycology
K. Physician's office laboratories (POLs)
L. Procurement stations
M. Urinalysis

___ 1. This laboratory department performs blood typing procedures, cross-matching, and the separation and storage of blood components for transfusion, as well as antibody-antigen reactions.

___ 2. This subdivision of the microbiology department detects the presence of disease-producing human parasites or ova present in patient specimens such as feces and blood.

___ 3. Independent laboratories often have smaller satellites or these stations located near isolated medical facilities or in areas convenient to patients.

____ 4. This laboratory department performs qualitative and quantitative tests on blood and blood components.

____ 5. This subdivision of the microbiology department is where fungi are grown and identified.

____ 6. These laboratories are independent, regionally located, and used by hospitals and providers for complex, expensive, or specialized tests.

____ 7. Some procedures performed by this department include assays of enzymes in the serum, serum glucose, or electrolyte levels.

____ 8. This laboratory department analyzes patient specimens for the presence of disease-producing microorganisms.

____ 9. These laboratories perform medical laboratory tests easily and inexpensively in the office by the medical assistant.

____ 10. These laboratories perform most of the tests required in inpatient settings and hospitals.

____ 11. This is the microscopic study of the form and structure of the various tissues making up living organisms. Tissue analysis and biopsy studies are performed in this area of the laboratory.

____ 12. This laboratory department performs microscopic examinations of cells to detect irregularities in growth and development.

____ 13. This involves the physical, chemical, and microscopic examination of urine as a diagnostic tool for physicians.

Short Answer

1. Identify each test named below.

   Hgb ______________________________

   Diff ______________________________

   ESR ______________________________

   Hct ______________________________

2. Name three electrolytes.

   ____

   ____

   ____

3. Name two types of tests performed in the cytology laboratory department.

   ____

   ____

4. Physicians depend on medical laboratories to help them ascertain a patient's state of health or state of disease. There are eight main reasons why a physician might need a laboratory test performed. Identify the proper reason laboratory testing is required for each example given.

   A. After feeling the abdomen for bladder distention and performing a rectal examination, Charles Williams's symptoms suggest to Dr. Lewis that Charles may be suffering from an enlarged prostate. Dr. Lewis orders blood tests and a urinalysis to confirm his diagnosis.

   ____

   ____

B. Patient Janet Renquiz, a retired homemaker, complies with the treatment plan for her diagnosed case of chronic lymphocytic leukemia by submitting to a regular testing of her blood for the presence of leukemic cells, which monitors the progress of the disease.

____

____

C. Anna Ortiz, who is pregnant, has had genital herpes for several years. In the week before her child is to be born, Dr. King takes a culture of Anna's cervical and vaginal mucosa to determine whether her baby is at risk for contracting herpes in the birth canal.

____

____

D. Dr. Mark Woo has been treating Edith Leonard, who describes having poor vision and fainting spells. Because Edith's symptoms are vague and he cannot make a firm diagnosis, Dr. Woo orders a complete blood profile to give him additional information about Edith's case.

____

____

E. Louise Kipperly comes to Inner City Health Care for her yearly medical checkup. Dr. Esposito orders a series of blood tests to make sure that Louise's cholesterol level is within a normal, healthy range.

____

____

F. Fifteen-year-old Hung Chu comes to Inner City Health Care with a severe sore throat. A physical examination detects the presence of fever, headache, difficulty swallowing, and inflamed tonsils. Dr. Whitney orders a complete blood cell count (CBC) and a heterophil antibodies test to confirm a diagnosis of either tonsillitis or infectious mononucleosis. When the results of Hung's blood tests come back from the laboratory, however, atypical lymphocytes in the blood indicate the early onset of infectious mononucleosis.

____

____

G. When Naoki Tamura's laboratory tests come back positive for *Herpesvirus hominis*, his girlfriend Eleanor is instructed to come into Inner City Health Care for testing. Eleanor, who has no symptoms, is tested for herpes simplex and nonspecific urethritis.

____

____

H. Maria Jover, who was diagnosed with HIV, takes protease inhibitors to help her immune system fight the disease. Dr. King orders blood tests to determine how Maria is responding to the treatment.

____

____

5. Name five tests commonly performed in a physician's office laboratory (POL).

____

____

____

6. Name three criteria that would justify using point-of-care testing.

____

____

7. Identify each entry that follows as a way an infectious agent leaves the body of a sick person (L), the way an organism may be transmitted (T), or the way an organism enters the body (E).

____ A. Discharges from infected eyes

____ B. Contaminated needles and syringes

____ C. Contaminated water in a river

____ D. Directly onto mucous membrane

____ E. Breast milk

____ F. Towels

____ G. Health care workers exposed to blood

____ H. Transplacentally to fetus

____ I. Contact with blood and body fluids

____ J. Discharges from respiratory tract

____ K. Feces and urine

____ L. Flies

____ M. Excreta from intestinal tract

____ N. Directly on the conjunctiva

8. The accuracy of any laboratory test result depends on the performance of quality controls by all health care workers who handle a specimen. Medical assistants must have a thorough knowledge of quality controls and standards. List five factors that can compromise the accuracy of laboratory test results.

____

____

____

____

9. What is the reason for using a control test sample? Explain in detail.

____

____

____

____

____

____

____

____

____

10. Knowing how to perform tasks safely is critical when working in a medical laboratory. Medical assistants must understand the different types of hazards present in a medical laboratory and know how to protect themselves and other health care professionals from possible harm.

    A. It is important to avoid ingestion or exposure to chemicals and pathogens. Name four ways this can be avoided.

    ____

    ____

    ____

    ____

    B. What is the first action to take when a surface becomes contaminated?

    ____

    ____

    C. Explain why it is important to avoid wearing loose clothing or accessories in the laboratory.

    ____

    ____

    ____

    D. In terms of safety issues, why is it important to properly maintain laboratory equipment?

    ____

    ____

    ____

11. For each method of exposure, list one circumstance in which pathogens may be transmitted in the ambulatory care setting and Standard Precautions that are effective in reducing or preventing the transmission of pathogens under each circumstance.

    A. Direct contact

    ____

    ____

    ____

    ____

    B. Ingestion

    ____

    ____

    ____

    ____

    ____

    C. Mucous membranes

    ____

    ____

    ____

    ____

12. What is the purpose of a microscope?

13. Name the five parts of a microscope.

14. What type of microscope is the most commonly used in a medical laboratory?

15. Name three other types of microscopes and explain what each is designed for viewing.

16. Name the two adjustments found on a microscope and explain the purpose of each.

17. Name six practices that should always be followed to properly care for a microscope.

CERTIFICATION REVIEW

These questions are designed to mimic the certification examination. Select the best response.

1. Choosing to perform the simplest and least invasive procedure to rule out a particular disease before requiring more extensive testing is known as a:
   a. clinical diagnosis
   b. cumulative diagnosis
   c. developmental diagnosis
   d. differential diagnosis

2. ___________ involve actual number counts such as are done in WBC counts, RBC counts, and platelet levels.
   a. Qualitative tests
   b. Quantitative tests
   c. CLIA waived tests
   d. Functional tests
3. The area of the clinical laboratory where organisms such as bacteria and fungi are grown and identified is called the:
   a. cytology department
   b. chemistry department
   c. microbiology department
   d. histology department
4. A hepatic function panel will include a:
   a. creatinine level
   b. rheumatoid factor
   c. cholesterol level
   d. bilirubin level
5. Serum separator tubes used in hematology may not be used when collecting blood for a:
   a. lipid profile
   b. thyroid profile
   c. cardiac profile
   d. toxicologic study

LEARNING APPLICATION

Hands-on Activity

At Abigail Johnson's annual physical examination on June 5, 20xx, at 2 PM, Dr. Elizabeth King orders several laboratory tests to monitor Abigail's diagnosed conditions of hypertension, diabetes mellitus, and moderate angina pectoris. Dr. Frank Jones, Abigail's cardiologist, will also receive a copy of the final laboratory report. Ellen Armstrong, CMA (AAMA), prepares the laboratory requisition form. Complete Ellen's laboratory requisition form for Abigail's laboratory work.

Patient:
Abigail Johnson
225 River Street
Northborough, OH 12336
Phone: 389-2631
Date of Birth: March 1, 1920
Social Security Number: 011-11-1231
Medicare #: 021-45-6712-D

Physicians:
Dr. Elizabeth King
Northborough Family Medical Group
2501 Center Street
Northborough, OH 12345
Phone: 651-8000

Dr. Frank Jones
815 Heart Health Blvd
Northborough, OH 12339
Phone 655-7000

Physician's Order for Laboratory Testing: Blood profile to include BUN, chloride, cholesterol, creatinine, glucose, LDH, potassium, SGOT, SGPT, sodium, triglycerides.

NORTHBOROUGH REFERENCE LABORATORIES

128 Analysis Way
Northborough, OH 12468

❑ GROUP ACCOUNT ❑ PATIENT

Ordering Physician Signature

LAST NAME	FIRST NAME	MI	SEX	DATE OF BIRTH
ADDRESS	CITY		STATE	ZIP
PHONE # Home / Work	SOC. SEC #			

COMPLETE SHADED BOX BELOW FOR PATIENT AND THIRD PARTY BILL ONLY

RESPONSIBLE PARTY	LAST NAME	FIRST NAME	MI	MEDICARE ❑ AMERICAID ❑ # 021-45-6712-D
ADDRESS	CITY	STATE	ZIP	PHONE #
INSURED NAME	INSURANCE CO. NAME/ADDRESS			
INSURED'S EMPLOYER	RELATIONSHIP TO PATIENT ❑ Self ❑ Spouse ❑ Dependent		CONTRACT #	GROUP #

REASON FOR TEST (A DIAGNOSIS IS NECESSARY FOR ALL INSURANCE CLAIMS) *SEE REVERSE FOR CODES*

PRIMARY CARE PHYSICIAN

SPECIMEN INFORMATION

❑ STAT
Date of Collection ________
Time of Collection ________

❑ Serum ❑ Plasma
❑ Urine (Volume) ________
Hours ________
❑ Other ________

CALL RESULTS TO:
____
Phone #:( ) ________
Copy Results to:
____
____
____

SPECIMEN CODES: G - GEL, L - LAVENDER, R - RED, B - BLUE, BK - BLACK, U - URINE

PROFILES

Test	Code	Test	Code	Test	Code	Test	Code
❑ BIOCHEM BASIC	1G	❑ BIOCHEM PROFILE III	2G, 1L	❑ LIPID 12-16 HOUR FAST REQUIRED	1G	❑ THYROID	1G
❑ BIOCHEM PROFILE I	1G, 1L	❑ ARTHRITIS	2G,1BK	❑ LIVER	1G	❑ HYPERTHYROID	1G
❑ BIOCHEM PROFILE II	1G, 1L	❑ HEPATITIS	1G	❑ PRENATAL	1G, 1L, 1R	❑ HYPOTHYROID	1G
						❑ TORCH PROFILE	1G

INDIVIDUAL TESTS

Test	Code	Test	Code	Test	Code
❑ ALBUMIN	G	❑ FSH	G	❑ PROSTATE SPECIFIC ANTIGEN	G
❑ ALK. PHOSPHATASE	G	❑ GC CULTURE, SOURCE ________		❑ PT W/INR	B
❑ AMYLASE	G	❑ GLUCOSE	G	❑ PTT	B
❑ ANA SCREEN	G	❑ GLYCATED HEMOGLOBIN	L	❑ RHEUMATOID FACTOR	G
❑ BILIRUBIN, TOTAL	G	❑ hCG, BETA SUBUNIT QUANT.	G	❑ RPR	G
❑ BILIRUBIN, TOTAL + DIRECT	G	❑ HDL	G	❑ RUBELLA IgG ANTIBODY	G
❑ BILIRUBIN, NEONATAL	G	❑ HEPATITIS B SURF. ANTIBODY	G	❑ SEDIMENTATION RATE	BK
❑ BUN	G	❑ HEPATITIS B SURF. ANTIGEN	G	❑ SGOT	G
❑ CALCIUM, TOTAL	G	❑ HEPATITIS C ANTIBODY	G	❑ SGPT	G
❑ CBC W/AUTOMATED DIFF	L	❑ HIV ANTIBODY (SIGNED CONSENT REQUIRED)	G	❑ SPUTUM CULTURE	
❑ CBC W/MANUAL DIFF	L	❑ LACTIC DEHYDROGENASE	G	❑ STOOL CULTURE	
❑ CHLAMYDIA SCREEN, SOURCE ________		❑ LEAD, PEDIATRIC	L	❑ THROAT, GROUP A STREP CULTURE	
❑ CHOLESTEROL	G	❑ LH	G	❑ TOTAL PROTEIN	G
❑ CREATININE	G	❑ LIPASE	G	❑ TSH	G
❑ CULTURE, SOURCE ________		❑ LITHIUM	G	❑ URIC ACID	G
❑ ELECTROLYTES	G	❑ OVA & PARASITE PREP.		❑ URINALYSIS	U
❑ ESTRADIOL	G	❑ PHOSPHORUS	G	❑ URINE CULTURE	U
❑ FERRITIN	G	❑ PREGNANCY TEST, BLOOD	G	❑ VITAMIN B12	G
❑ FOLIC ACID	G	❑ PROGESTERONE	G		
❑ FREE T4	G	❑ PROLACTIN	G		

ICD-9-CM DIAGNOSIS CODES

- ☐ 648.80 ABN GLUC TOL/PREG OR PP
- ☐ 682.9 ABSCESS
- ☐ 042 AIDS
- ☐ 477.9 ALLERGIC RHINITIS
- ☐ 626.0 AMENORRHEA
- ☐ 285.9 ANEMIA
- ☐ 413.9 ANGINA
- ☐ 716.90 ARTHRITIS
- ☐ 414.00 ASHD
- ☐ 493.90 ASTHMA
- ☐ 600 BENIGN PROSTATIC HYPERTROPHY
- ☐ 466.0 BRONCHITIS
- ☐ 199.1 CA SPECIFY SITE:________
- ☐ 428.0 CHF
- ☐ 496 COPD
- ☐ 436 CVA
- ☐ E934.9 COUMADIN THERAPY
- ☐ 250.00 DIABETES
- ☐ 558.9 DIARRHEA
- ☐ 562.11 DIVERTICULITIS
- ☐ 780.4 DIZZINESS
- ☐ 276.9 ELECTROLYTE IMBALANCE
- ☐ 259.9 ENDOCRINE DISORDERS
- ☐ 530.10 ESOPHAGITIS
- ☐ 780.6 FEVER
- ☐ 558.9 GASTROENTERITIS
- ☐ 784.0 HEADACHE
- ☐ 599.7 HEMATURIA
- ☐ 573.3 HEPATITIS
- ☐ 070.9 HEPATITIS, VIRAL
- ☐ 272.4 HYPERLIPIDEMIA
- ☐ 401.9 HYPERTENSION
- ☐ 244.9 HYPOTHYROID
- ☐ 628.9 INFERTILITY, FEMALE
- ☐ 487.1 INFLUENZA
- ☐ 774.6 JAUNDICE OF NEWBORN
- ☐ 782.4 JAUNDICE NOT NEWBORN
- ☐ V72.6 LAB EXAMINATION
- ☐ 709.8 LESION, SKIN
- ☐ 573.9 LIVER DISEASE
- ☐ 785.6 LYMPHADENOPATHY
- ☐ 780.7 MALAISE & FATIGUE
- ☐ 382.9 OTITIS MEDIA
- ☐ 789.0 PAIN, ABDOMEN
- ☐ 724.5 PAIN, BACK
- ☐ 723.1 PAIN, CERVICAL NECK
- ☐ 786.50 PAIN, CHEST
- ☐ 719.40 PAIN, JOINT
- ☐ V76.2 PAP SMEAR
- ☐ 614.9 PID
- ☐ 462 PHARYNGITIS
- ☐ 486 PNEUMONIA
- ☐ V22.2 PREGNANCY, NORMAL
- ☐ 593.9 RENAL DISEASE
- ☐ 461.9 SINUSITIS
- ☐ 462 SORE THROAT
- ☐ V67.0 SURGICAL FOLLOW UP
- ☐ 780.2 SYNCOPE
- ☐ 465.9 URI
- ☐ 599.0 UTI
- ☐ 616.10 VAGINITIS
- ☐ 079.9 VIRAL SYNDROME
- ☐ 998.5 WOUND INFECTION
- ☐ OTHER:________
- ☐ ________
- ☐ ________
- ☐ ________

PROFILES / CPT CODES

BIOCHEM BASIC / 80019

Albumin
Alkaline Phosphatase
Anion Gap
Bicarbonate
Bilirubin, Total
BUN
Calcium
Chloride
Cholesterol
Creatinine
GGTP
Glucose
LDH
Phosphorus
Potassium
Protein, Total
SGOT (AST)
SGPT (ALT)
Sodium
Triglycerides
Uric Acid

BIOCHEM PROFILE I / 80019, 85025, 85029

Biochem Basic
CBC w/Automated Diff

BIOCHEM PROFILE II / 80019, 85025, 85029, 83718

Biochem Basic
CBC w/Automated Diff
Lipid Profile

BIOCHEM PROFILE III / 80019, 85025, 85029 83718, 80091

Biochem Basic
CBC w/Automated Diff
Lipid Profile
Thyroid Profile

ARTHRITIS PROFILE / 80072

ANA
Rheumatoid Factor
Sed Rate
Uric Acid

HEPATITIS PROFILE / 80059

Hepatitis A Ab (HAAB)
Hepatitis B Core Ab (HBCAB)
Hepatitis B Surf Ab (HBSAB)
Hepatitis B Surf Ag (HBSAG)
Hepatitis C Ab (HCAB)

LIPID PROFILE / 80061
12-16 Hour Fast Required

Cholesterol
HDL
LDL
Triglycerides

LIVER PROFILE / 80058

Albumin
Alkaline Phosphatase
Bilirubin, Total
SGOT (AST)
SGPT (ALT)

PRENATAL PROFILE / 80055

ABO/Rh type
Antibody Screen
CBC w/Automated Diff
Hepatitis B Surf Antigen
Rubella IgG Antibody
RPR

THYROID PROFILE / 80091

Free Thyroxine Index
T_3 Uptake
T_4

HYPERTHYROID PROFILE / 80091, 84480

Thyroid Profile
T_3 Total

HYPOTHYROID PROFILE / 80092

Thyroid Profile
TSH

TORCH PROFILE / 80090

CMV IgG Ab
Herpes I and II Ab
Rubella IgG Antibody
Toxoplasma IgG Ab

CHAPTER POST-TEST

Perform this test without looking at your book. If an answer is "false," rewrite the sentence to make it true.

1. True or False? Histology is the study of cells.

____

____

2. A urine culture would be performed in which department of a regional laboratory?
   a. Urinalysis department
   b. Bacteriology department
   c. Culture department
   d. Cytology department
3. True or False? NPO means that the patient may have water but nothing else by mouth for 12 hours.

____

____

4. Which of the following is a description of a profile?
   a. All the tests for one patient during one calendar year
   b. All the tests a doctor orders consistently throughout his or her practice
   c. Many tests all billed together at one time
   d. A related set of tests about an organ, system, or function
5. True or False? Proficiency tests are required by CLIA.

____

____

SELF-ASSESSMENT

Working in a medical laboratory requires spending large amounts of time performing extremely detail-oriented procedures, such as observing specimens through a microscope for signs of disease. Laboratory analysis also involves maintaining high-quality controls and safety standards to ensure the accuracy and reliability of results. The way you deal with details in your everyday life can reveal much about your predisposition for detail-oriented analytic tasks. For each statement, circle the response that best describes you.

1. When walking along a city street, I:
   a. notice each person who passes me, remember details from storefronts, and even recognize the make and model of cars as they drive by
   b. like to listen to other people's conversations and enjoy interacting with friends who are accompanying me
   c. usually spend my time daydreaming
2. If I think about the way a pine tree looks, I:
   a. visualize the rough texture of its bark and see its long, thin leaves perfectly in my head
   b. think about the great Christmas trees my family always had when I was a kid
   c. see two blobs of color, green and brown

3. I prefer working in an atmosphere:
   a. that is structured and involves analytic thinking
   b. where the decision-making process is cut-and-dry and the options are well defined
   c. where I do not have to make decisions or interpret anything
4. When preparing a meal or recipe, I:
   a. am very careful to make sure I read the recipe over twice before I start and have each of the ingredients on hand
   b. read the recipe quickly just to make sure I understand the basics
   c. just wing it; I cook by intuition
5. When preparing for a trip or vacation, I:
   a. know exactly where my passport and other important papers are located, make a list of all essential items to bring and check off the list as each is packed, and leave detailed written instructions for the housesitter
   b. know pretty much what I need and where I can find it; but I wait until the day before to get it all together
   c. let someone else do all the packing and handle all the arrangements; too many details for me
6. After a conversation with someone I have just met, I:
   a. remember the exact color of his or her eyes
   b. would be able to make a pretty good guess about what color his or her eyes are
   c. have no idea what color his or her eyes are
7. When giving people driving directions to a destination, I:
   a. make sure to give detailed instructions, using at least two different routes, noting landmarks and the location of gas stations along the way
   b. say basically what area of town they need to head toward and the street address; I know they can figure out the rest on their own
   c. usually give people the wrong directions, so I tell them to ask someone else
8. In regard to friends' birthdays, I:
   a. have them all written down in my calendar, and I send cards out four days before the date
   b. know what month they fall in, and make sure to wish them a happy birthday somewhere around the middle of the month
   c. am usually embarrassed when I find out a friend's birthday has passed; I can never remember dates

Scoring: If most of your answers were A's, you are an extremely detail-oriented and observant person. You are well suited to the tasks performed in the medical laboratory. If your answers were mostly B's, you can be observant, but you do not always pay close attention to details. If your answers were mostly C's, you will need to work on your observation skills.

Name ______________________ Date __________ Score ______

CHAPTER 28

Phlebotomy: Venipuncture and Capillary Puncture

CHAPTER PRE-TEST

Perform this test without looking at your book.

1. Red blood cells (RBCs) are produced in the:
   a. liver
   b. lymph nodes
   c. spleen
   d. bone marrow
2. What type of blood is the most common for laboratory tests?
   a. Arterial blood
   b. Venous blood
   c. Capillary blood
   d. Coronary blood
3. What is a buffy coat made of?
   a. White blood cells (WBCs)
   b. RBCs
   c. Platelets
   d. a. and c.
4. Which way should the bevel of the needle be held when performing venipuncture?
   a. Up
   b. Down
   c. Sideways
   d. Any of the above

5. Which of the following tubes contains no anticoagulants?
   a. Green
   b. Red
   c. Gray
   d. Lavender
6. What position should patients be in while they are having their blood drawn?
   a. Standing
   b. Lying down
   c. Sitting
   d. Either b. or c.
7. What is the maximum amount of time a tourniquet should be left on?
   a. 30 seconds
   b. 60 seconds
   c. 90 seconds
   d. 120 seconds
8. What is the most common method used to draw blood from an adult?
   a. Syringe
   b. Vacuum tube
   c. Butterfly
   d. Intravenous needle

VOCABULARY BUILDER

Misspelled Words I

Find the words in Column A that are misspelled; circle them, and correctly spell them in the spaces provided. Then match each of the vocabulary terms below with the correct definition in Column B.

	Column A	Correct Spelling	Column B
____	1. Aliquot	______________	A. WBCs
____	2. Hemololysis	______________	B. A portion of a specimen that has been taken for storage
____	3. Phlebotomy	______________	C. Swollen from abnormal fluid accumulation
____	4. Anticoagulant	______________	D. RBCs
____	5. Leukocytes	______________	E. A tube used for insertion into a body cavity
____	6. Therapeutic	______________	F. Device that screws into an evacuated tube holder
____	7. Canulla	______________	G. Destruction of red blood cell membrane
____	8. Luer-Lok	______________	H. A band to be applied around a limb to restrict blood flow and distend the veins
____	9. Torniquet	______________	I. Thickness or stickiness, resistance to flow
____	10. Edematous	______________	J. The act of feeling with the hand or fingers

____ 11. Lipemia ______________

____ 12. Viscosity ______________

____ 13. Erythrocytes ______________

____ 14. Palpitate ______________

K. A condition in which there are increased amounts of lipids in the blood

L. Puncture or the incision of a vein

M. Used in the treatment of disease

N. A substance used to prevent blood clotting

Misspelled Words II

Find the words listed below that are misspelled; circle them, and correctly spell them in the spaces provided. Then match the vocabulary terms with the correct definitions below.

additive	hypoglycemia	thrombocytes
diurnal	plasma	venipuncture
hemoconcentration	serum	
hemotoma	thirotrophic gel	

______________ ______________

______________ 1. The fluid portion of blood from an anticoagulated tube

______________ 2. The state of having a lower than normal blood glucose level

______________ 3. The process of collecting blood

______________ 4. Any material placed in a tube that maintains or facilitates the integrity and function of the specimen

______________ 5. The body's daily cycle; levels fluctuate during this cycle

______________ 6. An accumulation of blood around the venipuncture site during or after venipuncture, caused by the leakage of blood from where the needle punctured the vein

______________ 7. The fluid portion of the blood after clotting has taken place

______________ 8. A gel material capable of forming an interface between the cells and fluid portion of the blood as a result of centrifugation

______________ 9. Platelets

______________ 10. Leaving a tourniquet on the arm longer than 1 minute, causing an increased concentration of constituents in the blood sample, resulting in inaccurate test results

Definitions

Write a brief definition of the following vocabulary words.

1. Integrity ______________
2. Oxygenated ______________
3. Primary container ______________
4. Dilate ______________
5. Centrifuge ______________

____

6. Buffy coat ____

____

7. Constrict ____

LEARNING REVIEW

Short Answer

1. Identify and describe the first, second, and third choices of sites on the human body used to perform venipuncture.

____

____

____

____

____

____

2. Tourniquets play a critical role in venipuncture and must be applied and used properly to obtain a blood specimen for analysis.

   A. What is the purpose of a tourniquet?

   ____

   ____

   B. Where is the tourniquet placed?

   ____

   ____

   C. How long should the tourniquet remain on the arm during the procedure?

   ____

   ____

   D. At what point during the procedure should the tourniquet be removed? Why is the timing of removal so important?

   ____

   ____

   ____

   ____

3. Match the collection tubes containing anticoagulants with their corresponding color stoppers: green, gray, blue, and lavender.

   A. Coagulation "citrate" tube: ____________

   B. EDTA tube: __________

   C. Oxalate/fluoride tube: ____________

   D. Heparin tube: ____________

4. Discuss how the five factors listed below might have an effect on blood test results.

   Exercise ______________________________

   Tourniquet ______________________________

   Volume of blood drawn ______________________________

   Heparin ______________________________

   Temperature of specimen ______________________________

5. Vein stimulation refers to techniques used when initial attempts to obtain a blood sample are not successful. What are five techniques used to stimulate veins?

   ____

6. What is the purpose of additives? How do they differ from anticoagulants? Give examples of each.

   ____

7. How can medical assistants be sure they have found a vein and not an artery or a tendon when preparing to draw blood from a patient? Describe the characteristics of each.

____

____

____

____

____

____

____

____

____

8. Identify the recommended venipuncture method for each of the situations listed below.
   A. When drawing blood from a 75-year-old patient with thin veins _______________
   B. For collecting a blood specimen from children, who have small veins and a tendency to move during the venipuncture procedure _______________
   C. When multiple blood samples must be obtained from one venipuncture procedure _______________

Matching

Arteries and veins are crucial elements of the circulatory system. Indicate which of the following are functions or characteristics of arteries (A) and which are functions of veins (V).

____ 1. Normally brighter in color

____ 2. No pulse

____ 3. Carry blood to heart; carry deoxygenated blood (except pulmonary)

____ 4. Thin wall and less elastic

____ 5. Carry blood from heart; carry oxygenated blood (except pulmonary)

____ 6. No valves

CERTIFICATION REVIEW

These questions are designed to mimic the certification examination. Select the best response.

1. To speed removal of serum from a tube of blood, an instrument called a(n) _____________ is used.
   a. autoclave
   b. centrifuge
   c. calibrator
   d. incubator

2. Plasma contains:
   a. fibrinogen
   b. a buffy coat
   c. RBCs
   d. a clot
3. Needle insertion for venipuncture should be at an angle of:
   a. 90 degrees
   b. 30 degrees
   c. 45 degrees
   d. 15 degrees
4. The first step in a successful venipuncture is to:
   a. select the site
   b. put the patient at ease
   c. tie the tourniquet appropriately
   d. apply gloves
5. Syncope refers to:
   a. fasting
   b. relaxation
   c. fainting
   d. reclining

LEARNING APPLICATION

1. Make your own flashcards using the form on the last page of this chapter. Tear out the page of flashcards and copy them double-sided onto a cardstock or heavy-weight paper. Cut them apart. Color in the "O" with the same color as the vacuum tube tops (brick red, lavender, green, blue, etc.) and fill in the information. Use the cards to drill yourself and your classmates.

CASE STUDY

Wanda Slawson, CMA (AAMA), performs a successful venipuncture on Jaime Carrera using the vacuum tube system and a 21-gauge needle. Wanda is now preparing to label the tubes for laboratory analysis. She is careful to label all tubes at the patient's side before leaving the examination room.

CASE STUDY REVIEW QUESTIONS

1. What information must be included on the specimen labels for the specimen to be accepted for analysis?

____

____

____

____

____

2. What guidelines must Wanda follow during the venipuncture procedure to ensure that anticoagulated blood specimens are acceptable for analysis?

____

____

____

____

3. Once Wanda has followed all procedures for correct labeling and processing of the blood specimens, what Standard Precautions must she perform?

____

____

____

____

CHAPTER POST-TEST

Perform this test without looking at your book.

1. Red blood cells are produced in the:

   a. liver

   b. lymph nodes

   c. spleen

   d. bone marrow

2. The most common type of blood for laboratory tests is:
   a. capillary blood
   b. venous blood
   c. arterial blood
   d. coronary blood
3. A buffy coat is a combination of:
   a. RBCs
   b. WBCs
   c. platelets
   d. b. and c.
4. The bevel of the needle should be held in which of the following positions when performing venipuncture?
   a. Down
   b. Up
   c. Sideways
   d. Any of the above
5. Which tube color contains no anticoagulants?
   a. Red top
   b. Gray top
   c. Green top
   d. Lavender top
6. Which of the following position(s) should patients be in while they are having their blood drawn?
   a. Lying down
   b. Standing
   c. Sitting
   d. Either a. or c.
7. What is the maximum amount of time a tourniquet should be left on?
   a. 30 seconds
   b. 60 seconds
   c. 90 seconds
   d. 120 seconds
8. The most common method used to draw blood from an adult is:
   a. syringe
   b. butterfly
   c. vacuum tube
   d. intravenous needle

SELF-ASSESSMENT

During your career as a medical assistant, you will probably run into a patient who refuses to have his or her blood drawn.

a. How will you calm the patient?

b. What measures will you take that might be different from typical blood draws?

c. What would make you decide not to continue with a blood draw?

d. How would you chart each situation? In the first situation, you are able to convince the patient and end up with a successful blood draw. In the other situation, you decide to stop the procedures without obtaining a blood draw. On the lines below, chart both situations.

	Color: Additive: Specimen type: Tests:
	Color: Additive: Specimen type: Tests:
	Color: Additive: Specimen type: Tests:
	Color: Additive: Specimen type: Tests:
	Color: Additive: Specimen type: Tests:
	Color: Additive: Specimen type: Tests:
	Color: Additive: Specimen type: Tests:
	Color: Additive: Specimen type: Tests:

Name ______ Date ______ Score ______

CHAPTER 29

Hematology

CHAPTER PRE-TEST

Perform this test without looking at your book. If an answer is "false," rewrite the sentence to make it true.

1. True or False? Hematology is the study of blood cells and coagulation.

2. True or False? Hematopoiesis is the formation of blood cells.

3. True or False? An increase in neutrophils is indicative of a bacterial infection.

4. True or False? White blood cells (WBCs) are responsible for carrying oxygen to the body's cells.

5. True or False? Platelets assist with clotting.

6. True or False? Red blood cells (RBCs) are the most numerous of all the body's blood cell components.

VOCABULARY BUILDER

Misspelled Words

Find the words in Column A that are misspelled; circle them, and correctly spell them in the spaces provided. Then match each of the vocabulary terms below with the correct definition in Column B.

	Column A	Correct Spelling
____	1. Complete blood count	________________
____	2. Erythrocysts	________________
____	3. Esinophil	________________
____	4. Microcytic	________________
____	5. Luekocytes	________________
____	6. Hematacrit	________________
____	7. Hemaglobin	________________
____	8. Basophil	________________
____	9. Thrombocytes	________________
____	10. Lymphocytes	________________
____	11. Monocytes	________________
____	12. Macrocytic	________________
____	13. Hypochromic	________________
____	14. Erythropotin	________________

Column B

A. A hormone triggered by the kidneys that helps produce RBCs

B. Having less color than normal

C. A larger than normal cell

D. A WBC without cytoplasmic granules that has a large, convoluted, nonsegmented nucleus

E. A smaller than normal cell

F. WBCs, one of the formed elements of blood

G. WBC with a dense, nonsegmented nucleus that lacks granules in the cytoplasm

H. Platelets

I. Granulocytic WBC with dark purple cytoplasmic granules

J. Molecule of the RBC that transports oxygen

K. Percentage of RBCs within a specimen of anticoagulated whole blood

L. A granulocytic WBC with red-stained granules in the cytoplasm that is increased with allergies

M. RBCs, one of the formed elements of blood

N. Hematologic test consisting of Hct, Hgb, RBC and WBC counts, differential WBC count, and the erythrocyte indices

LEARNING REVIEW

Short Answer

1. When Dr. Winston Lewis orders CBCs on his patients, what are the general tests the provider will study to help him make a diagnosis?

____

____

____

2. While Dr. Elizabeth King is reviewing blood tests drawn on one of her patients, she notes the hematocrit is normal, yet the hemoglobin is low. This is an indication of what disease?

____

____

3. What two WBC features on a stained differential slide are studied to assist in the identification of the cell?

____

____

4. Identify the following erythrocyte indices and list the correct formula for determining each one.

MCH ____________________ ____________________________

MCHC ____________________ ____________________________

____

MCV ____________________ ____________________________

5. In Dr. Lewis's office, Larry Dykstra, CMA (AAMA), performs a test of erythrocyte sedimentation rate (ESR) using the Wintrobe method, whereas at Inner City Health Care, Cole Kozloff, CMA (AAMA), uses the Westergren method. Describe the difference between the two procedures.

____

____

____

6. Sedimentation-rate results vary with different states of health. Name two factors that influence the sedimentation rate. Why is the ESR a more accurate tool in diagnosing the onset of a disease than in checking on the progress of treatment?

____

____

____

____

____

____

7. At Inner City Health Care, Mary Kilmer-Tice, CMA (AAMA), uses automated hematology instruments. Automated hematology procedures have many advantages over the manual methods. List five of these advantages.

____

____

____

____

8. Name three procedures required by CLIA '88 regulations for automated hematology instruments.

____

____

____

____

____

Matching

Match the appropriate adult parameters with the following blood tests.

____	1. 36–55%	A. Hemoglobin
____	2. 80–100 fl	B. WBC count
____	3. 4,500–11,000/mm^3	C. Mean corpuscular volume
____	4. 32–36 g/dL	D. Hematocrit
____	5. 4.0–6.0 million/mm^3	E. Mean corpuscular hemoglobin concentration
____	6. 12–18 g/dL	F. RBC count
____	7. 27–33 pg	G. Mean corpuscular hemoglobin

CERTIFICATION REVIEW

These questions are designed to mimic the certification examination. Select the best response.

1. When a provider collects a bone marrow sample in an adult, the site chosen is the iliac crest or the:
   a. femur
   b. sternum
   c. tibia
   d. scapula
2. The central ion of each heme group is:
   a. magnesium
   b. calcium
   c. potassium
   d. iron
3. A buffy coat contains WBCs and:
   a. RBCs
   b. plasma
   c. platelets
   d. serum
4. When a patient has iron deficiency anemia, the erythrocytes will appear:
   a. hyperchromic
   b. hypochromic
   c. polychromic
   d. bichromic

5. Increased eosinophils may indicate:
   a. hay fever or other allergic conditions
   b. leukemia
   c. appendicitis
   d. tuberculosis

LEARNING APPLICATION

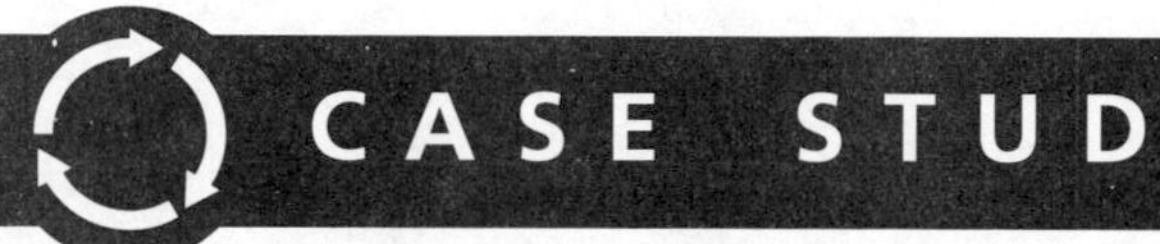

Wayne Elder is a regular patient at Inner City Health Care. Two days ago, he began to feel fatigued, experiencing development of a cough, fever, and chills. Dr. Ray Rehnolds has examined Mr. Elder and, based on the presented symptoms, makes a clinical diagnosis of influenza.

CASE STUDY REVIEW QUESTIONS

1. What type of blood test will Dr. Reynolds order to confirm his diagnosis?

____

____

2. What type of results are to be expected based on a diagnosis confirming clinical data?

____

____

____

____

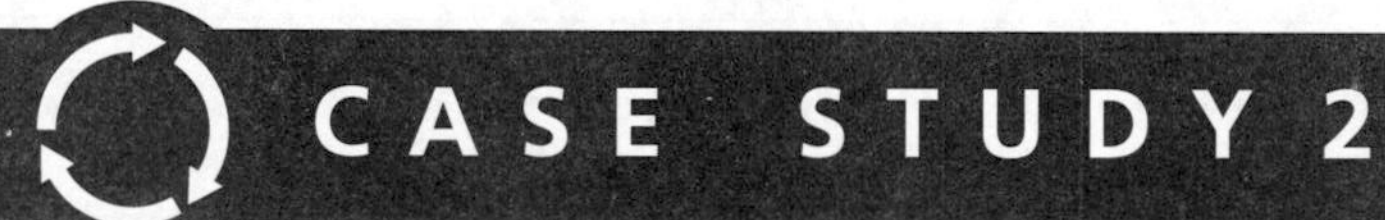

Maria Jover is describing a constant rundown feeling. After examining her, Dr. Elizabeth King has ordered a hemoglobin determination. Also, because of a past history of blood transfusion, she has also ordered an HIV test to be done at an outside reference laboratory. Dr. King asks Ellen Armstrong, CMA (AAMA), to perform the venipuncture procedure on Maria to obtain the blood specimens for analysis.

CASE STUDY REVIEW QUESTIONS

1. What tube will Ellen use to collect the blood sample to be used for the hemoglobin determination test?

____

____

continues

2. What is Dr. King hoping to learn from the hemoglobin test results?

3. With the fact that HIV infection cannot yet be ruled out, what Standard Precautions should Ellen follow in performing the venipuncture and the automated hemoglobin determination test?

CHAPTER POST-TEST

Perform this test without looking at your book. If an answer is "false," rewrite the sentence to make it true.

1. True or False? Hematology is the study of blood cells, coagulation, and chemistry.

2. True or False? Hematosis is the formation of blood cells.

3. True or False? An increase in lymphocytes is indicative of a bacterial infection.

4. True or False? RBCs are responsible for carrying oxygen to the body's cells.

5. True or False? Thrombocytes assist with clotting.

6. True or False? RBCs are the least numerous of all the body's blood cell components.

SELF-ASSESSMENT

What are your personal feelings about performing venipuncture and testing the blood of individuals who may be infected with HIV?

1. Do you think you will be more cautious than with a non–HIV infected patient?

2. Do you think you should be notified if the blood you are drawing or testing is known to be HIV positive?

3. Do you have the same concerns with hepatitis-infected specimens?

Name ______________________ Date __________ Score ______

CHAPTER **30**

Urinalysis

CHAPTER PRE-TEST

Perform this test without looking at your book. If an answer is "false," rewrite the sentence to make it true.

1. Which part of the urinalysis is to be performed by the provider?
   a. The chemical examination
   b. The physical examination
   c. The specific gravity
   d. The microscopic examination
2. Ketones in urine indicate:
   a. diabetes
   b. glomerulonephritis
   c. cystitis
   d. lipolysis
3. If the patient brings a urine sample in a household container from home for a complete urinalysis, you would:
   a. accept it this time, but after this, you will give them a proper container
   b. provide the patient with an appropriate container and ask for a fresh sample
   c. carefully and politely explain to the patient why you require a freshly voided specimen in a sterile container.
   d. b. and c.
4. The most common urine specimen type in the provider's office laboratory (POL) is the:
   a. sterile specimen
   b. timed specimen
   c. random specimen
   d. a. and c.

5. The written patient instructions for a midstream, clean catch urine specimen should be:
   a. posted in the restroom behind the toilet
   b. posted in the restroom beside the toilet
   c. posted in the restroom behind the door
   d. both a. (for male patients) and b. (for female patients)
6. True or False? The minimum amount of urine needed for a complete urinalysis is 10 mL.

____

____

7. Pyridium, a bladder analgesic, can:
   a. increase urine flow
   b. turn the urine a bright orange to red and may stain clothes
   c. calm bladder irritation
   d. both b. and c.

VOCABULARY BUILDER

Misspelled Words

Find the words in Column A that are misspelled; circle them, and then correctly spell them in the spaces provided. Then match each of the vocabulary terms below with the correct definition in Column B.

	Column A	Correct Spelling
____	1. Ketones	____________
____	2. pH	____________
____	3. Urochrome	____________
____	4. Sedament	____________
____	5. Amorphus	____________
____	6. Cultures	____________
____	7. Casts	____________
____	8. Urinalysis	____________
____	9. Quality control	____________
____	10. Specific gravity	____________
____	11. Hyline	____________
____	12. Crystals	____________
____	13. Midstream collection	____________
____	14. Supernatant	____________
____	15. Reagent test strips	____________
____	16. Urea	____________
____	17. Meniscus	____________
____	18. Turbid	____________
____	19. Screaning	____________

Column B

A. Urine testing that includes physical, chemical, and microscopic testing of a urine sample

B. Crystalline material found in urine sediment; shapeless; possessing no definite form

C. Tiny structures usually formed by deposits of protein (or other substances) within the walls of renal tubules

D. Compounds produced during increased fat metabolism; can be tested on a reagent strip

E. Found in normal urine sediment, these structures generally have no particular significance; the presence of a few should be noted because they may indicate disease states.

F. Microorganisms grown in a nutrient medium

G. Transparent, clear casts that are often hard to see in urine; these casts should be examined under subdued lighting

H. The liquid (top) portion of centrifuged urine that is disposed of

I. The part of the urinalysis that determines amount, color, clarity, and general characteristics

J. Curvature appearing in a liquid's upper surface when the liquid is placed in a container

____ 20. Acid-base balance ______________

____ 21. Physical examination ______________

____ 22. UTI ______________

____ 23. CLIA ______________

K. Urine sample collected in the middle of the flow of urine

L. The abbreviation for an infection of the urinary system

M. Scale that indicates the relative alkalinity or acidity of a solution; measurement of hydrogen ion concentration

N. Program that ensures accurate and dependable test results

O. Narrow strip of plastic on which pads containing reagents are attached; used in urinalysis to detect a variety of substances and values

P. Insoluble matter that settles to the bottom of a liquid; material examined in the urinalysis microscopic examination

Q. Ratio of weight of a given volume of a substance to the weight of the same volume of distilled water at the same temperature; test often performed during the urinalysis physical examination (can also appear on the reagent strip)

R. Opaque; lack of clarity

S. The governing body that determines which parts of the urinalysis can be waived

T. Principal end product of protein metabolism

U. Yellow pigment that provides color to urine

V. Condition that occurs when the net rate at which the body produces acids or bases is equal to the net rate at which acids or bases are excreted

W. Preliminary examination used to detect the most characteristic signs of a disorder that may eliminate or indicate the need for further investigation

Urinalysis Terms

Fill in the proper terms relating to urinalysis.

__________ 1. Orange-yellow pigment that forms from the breakdown of hemoglobin in red blood cells. It usually travels in the bloodstream to the liver, where it is converted to a water-soluble form and excreted into the bile.

__________ 2. Abnormal presence of blood in urine, symptomatic of many disorders of the genitourinary system and renal diseases

__________ 3. Simple sugar that is a major source of energy in the human body; monitoring of its levels in the urine and blood is a vital diagnostic test in diabetes and other disorders; a test on a reagent strip.

__________ 4. Test on a reagent strip that indicates the presence of white blood cells in the urinary tract

__________ 5. Colorless compound produced in the intestine after the breakdown by bacteria of bilirubin

__________ 6. Chemical substances that detect or synthesize other substances in a chemical reaction and are used in laboratory analyses because they are known to react in a specific way

__________ 7. Accumulation of ketones in the body, occurring primarily as a compilation of diabetes mellitus; if left untreated, it could cause coma.

__________ 8. Pattern based on 24-hour cycle that emphasizes the repetition of certain physiologic phenomena such as eating and sleeping

__________ 9. Waste product formed in muscle that is excreted by the kidneys; increased in blood and urine when kidney function is abnormal

__________ 10. Instrument that measures the refractive index of a substance or solution; used in the urinalysis chemical examination to measure the urine specimen's specific gravity

__________ 11. Device used to measure specific gravity; consists of a float with a calibrated stem. May be replaced by a refractometer or reagent strips

__________ 12. Urine that appears to be above the sediment when centrifuged; poured off before sediment is examined in the urinalysis microscopic examination

__________ 13. Mucoprotein excreted by the epithelial cells of the renal tubules.

LEARNING REVIEW

Fill in the Blanks

Fill in the blanks in the following paragraphs with the appropriate term(s).

A.

electrolytes	metabolism	tubule
excess fluid	milliliters	urea
filtration	nephron	urine
glomerulus	salts	waste products
homeostasis	soluble	

The formation and excretion of ______________________ is the principal method by which the body excretes water and the dissolved, or ______________________, waste products of the body's ______________________. The kidneys control this process and also regulate the fluids outside the cells of the body, carefully maintaining the body's balance of fluids eliminated or retained. This balance, or ______________________, of body fluids is important to our overall health. The kidneys are responsible for the ______________________ of ______________________, ______________________, and ______________________ from the blood. Substances filtered out of the body can include water, ammonia, ______________________, glucose, amino acids, creatinine, and ______________. These wastes leave the body through the eliminated urine. The filtering unit of the kidney is called the ______________________. The ______________________ is the long, curved part of the nephron that concentrates the filtered material. The filtering unit of the kidney is called the ______________. Each minute, more than 1,000 ______________________ of blood flows through the kidney to be cleansed.

B.

amino acids	creatinine	protein
blood	glucose	thresholds
concentration	kidney	

While passing through the ____________________, some substances, such as ____________________ and ____________________, need to be reabsorbed into the ____________________. These substances are reabsorbed in relation to their ____________________ in the blood and those levels are known as ________________. Some of these substances need only be partially reabsorbed, such as ____________ and ______________________.

C.

ammonium	hydrogen	secreted
blood	kidney	urine
drugs		

Toward the end of the __________________'s journey through the __________________, other substances that have not already been filtered out are __________________ into the __________________—for instance, substances such as __________________ and __________________ ions. In addition, certain __________________ in the blood at this point may also be secreted into the urine.

Multiple Choice

Circle the correct response for each multiple choice question below.

1. QC programs:
   a. provide a random spot-check of accuracy
   b. ensure accurate and reliable results for the patient
   c. provide comparisons with patient specimens necessary to interpret urinalysis test results
2. Equipment and instruments used for urine testing:
   a. must be disposed of properly in biohazard containers after each procedure
   b. are self-calibrating and require no adjustment
   c. should be checked daily for proper calibration
3. QC procedures on control samples should be performed:
   a. exactly as procedures are performed on patient specimens
   b. on every other urine specimen tested
   c. only by a licensed health care professional trained to interpret the results
4. Urine control samples:
   a. have no special storage requirements
   b. are purchased commercially from manufacturers
   c. are used to obtain baseline urinalysis results from healthy patients
5. Documentation of QC testing:
   a. must be recorded in a daily urinalysis QC log and kept for at least 3 years
   b. is not necessary unless the equipment is malfunctioning
   c. should be recorded in the patient's medical record

Short Answer

1. After passing through a healthy kidney, urine composition is approximately _____ perrcent water and _____ percent dissolved substances, which generally come from dietary intake or metabolic waste products.
2. Identify each substance below as a normal (N) or an abnormal (AB) substance found in urine.

Urobilinogen ______

Potassium ______

Uric acid ______

White blood cells ______

Fat ______

1+ Protein ______

Blood ______

Creatinine ______

Chloride ______

3. When handling urine specimens, Standard Precautions must be followed to ensure that proper infection control standards are observed. In the spaces provided below, list five precautions used when handling urine specimens.

4. List seven regulations of the Clinical Laboratory Improvement Act (CLIA) that apply to the clinical medical assistant performing urine testing.

5. Name the four types of urine specimens frequently ordered by providers.

6. Name the two methods of urine collection.

7. What are the four steps in a physical examination of a urine specimen?

8. What does the specific gravity of urine indicate?

9. Name three methods of measuring the specific gravity of a urine specimen and state the advantages and disadvantages of each. Indicate the method that is available in conjunction with chemical testing.

10. How should reagent test strips be handled and stored?

____

____

____

____

____

____

11. Crystals are the most insignificant part of urinary sediment and are not usually an important element of microscopic analysis, though many laboratories do report them. However, a few crystals may indicate disease states; name three.

____

____

12. Casts are formed when protein accumulates and precipitates in the kidney tubules and are then washed into the urine. Identify each cast below and draw an example in the square provided.

Description	**Cast Name**	**Drawing**
These casts contain remnants of disintegrated cells that have a fine or coarse appearance.	____________	
These casts contain leukocytes, erythrocytes, or skin cells.	____________	
These casts are difficult to see under the microscope without some light adjustment because of their near transparency.	____________	

13. In the squares below, draw an example of the sediment as seen under a microscope.

Drawing	**Sediment**
	Spermatoza, cotton fibers, and starch granules
	Yeast
	Squamous epithelial cells
	Bacteria

Matching I

Reagent test strips, or dipsticks, are used to test urine for many metabolic processes, including kidney and liver functions, urinary tract infection, and pH balance. Match each test below to the information that best describes it.

____ 1. Glucose

____ 2. pH

____ 3. Urobilinogen

____ 4. Blood

____ 5. Nitrites

____ 6. Leukocyte esterase

____ 7. Specific gravity

____ 8. Ketones

____ 9. Protein

____ 10. Bilirubin

A. These occur during prolonged fasting. They appear when excessive amounts of fatty acids are broken down into simpler compounds and when glucose availability is limited.

B. Increased levels of this substance suggest liver disease or bleeding disorders. It is a degradation product of bilirubin formed by intestinal bacteria.

C. This substance in a urine sample indicates infection, urinary tract trauma, kidney bleeding, and menses.

D. This substance can increase during a high fever and also indicates injury to the kidney, specifically to the glomerular membrane.

E. This test indicates white blood cells in the urinary tract, presumably attracted by invading bacteria.

F. This test detects unsuspected diabetes or is used to check the efficiency of insulin therapy in patients with diabetes.

G. This test changes color, depending on the ion concentration in urine. The highest reading available on the test is 1.030.

H. This test has a range of 4.6 to 8.0 and measures the acidity or alkalinity of the urine. A reading less than 7.0 indicates increased acidity; greater than 7.0 indicates increased alkalinity.

I. The presence of this substance indicates a urinary tract infection, because it is normally absent from urine. It is formed from the conversion of nitrates by certain species of bacteria.

J. This substance, a product of the breakdown of hemoglobin, breaks down in the light; a urine sample should be protected from light during testing.

Matching II

Microscopic examination of urine sediment is also a valuable diagnostic tool for providers. Match each type of sediment listed to the statement that best describes it.

A. White blood cells
B. Yeast
C. Squamous epithelial cells
D. Renal epithelial cells
E. Bacteria
F. Artifacts
G. Red blood cells
H. Parasite
I. Sperm

____ 1. Hair, fiber, air bubbles, and oil are common examples.

____ 2. These skin cells are not medically significant and are sloughed off continuously in urine.

____ 3. *Trichomonas vaginalis* is the most common example.

____ 4. Cocci, bacilli, and spirilla

____ 5. These non-nucleated cells appear as pale, light-refractive disks; they are counted in a microscopic field and reported as cells per high-power field (HPF)

____ 6. These cells are larger than erythrocytes, have a visible nucleus, and may appear granular; they are reported as cells per HPF.

____ 7. These are reported when seen in urine, although they do not necessarily indicate a disorder.

____ 8. *Candida albicans* is the most common example.

____ 9. These cells can indicate kidney disease if present in large numbers and are easily confused with other surface cells. If suspected, the slide should be reviewed by the provider. They are reported as cells per HPF.

CERTIFICATION REVIEW

These questions are designed to mimic the certification examination. Select the best response.

1. The filtering unit of the kidney is called the:

   a. meatus

   b. glomerulus

   c. ureter

   d. urethra

2. A common medication used to treat bladder infections and that turns the urine bright orange is:

   a. Pyridium®

   b. Zestoretic®

   c. propranolol

   d. Neurontin

3. The urine of a diabetic patient with ketoacidosis may smell:

   a. musty

   b. sour

   c. putrid

   d. sweet

4. The curvature that appears in a liquid's upper surface when placed in a container is the:

   a. specific gravity

   b. urobilinogen

   c. meniscus

   d. buffy coat

5. The most common type of cast seen in urine sediment is:

   a. hyaline

   b. granular

   c. waxy

   d. cellular

LEARNING APPLICATION

Labeling Activity

1. One of the most important steps in the collection of urine specimens is to correctly identify the specimen through proper labeling. Make up your own identification number, using Dr. Mark Woo as your provider, and write out complete labeling information for a specimen of your own urine below.

2. What is the proper procedure for testing an unlabeled or incorrectly labeled specimen?

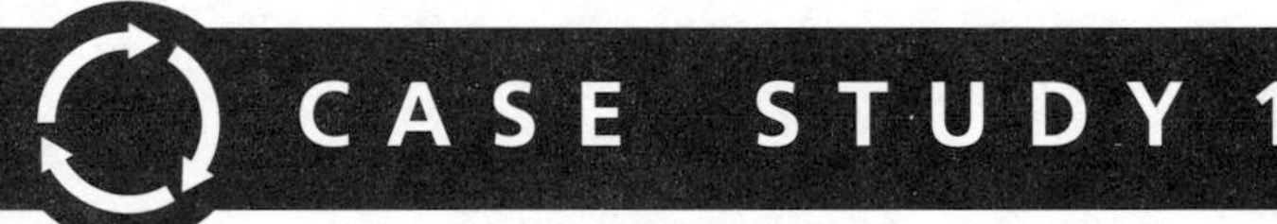

CASE STUDY 1

At Inner City Health Care, Wanda Slawson, CMA (AAMA), gives patient Wendy Janus written directions for a 24-hour urine collection to be performed at home, but Wendy misplaces them. Wanda must give directions to Wendy over the telephone.

CASE STUDY REVIEW QUESTIONS

1. What directions should be given to the patient to correctly perform the urine collection?

continues

2. What communication techniques should Wendy use to make sure the patient understands the collection procedures? What other potential alternatives for communicating the information, besides the telephone, are available?

CASE STUDY 2

Wanda Slawson, CMA (AAMA), is asked to give a male adolescent patient the proper procedure for a clean-catch specimen. The 15-year-old boy is visibly embarrassed and will not hold eye contact with Wanda as she relates the instructions for collection to him.

CASE STUDY REVIEW QUESTIONS

1. What instructions are relevant for a clean-catch specimen for this patient?

2. What communication techniques should Wanda use when working with this patient?

CHAPTER POST-TEST

Perform this test without looking at your book. If an answer is "false," rewrite the sentence to make it true.

1. Which part of the urinalysis is to be performed by the medical assistant?

   a. The chemical examination

   b. The physical examination

   c. The specific gravity

   d. All of the above

2. Fat lipolysis is indicated by what in the urine?

   a. Sugar

   b. Bacteria

   c. Protein

   d. Ketones

3. If the patient brought a urine sample in a mayonnaise jar from home, you would:

   a. provide the patient with an appropriate container and ask for a fresh sample

   b. politely accept it this time, but after this, you will give the patient a proper container

   c. accept it if it is a first morning voided specimen for pregnancy testing and the container is clean

   d. a. and c.

4. The most common urine specimen type in the POL is the:

   a. clean-catch, midstream specimen collection

   b. random collection

   c. timed specimen

   d. a. and b.

5. The written patient instructions for a midstream, clean catch should be:

   a. posted in the restroom beside the toilet

   b. posted in the restroom above the sink

   c. posted in the restroom behind the door

   d. handed to the patient as he or she enters

6. True or False? The minimum amount of urine needed for a complete urinalysis is 20 mL.

   ____

   ____

7. Pyridium, a bladder analgesic, can:

   a. turn the urine a bright orange to red and may stain clothes

   b. decrease urine flow

   c. calm bladder irritation

   d. a. and c.

SELF-ASSESSMENT

1. Have you ever had a urinalysis performed?

2. Were you ever given proper instructions? If not, why do you think you were not instructed properly. If you were, did you understand clearly what you were to do?

3. Were instructions clearly written and posted in the restroom at a location that was readable during the collection?

4. Do you think that good patient preparation and instructions influence the result of the test performed? In what way?

5. Now that you know the importance of proper patient teaching, how will your experience and training influence your work as a medical assistant in other areas of patient education?

CERTIFICATION REVIEW

These questions are designed to mimic the certification examination. Select the best response.

1. Common nosocomial infections are caused by:
   a. salmonella
   b. *Staphylococcus*
   c. *Shigella*
   d. *Protista*
2. Some bacteria produce ____________, which are so resistant that they can live 150,000 years.
   a. flagella
   b. cell walls
   c. nuclei
   d. spores
3. Septicemia is a:
   a. blood infection
   b. throat infection
   c. urinary tract infection
   d. respiratory infection
4. Bacilli are:
   a. rod shaped
   b. round
   c. spiral shaped
   d. found in clusters
5. Gram-negative bacteria stain:
   a. purple
   b. pink
   c. red
   d. green

LEARNING APPLICATION

Research Activity

Make a list of all the things that are done to keep your food and environment free of pathogens. This would include water purification, food processing, homogenization, use of antibacterial soap and cleansers, immunizations, and any other process you can think of.

1. After each item on the list, place a check mark by those that are available only to certain populations but not to underdeveloped countries and areas.

2. Discuss with fellow students which of the things on your lists could be implemented fairly simply and inexpensively.

3. Reorganize the lists starting with the easiest to implement and going toward the most expensive/difficult.

4. List other items or processes that would need to be done to implement each item on your list.

CASE STUDY

Winston Lewis, M.D., has ordered a series of three sputum cultures for Herb Fowler, who has been suffering with a productive cough for several months and extreme fatigue. Audrey Jones, CMA (AAMA), is assigned to obtain the cultures. When each culture is obtained from Mr. Fowler, Audrey brings it to the POL for culturing.

CASE STUDY REVIEW QUESTIONS

1. What is the procedure for obtaining a sputum specimen? Why are detailed patient instructions critical?

2. Mr. Fowler wishes to give all three specimens in one day to save on the transportation to and from the provider's office. Audrey explains that the specimens must be obtained one each day, on awakening, for three days. What is the reason for this?

3. What microorganisms might the provider suspect, and how should the specimen be treated in the POL? Under what circumstances should the specimen be sent to an outside reference laboratory for further testing?

CHAPTER POST-TEST

Perform this test without looking at your book. If an answer is "false," rewrite the sentence to make it true.

1. The field of microbiology includes:
   a. bacteria, fungi, vectors, and parasites
   b. mice, their parasites, and bacteria
   c. fungi, bacteria, viruses, and other microbes
   d. parasites, fungi, viruses, bacteria, and vectors
2. True or False? Many bacteria are normal in our bodies.

   ____

   ____

3. Media is:
   a. the laboratory chemical that is used in testing
   b. the microscopic slide that is smeared with a specimen
   c. a sample of body secretions that contains harmful pathogens
   d. a nutritional mixture specifically created for a particular type of bacteria
4. True or False? Mycology is the study of fungi.

   ____

   ____

5. True or False? An incubator is part of the medical assistant's protective equipment.

   ____

   ____

6. True or False? Anaerobic organisms grow well in the presence of oxygen.

   ____

   ____

7. Appropriate handling of specimens includes:
   a. wearing PPE
   b. wearing gloves
   c. washing hands often
   d. all of the above
8. True or False? Microbial waste should not be thrown out with the regular waste.

   ____

   ____

9. Which of the following is not an important quality control measure?
   a. OSHA manuals have to be updated periodically.
   b. Check the refrigerator temperatures daily.
   c. Culture media should be checked for accuracy with positive and negative controls.
   d. Respect the expiration date of testing materials.

10. True or False? The Rapid Strep Test is popular because it is easy to read and is available in minutes, but it does often result in false positives.

SELF-ASSESSMENT

Describe how you feel about working with patients who have infections that are possibly communicable. What, if anything, concerns you? What resources do you have in addressing your concerns?

Name ______________________ Date ____________ Score ______

CHAPTER 32

Specialty Laboratory Tests

CHAPTER PRE-TEST

Perform this test without looking at your book. If an answer is "false," rewrite the sentence to make it true.

1. How many different blood types are there?
   a. 3
   b. 5
   c. 4
   d. 8
2. True or False? The phenylketonuria (PKU) test is mandatory for all infants in all states.

   ____

   ____

3. True or False? During pregnancy, human chorionic gonadotropin (hCG) levels peak at 8 weeks.

   ____

   ____

4. True or False? About 15 percent of the general population is Rh negative.

   ____

   ____

5. True or False? The Rh system was named for the rhesus monkeys used in the experiments that led to the discovery of an Rh factor.

   ____

   ____

6. True or False? Insulin helps regulate glucose levels in the blood.

   ____

   ____

7. True or False? A purified protein derivative (PPD) is administered with an intradermal injection.

   ____

   ____

8. True or False? The urine hCG test is more accurate than the blood enzyme immunoassay.

____

____

VOCABULARY BUILDER

Find the words listed below that are misspelled; circle them, and correctly spell them in the spaces provided. Then insert the following correct vocabulary terms into the sentences that follow.

ABO blood group	Epstein-Barr virus	infectious mononucleosis
agglutinition	eptopic	insulin
antibody	Guthrie screening test	latex beads
antigen	hemolytic anemia	low-density lipoprotein
antiserum	heterophile antibodies	Mantous test
billirubin	high-density lipoprotein	phenylketonuria (PKU)
blood urea nitrogen	human chorionic gonadotropin (hCG)	purified protein derivative (PPD)
cholesterol	hydatidiform	Rh factor
choriocarcinoma	hyperglycemia	semen
Cushing's syndrome	hypoglycemia	triglyceride
diabetes melitis	immunoessay	tuberculosis

________________ ________________ ________________

________________ ________________ ________________

1. Although PPD is used to test for ________________, it is called the Mantoux test after the physician who developed it.

2. When a patient's glucose levels test high, Audrey Jones, CMA (AAMA), knows it could be an indication of diabetes mellitus. She understands, however, that the high glucose levels could also be a sign of ________ ________________, a hormonal disorder caused by an excess of corticosteroid hormones secreted by the adrenal glands, or a sign of acute stress response. A glucose tolerance test should be performed.

3. When Mary O'Keefe's enzyme ________________ test is positive, Ellen Armstrong, CMA (AAMA), assumes that this positive reaction indicates a normal pregnancy. However, detection of hCG, ________________, can also indicate abnormal conditions such as an ________________ pregnancy; a developing ________________ mole of the uterus; or ________________, a rare malignant neoplasm, usually of the uterus.

4. When Ellen Armstrong, CMA (AAMA), performs a test for pregnancy using a slide test, she makes sure that after she adds hCG ________________ (which is an antibody to hCG) to the urine on a microscope slide, she then adds an ________________ reagent containing ________________ coated with hCG to the mixture.

5. Bruce Goldman, CMA (AAMA), commonly performs tests for blood glucose levels at Inner City Health Care. The results are used to screen for carbohydrate disorders such as ________________, in which a patient has a low blood glucose level.

6. Joe Guerrero, CMA (AAMA), performs a slide test for pregnancy, remembering that negative ________________ indicates positive pregnancy.

7. When renal disease is suspected, a physician will order, as one of several tests, a BUN, or ________________ ________________, test, which measures the concentration of urea in the blood.

8. Abigail Johnson has been diagnosed with ______________________, which is a type of carbohydrate disorder usually characterized by a deficiency of ______________________, a hormone secreted by the pancreas.

9. High levels of ______________________, the "bad" cholesterol, are associated with an increased risk for coronary artery disease. Cholesterol bound to ______________________, the "good" cholesterol, is transported to the liver, where it is excreted in the form of bile.

10. To determine the severity of ______________________, the quantity of bilirubin in the amniotic fluid of pregnant women is evaluated.

11. Serum ______________________ concentration will increase moderately after ingesting a meal containing fat, peaking 4 to 5 hours later.

12. When a ______________________ sample is required of a male patient for analysis, Wanda Slawson, CMA (AAMA), instructs patients to avoid ejaculation for 3 days before collection of the sample.

13. Liz Corbin performs a ______________________ on Lenny Taylor's arm, raising a wheal where 0.1 mL PPD was administered properly with an intradermal injection.

14. Bruce Goldman, CMA (AAMA), explains to Corey Boyer that his case of IM, ______________________, is a result of infection of the lymphocytes by the ______________________. Dr. Whitney confirmed the diagnosis from hematologic and clinical findings combined with the detection of ______________________.

15. Nora Fowler was born with ______________________, an inherited condition in which the amino acid phenylalanine is not metabolized.

16. To evaluate a newborn for PKU, Audrey Jones, CMA (AAMA), uses the ______________________ to evaluate the baby's blood.

17. The symptoms of ______________________ are similar to those of diabetes mellitus: excessive thirst; passing large amounts of urine; glycosuria, high levels of glucose in the urine; and ketosis, high levels of ketones.

18. Patients exhibiting a positive or questionable ______________________ reaction should have a chest X-ray to examine for tubercules, and a sputum sample should be stained to search for acid-fast rods. The presence of tubercules and acid-fast rods confirms active tuberculosis.

19. Two categories of blood typing are for the ______________________ and the ______________________.

LEARNING REVIEW

Short Answer

1. Name three reasons for performing a semen analysis on a male patient.

____

____

____

____

2. When a semen analysis is performed as part of a fertility workup, seminal fluid is analyzed to determine what four factors?

____

____

____

3. Name the four blood group categories.

____

____

4. Fill in the missing information in the chart below.

Blood Group/Type	Antigen on RBC	Serum Antibodies
AB	________	________
________	B	________
________	________	No anti-D

5. How can most cases of hemolytic disease of the newborn (HDN) be prevented?

____

____

____

6. To ensure an accurate reading, what precautions should be taken when performing a pregnancy test?

____

____

____

7. Describe the cholesterol molecule.

____

____

____

8. Explain the difference between saturated, monounsaturated, and polyunsaturated fats and give an example of each.

____

____

____

____

____

9. Describe the function of cholesterol.

____

____

____

Fill in the Blanks

Fill in the blanks with the correct term.

1. The Rh type of most North Americans is ____________________.
2. Glucose is the principal carbohydrate found circulating in the ____________________.
3. In glucose analyzers based on ____________________, the glucose in the sample reacts with the reagents in the pad, causing a color to develop.
4. Excess glucose is converted into ____________________ for short-term storage in the liver and muscle cells.

5. The blood glucose level of ______________________________ patients usually peaks 30 to 60 minutes after consumption of the glucose test solution, leading to a level of 160 to 180 mg/dL, and then returns to the fasting level after 2 to 3 hours.

6. A patient should be instructed to eat a diet high in ________________________________ for 3 days before the glucose tolerance test.

7. To determine whether diabetic patients are consistently adhering to their diets, providers can administer the ____.

CERTIFICATION REVIEW

These questions are designed to mimic the certification examination. Select the best response.

1. Antigens present or absent on the surface of the red blood cell (RBC) are used to determine blood types. These are ____________ molecules.

   a. carbohydrate

   b. protein

   c. fat

   d. electrolyte

2. A potentially life-threatening situation during incompatible blood transfusion is called:

   a. Epstein-Barr

   b. intravascular hemolysis

   c. hydatidiform mole

   d. phenylketonuria

3. Men with oligospermia should be evaluated for which type of disorder?

   a. Pancreatic

   b. Liver

   c. Thyroid

   d. Kidney

4. A negative reaction to a Mantoux test would include an induration of:

   a. 10 mm or more

   b. 5–9 mm

   c. 12–15 mm

   d. less than 5 mm

5. Postprandial refers to:

   a. after eating

   b. after medication

   c. after sleeping

   d. after urinating

6. Insulin is secreted by which organ?

   a. Liver

   b. Spleen

   c. Kidney

   d. Pancreas

7. When performing the Mantoux test, what size needle would you choose?

   a. 25 gauge, ½ inch

   b. 26 gauge, ⅜ inch

   c. 27–28 gauge, ½ inch

   d. 29–30 gauge, ⅜ inch

8. Which of the following factors can alter the results of semen analysis?

   a. Eating foods containing garlic

   b. Smoking cigarettes

   c. Riding a bicycle on the day of the analysis

   d. Drinking milk

9. The wheal produced on a patient's arm in response to a Mantoux test is positive for a past or present infection of *Mycobacterium* tuberculosis if it is:

   a. almost invisible

   b. 15 mm or more of induration

   c. 10 mm or more of induration

   d. exactly 2 mm of induration

LEARNING APPLICATION

Research Activities

1. Do an Internet investigation to see if your state requires PKU testing on newborns.

   A. If not, why do you think it is not required? Is the test recommended? How much does it cost? What can you do to change the law?

   B. If your state does require it, are parents allowed to refuse? Why would a parent refuse?

   C. Role-play with another student: How would you react if a parent refused?

2. Look at Table 32-4 in your textbook (Values for Cholesterol, HDL, LDL, and Triglycerides). What are the normal ranges of each for your gender?

   ____

   ____

CASE STUDY

Mary Alexander is an established patient of Dr. Esposito's at Inner City Health Care. Mary, 32 years old, is about 10 pounds overweight for her height. Mary has been diagnosed with type 1 insulin-dependent diabetes mellitus since childhood. Dr. Esposito's treatment plan includes administration of 30 units of U-100 NPH insulin by injection every day. Dr. Esposito knows that Mary has trouble complying with the dietary restrictions included in her treatment plan and in observing regular mealtimes. Every now and then, the lifetime rigor of the diet wears Mary down and she begins to eat whatever she likes, whenever she feels like it. To guard against this, Mary must report her average glucose levels to Bruce Goldman, CMA (AAMA), twice monthly as a safeguard. At her next regular follow-up examination with Dr. Esposito, the physician orders a glycosated hemoglobin determination and discovers that Mary has been cheating on her diet again and has been reporting inaccurate glucose levels to the physician's office, hoping she would not get caught.

CASE STUDY REVIEW QUESTIONS

1. How is Dr. Esposito able to tell from the glycosated hemoglobin determination that Mary is not adhering to her diet and health guidelines?

____

____

____

____

____

____

2. What is glycosated hemoglobin?

____

____

____

3. What is the role of the medical assistant in this situation?

____

____

____

____

____

____

____

____

____

____

____

CHAPTER POST-TEST

Perform this test without looking at your book. If an answer is "false," rewrite the sentence to make it true.

1. What are the different blood types?
   a. A, B, O, and AB
   b. B, O, A, and OB
   c. A, B, C, and O
   d. O, B, A, and AC
2. True or False? The PKU test is not mandatory for all infants in all states.

3. True or False? During pregnancy, hCG levels peak at 22 weeks.

4. True or False? About 85 percent of the general population is Rh negative.

5. True or False? The Rh system was named for the rhesus rats used in the experiments that led to the discovery of an Rh factor.

6. True or False? Insulin helps regulate glucose levels in the urine.

7. True or False? A PPD is administered with a subcutaneous injection.

8. True or False? The urine hCG test is more accurate than the blood enzyme immunoassay.

SELF-ASSESSMENT

1. Do you think all states should require PKU testing on all newborns? List three advantages and three disadvantages of each.

Name ____________ Date ____________ Score ______

CHAPTER 33

The Medical Assistant as Office Manager

CHAPTER PRE-TEST

Perform this test without looking at your book. If an answer is "false," rewrite the sentence to make it true.

1. True or False? Teamwork results in getting more accomplished with the resources available.

2. True or False? Office managers do not need effective communication skills.

3. True or False? It is not necessary to update the office procedures manual.

4. True or False? Minutes should be sent only to the team members who attended the meeting.

5. True or False? When working with an externing student, each step should be explained together with the rationale.

6. True or False? Office managers need to be able to accept and offer criticism constructively.

7. True or False? The office manager will always serve as the human resources director.

VOCABULARY BUILDER

Misspelled Words

Find the words listed below that are misspelled; circle them, and correctly spell them in the spaces provided. Then insert the correct vocabulary terms beside the sentences that follow.

agenda
ancilliary services
benchmarking
benefits
bond
embezzel
externs
"going bare"
itinerary
liability
marketing
minutes
negligance
practicum
procedures manual
professional liability insurance
risk management
teamwork
work statement

____________________ ____________________ ____________________

____________________ 1. Professional occupational companies hired to complete a specific job such as janitorial services, laundry, or disposal of hazardous materials

____________________ 2. The situation of a provider who does not carry insurance to protect the provider's assets in the event of a liability claim

____________________ 3. Making a comparison between different organizations relative to how they accomplish tasks, remunerate employees, and so on

____________________ 4. Designed to protect assets in the event a liability claim is filed and awarded

____________________ 5. A written record of topics discussed and actions taken during meeting sessions

____________________ 6. This provides a concise description of the work you plan to accomplish

____________________ 7. A binding agreement with an employee ensuring recovery of financial loss should funds be stolen or embezzled

____________________ 8. A printed list of topics to be discussed during a meeting

____________________ 9. The process by which the provider of services makes the consumer aware of the scope and quality of those services. Examples might include public relations, brochures, patient education seminars, and newsletters.

____________________ 10. Involves persons synergistically working together

____________________ 11. A transitional stage providing an opportunity to apply theory learned in the classroom to a health care setting through practical, hands-on experience

____________________ 12. Remuneration that is in addition to a salary

____________________ 13. To appropriate fraudulently for one's own use

____________________ 14. Involves the identification, analysis, and treatment of risks within the medical office or facility

______________ 15. Performing an act that a reasonable and prudent provider would not perform.

______________ 16. Provides detailed information relative to the performance of tasks within the facility in which one is employed

______________ 17. A detailed plan for a proposed trip

LEARNING REVIEW

Short Answer

1. The office manager of a medical office or ambulatory care facility can have many varied responsibilities based on individual facility needs. What are five duties that are the responsibility of the office manager in a health care setting?

2. What are five attributes needed to perform as a quality manager in any office setting?

3. What is the difference between authoritarian and participatory management styles?

4. What does "management by walking around" mean, and why would it be useful in a medical office setting?

5. The table below discusses some of the common risks for medical offices, as well as risk control measures for each one. Fill in any missing information.

Risk	**Risk Control Measures**
______________________	Train various employees to assume other duties and perform them when an employee is ill, on vacation, etc.
Failure of a supplier or contractor	______________________
______________________	Have protocols in place for handling this situation and make patients aware of the protocols; notify patients immediately if confidential information is disclosed and work with them toward resolution.
Computer failure	______________________
______________________	Continually review safety procedures; conduct safety surveys; always carry liability insurance; complete an Incident Report to signal risk manager to implement existing protocols to minimize risk

6. Define harassment in the workplace.

____

7. List the steps that a manager should take if he or she is made aware of harassment in the medical office.

____

8. Why do some employers put new employees on probation? What is the usual length of an employee's probationary period?

____

Ordering Activity

All administrative and clinical supplies and equipment in the facility must be inventoried. The following tasks are performed when new supplies and/or equipment are received. Put the tasks steps in the correct order, from 1 to 5.

____ A. Unpack each item, checking against the packing slip.

____ B. Write the date the shipment was received and who verified it.

____ C. Stock each item appropriately.

____ D. Verify that no items have been substituted or backordered.

____ E. Find the packing slip listing the items ordered.

Matching

Most marketing tools used in a medical environment provide educational and office services information to patients, potential patients, and the local community. Match the following marketing tools with their potential use in the ambulatory care facility setting.

A. Seminars
B. Brochures
C. Newsletters
D. Press releases
E. Special events

____ 1. These are used for announcing new equipment, new staff, expanded or remodeled office space, and so on.

____ 2. These typically come in two types—patient education and office services—and present a professional image of the ambulatory care setting.

____ 3. These provide an effective way to join with other community organizations to promote wellness.

____ 4. These can educate patients and provide goodwill in the community. All facility staff can work as a team to organize these.

____ 5. These can include a wide range of information from health-related topics to staff introductions to insurance updates. They may form the nucleus of a marketing program.

CERTIFICATION REVIEW

These questions are designed to mimic the certification examination. Select the best response.

1. There is a direct correlation between a person's management style and his or her:
   a. technical expertise
   b. educational level
   c. personality
   d. salary
2. Most conflicts occur between employees and supervisors or providers because of:
   a. attitude
   b. poor communication
   c. a misunderstanding
   d. b. and c.

3. The person who applies the team-oriented management style is often comfortable with:
   a. teaching and coaching
   b. building, constructing, and modeling
   c. ideas, information, and data
   d. all of the above
4. A comprehensive safety program is essential to:
   a. marketing functions
   b. team building
   c. risk management
   d. equipment and supply maintenance
5. Leadership for the twenty-first century includes components of flexibility, mentoring, and:
   a. networking
   b. domination
   c. hierarchy
   d. rigidity
6. A rule that defines almost all of the ethical qualities of a manager is:
   a. Murphy's law
   b. the Rule of Nines
   c. the Golden Rule
   d. none of the above
7. The ______ management style is based on the premise that the worker is capable and wants to do a good job.
   a. walking around
   b. participatory
   c. risk
   d. authoritarian
8. The most significant task(s) of the team leader or office manager is (are):
   a. getting the team members to understand and support the specifics of the problem they are asked to solve
   b. enabling the team to develop their own work statement where they will assume ownership of the goals and objectives
   c. establishing a timetable for achieving results and identifying the standards that must be maintained
   d. all of the above
9. The documentation of policies and procedures that make up the office HIPAA manual should be:
   a. filed in a locked cabinet
   b. kept for six years, even though wording has been changed or has been eliminated
   c. made available for all employees
   d. b. and c.

10. If malpractice litigation should occur, the best protocol to follow is to:
    a. be honest with the patients and insurance carriers
    b. let the HR person handle the situation
    c. notify the provider
    d. not get involved

LEARNING APPLICATION

Time Management Activity

To practice your time management skills, make a to-do list for tomorrow or the upcoming weekend. Prioritize the list by importance.

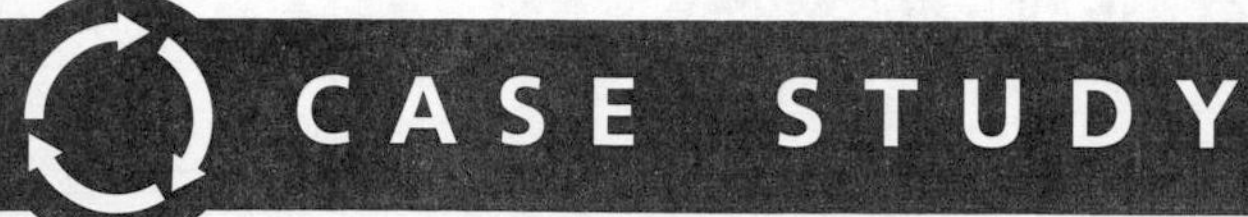

CASE STUDY

Office manager Shirley Brooks is responsible for the preparation and distribution of payroll checks at the offices of Drs. Lewis and King. Because the group practice is in the process of upgrading the computer system to accommodate a recent influx of new patients, Shirley is temporarily preparing the payroll using the manual write-it-once bookkeeping system. She is careful to consult payroll records for each employee, which include the employee's name, address, telephone number, and Social Security number; number of exemptions claimed on the W-4 form; gross salary; deductions withheld for all taxes, including Social Security, federal, state, local unemployment and disability; and date of employment.

CASE STUDY REVIEW QUESTIONS

1. As Shirley writes out the payroll check for Audrey Jones, CMA (AAMA), what information should be included on the paycheck stub?

2. What must the provider's office have to process payroll?

3. What responsibility does the office manager have with regard to the confidentiality of payroll records? How might employees' rights to privacy be maintained?

CHAPTER POST-TEST

Perform this test without looking at your book. If an answer is "false," rewrite the sentence to make it true.

1. True or False? Teamwork results in getting less accomplished with the resources available.

2. True or False? Office managers need effective communication skills.

3. True or False? It is necessary to update the office procedures manual.

4. True or False? Minutes should be sent to all team members, not just those who attended the meeting.

5. True or False? When working with externing students, each step does not need to be explained together with the rationale, because they already have training.

6. True or False? Office managers need to be able to offer criticism constructively, but they should not have to accept criticism.

7. True or False? The person who is the office manager is never the human resources director.

SELF-ASSESSMENT

Put yourself in the place of the office manager.

1. What type of management style do you think you are the most comfortable with?

2. Carefully read about each type of style and explain why you think you are that type.

____

____

____

____

3. What skills will come naturally to you?

____

____

____

____

4. What skills will you have to work on the most?

____

____

____

____

Name ______________________ Date ____________ Score ______

CHAPTER **34**

The Medical Assistant as Human Resources Manager

CHAPTER PRE-TEST

Perform this test without looking at your book. If an answer is "false," rewrite the sentence to make it true.

1. Which of the following is *not* a function of the human resources (HR) manager?
   a. Creating and updating a policy manual
   b. Recruiting and hiring office personnel
   c. Orienting new personnel
   d. Training new personnel
2. True or False? Wage and salary policies should be in writing.

   ____

   ____

3. True or False? A policy manual should contain daily step-by-step instructions.

   ____

   ____

4. True or False? Job descriptions are not always useful because they change so often.

   ____

   ____

5. True or False? All job applicants should be interviewed.

   ____

   ____

6. True or False? It is acceptable to ask job applicants about the last place they worked and a conflict they had there.

   ____

   ____

7. True or False? References are usually checked after the first interview.

____

____

8. True or False? The HR manager is responsible for dismissing employees.

____

____

9. True or False? Employees have a right to review their personnel files at any time.

____

____

10. True or False? Employers have the right to refuse to allow full-time employees to go on jury duty.

____

____

VOCABULARY BUILDER

Misspelled Words

Find the words listed below that are misspelled; circle them, and correctly spell them in the spaces provided. Then, insert the correct vocabulary terms into the following sentences.

exit interveiw	letter of referance	overtime
involuntary dismisal	letter of resignation	probation
job desciption	menter	résumés

_______________ _______________ _______________

_______________ _______________

1. Because of an unexpected staffing shortfall, Audrey Jones, CMA (AAMA), has volunteered to work _______________ this week. She will receive 1½ times the regular rate of pay for hours above her regular 40-hour week.
2. An _______________ has been scheduled for administrative/clinical medical assistant Liz Corbin before she leaves the clinic to continue her education. This session will give Liz an opportunity to provide her positive and negative opinions of the position and the facility.
3. Office manager Marilyn Johnson has received a _______________ from the former instructor of a current job applicant describing the applicant's performance, attitude, and qualifications.
4. The violation of office policies at Inner City Health Care led to the _______________ of one of the part-time employees.
5. Liz Corbin, CMA (AAMA), submitted a _______________ to her current employer when she decided to leave her present position to return to school to pursue an advanced degree.
6. Office manager Marilyn Johnson will inform all of the job applicants that they will be on _______________ for their first three months on the job. During this period, the employee and supervisory personnel can determine if the environment and the position are satisfactory for the employee.
7. Office manager Jane O'Hara, updating the employee manual, includes a _______________ for every position in the office, which details tasks, duties, and responsibilities.
8. Administrative medical assistant Ellen Armstrong looks upon office manager Marilyn Johnson as her _______________, since Marilyn has been instrumental in Ellen's training, coaching, and guidance in her newly acquired position.

LEARNING REVIEW

Short Answer

1. The manual that identifies clear guidelines and directions required of all employees is known as the policy manual. What are four topics that would be included in a policy manual regardless of the size of the practice identified in this chapter?

___

___

___

2. Office manager Marilyn Johnson has the responsibility of dismissing an employee for a serious violation of office policies. From the list below, select key points to keep in mind when dismissal is necessary by circling the letters of the statements that apply.

a. Have employee pack his or her belongings from desk.

b. The dismissal should be made in private.

c. Take no longer than 20 minutes for the dismissal.

d. Be direct, firm, and to the point in identifying reasons.

e. Explain terms of dismissal (keys, clearing out area, final paperwork).

f. Do not listen to the employee's opinion and emotions.

g. If he or she insists, allow the employee to finish the work of the day.

h. Do not engage in an in-depth discussion of performance.

3. Compare and contrast voluntary and involuntary separation.

___

___

___

___

___

___

4. The job description must have enough information to provide both the supervisor and the employee with a clear outline of what the job entails. Name four items that must be included in a job description.

___

___

___

5. The interview worksheet is an excellent tool to make certain that the interviews with each candidate are fair and equitable. Provide six items that should be included on any interview worksheet.

___

___

___

___

___

CERTIFICATION REVIEW

These questions are designed to mimic the certification examination. Select the best response.

1. A salary review is:
   a. usually conducted at the beginning of the new year
   b. virtually the same as the performance review
   c. conducted on the anniversary date of hire
   d. normally done every three years
2. Questions regarding drug use, arrest records, and medical history during an interview are:
   a. appropriate
   b. inappropriate
   c. illegal
   d. none of the above
3. Title VII of the Civil Rights Act addresses:
   a. overtime pay
   b. discrimination based on race, age, and sex
   c. hiring and firing practices
   d. sexual harassment
4. When a candidate accepts a position, the HR manager should write a letter outlining the specifics of the job. This letter is called a:
   a. confirmation letter
   b. congratulatory letter
   c. recommendation letter
   d. reference letter
5. A person with AIDS who satisfies the necessary skills for a job and has the experience and education required will be protected from discrimination by:
   a. OSHA
   b. CLIA
   c. AAMA
   d. ADA
6. A job description should be reviewed and updated:
   a. every 2 years
   b. every 90 days
   c. every year
   d. every 5 years

7. Voluntary separation usually occurs when:

   a. advancing to another position

   b. there is a violation of office policies

   c. the employee is relocating

   d. a. and c.

8. Verifying that all employees are authorized to work is done by

   a. asking for verbal clarification

   b. having the candidate complete an I-9 form

   c. having the candidate provide a notarized statement

   d. having the candidate fill out an attestation form

9. What documents should be included in the personnel file? *(circle all that apply)*

   a. Application

   b. Formal review

   c. Awards

   d. Employee handbook

10. What act was established to prevent injuries and illnesses resulting from unsafe and unhealthy working conditions?

    a. Americans with Disabilities Act

    b. Civil Rights Act

    c. OSHA

    d. Equal Pay Act

LEARNING APPLICATION

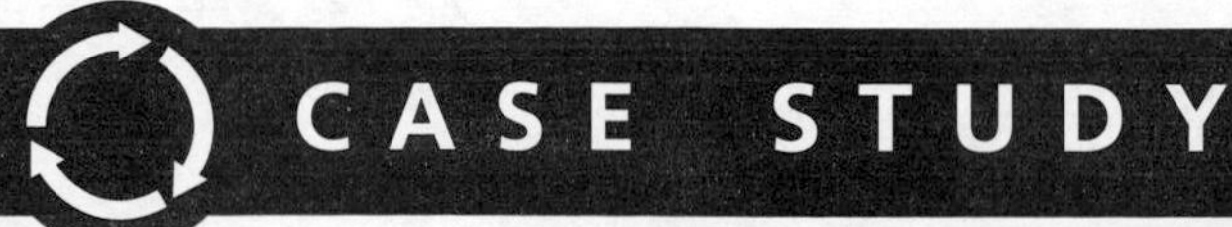

Since the offices of Drs. Lewis and King have expanded to cover a rapidly growing patient load, including the hiring of a co–office manager and a new clinical medical assistant, the work pace has been hectic, but challenging. At the suggestion of Dr. Lewis, the office managers decide to hold a staff meeting to talk about ways to keep the lines of communication open and to process the many changes occurring at the growing medical practice. Marilyn Johnson and Shirley Brooks encourage staff to be vocal with their feedback, suggestions, and concerns.

CASE STUDY REVIEW QUESTIONS

1. What other techniques can the office managers use to prevent or solve conflicts in the workplace during the period of growth and transition?

____

____

____

____

____

____

____

____

____

2. Why is effective communication one of the most important goals of the HR manager?

____

____

____

CHAPTER POST-TEST

Perform this test without looking at your book. If an answer is "false," rewrite the sentence to make it true.

1. Which of the following are functions of the HR manager? *(Circle all that apply)*
   a. Creating and updating a policy manual
   b. Training new personnel
   c. Recruiting and hiring office personnel
   d. Orienting new personnel
2. True or False? Wage and salary policies need not be in writing as long as both parties agree.
   ____
   ____
3. True or False? A policy manual should contain general policies and practices of the office.
   ____
   ____
4. True or False? Job descriptions are always useful and should be clearly written.
   ____
   ____
5. True or False? Only qualified job applicants should be interviewed.
   ____
   ____
6. True or False? It is good to ask job applicants about conflicts they have had and how they solved them.
   ____
   ____
7. True or False? References are usually checked before the first interview.
   ____
   ____
8. True or False? The HR manager is responsible for the exit interview, but usually not for dismissing employees.
   ____
   ____
9. True or False? Employees do not have the right to review their personnel files unless requested by an attorney.
   ____
   ____
10. True or False? Employers cannot condemn or discriminate against a full-time employee who is on jury duty.
    ____
    ____

SELF-ASSESSMENT

1. If you were put into the position of hiring a new employee, what attributes would you be looking for?

   a. Make a list of the technical skills your new employee would need.

   b. Make a list of the affective (behavior) skills your new employee would need, including a positive attitude, a good work ethic, and so forth.

   c. Determine how you could measure the technical skills you listed.

   d. Determine how you could quantify the affective (behavior) skills you listed in item b. above. How could you determine those qualities?

   e. Which is more difficult to measure: technical or behavioral qualities? Which is more difficult to train?

2. When you interview for a job, what technical and behavioral skills on your lists will you need to improve on?

Name ______________________ Date __________ Score ______

CHAPTER **35**

Preparing for Medical Assisting Credentials

CHAPTER PRE-TEST

Perform this test without looking at your book. If an answer is "false," rewrite the sentence to make it true.

1. True or False? A registered medical assistant (RMA) and a certified medical assistant (CMA [AAMA]) have the same bylaws and creed.

____

____

2. True or False? A CMA (AAMA) may work only in the state in which the credentials were received.

____

____

3. True or False? Three major areas included in the RMA examination are clinical, administrative, and general medical knowledge.

____

____

4. True or False? Medical assistants may be trained on the job; however, providers recognize that their offices operate much more efficiently and effectively with professionally trained and formally educated personnel.

____

____

5. True or False? On meeting CMA recertification requirements, the applicant will receive a new certificate.

____

____

6. True or False? Once a student has become a member of AAMA, he or she may stay at the student rate for one year after graduation.

____

____

7. True or False? The National Healthcare Association (NHA) does not offer continuing education programs and does not encourage recertification.

____

____

8. True or False? Retaking the RMA examination is not an option for reinstatement or recertification.

____

____

VOCABULARY BUILDER

Matching

Match each correct vocabulary term to the aspect of the certification process that best describes it.

____ 1. Certification examination

____ 2. Certified medical assistant (CMA [AAMA])

____ 3. Continuing education units (CEUs)

____ 4. Certified clinical medical assistant (CCMA)

____ 5. Recertification

____ 6. Registered medical assistant (RMA)

____ 7. Task Force for Test Construction

A. Method for earning points toward recertification

B. A standardized means of evaluating medical assistant competency

C. Maintaining current CMA (AAMA) status

D. Credential awarded for successfully passing the AAMA certification examination

E. Committee of professionals whose responsibility is to update the CMA (AAMA) examination annually to reflect changes in medical assistants' responsibilities and to include new developments in medical knowledge and technology

F. Credential awarded for successfully passing the AMT examination

G. One of the credentials awarded for passing the National Healthcare Association exam

LEARNING REVIEW

Short Answer

1. The AAMA certification examination is a comprehensive test of the knowledge based on tasks performed in today's medical office. The test is updated annually to include the latest changes in medical assistants' daily responsibilities. In addition, the updates include the latest developments in medical knowledge and technology. Name the three major areas tested in the AAMA certification examination and describe what each includes.

____

____

____

____

____

____

____

____

2. What are the addresses, telephone numbers, and Web sites for obtaining applications for the certification examinations of the AAMA, AMT, and NHA?

AAMA ________________________________

AMT ________________________________

NHA ________________________________

3. To keep their CMA (AAMA) credentials current, how often are individuals required to recertify? How many continuing education units (CEUs) are necessary to recertify?

4. In addition to the RMA credential, what is the credential that the AMT offers for those who primarily want to be employed in the front office of provider offices, clinics, or hospitals?

5. List the criteria an applicant must possess for taking the NHA certification exam.

CERTIFICATION REVIEW

These questions are designed to mimic the certification examination. Select the best response.

1. General medical assisting knowledge on the AMT certification examination includes anatomy and physiology, medical terminology, and:
   a. insurance and billing
   b. medical ethics
   c. bookkeeping and filing
   d. first aid

2. The AMT registration exam consists of:
   a. 300 multiple choice questions
   b. 250 multiple choice questions
   c. 200–210 four-option multiple choice questions
   d. 500 multiple choice questions
3. A total of how many questions are on the CMA (AAMA) certification examination?
   a. 100
   b. 200
   c. 1,000
   d. It varies year to year.
4. How often does an RMA need to recertify?
   a. Every year
   b. Every 6 years
   c. Every 5 years
   d. Every 3 years
5. A total of how many CEUs are required to recertify the CMA (AAMA) credential?
   a. 45
   b. 60
   c. 100
   d. 120
6. When recertifying through the AAMA, a minimum of __________ points is required in each of the three categories. The remaining __________ points may be accumulated in any of the three content areas or from any combination of the three categories.
   a. 15, 60
   b. 20, 40
   c. 10, 30
   d. 30, 60
7. The purpose of certification is that it:
   a. acknowledges that you are a professional with standard entry-level knowledge and skills
   b. builds your personal self-esteem and confidence in knowing that you can do the job asked of you
   c. helps in your career advancement and compensation
   d. All of the above

LEARNING APPLICATION

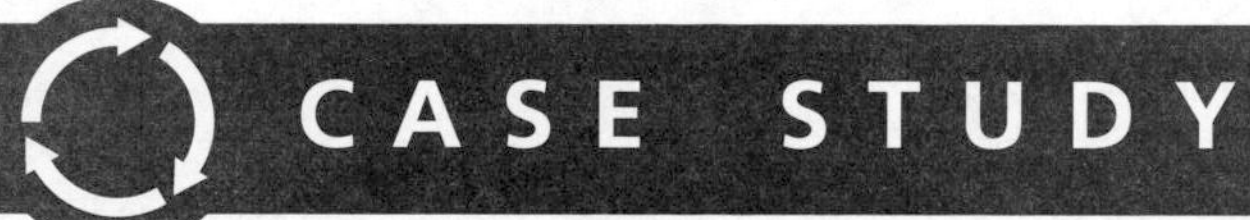

Michele Lucas is performing her practicum at Inner City Health Care under the direction of office manager Jane O'Hara. Michele has purchased a certification review study guide and has taken the sample 120-question certification examination available from the AAMA. From her studies, she has determined that she needs more work in the area of collections and insurance processing. Part-time administrative medical assistant Karen Ritter is responsible for these duties at Inner City Health Care, under Jane's supervision.

CASE STUDY REVIEW QUESTIONS

1. How can Michele use her practicum experience to help her concentrate on improving her skills in the area of collections and insurance processing?

____

____

____

____

____

____

2. What are your own personal strengths and weaknesses in preparing for a certification examination through AAMA, AMT, or NHA? What can you do to improve your areas of weakness?

____

____

____

CHAPTER POST-TEST

Perform this test without looking at your book. If an answer is "false," rewrite the sentence to make it true.

1. True or False? An RMA and a CMA (AAMA) have different bylaws and creeds.

____

____

2. True or False? A CMA (AAMA) has a national credential, so he or she may work in any state.

____

____

3. True or False? Three major areas included in the AMT's RMA examination are clinical, administrative, and general.

____

____

4. True or False? Providers recognize that their offices operate much more efficiently and effectively with professionally trained and formally educated personnel such as medical assistants.

____

____

5. True or False? Upon meeting recertification requirements, applicants receive an identification card which will indicate the year of recertification and the expiration date.

____

____

6. True or False? Once students have become members of AAMA, they may stay at the student rate for two years after graduation.

____

____

7. True or False? The NHA encourages recertification and offers CE programs.

____

____

8. True or False? Retaking the RMA examination is an option for reinstatement or recertification.

____

____

SELF-ASSESSMENT

1. Think of two different places where you could get continuing education credits.
   a. Investigate each one.
   b. Write a paragraph on the benefits and disadvantages of each method for you in your lifestyle.
2. Find out when and where your local chapter meetings are held.
   a. Attend a meeting with a classmate.
   b. Discuss what you learned from the meeting.
3. What can you do to prepare for the national certification examination?
   a. Write a plan in which you determine how much time you have to prepare and what you will accomplish each week/month in preparation.
   b. Make a calendar showing the steps toward your examination date.
   c. Try to stick with the plan as you progress closer to the examination date.

Name ______________________ Date __________ Score ______

CHAPTER 36

Employment Strategies

CHAPTER PRE-TEST

Perform this test without looking at your book. If an answer is "false," rewrite the sentence to make it true.

1. True or False? Positive thinking is one of the primary keys to success in planning your career and doing your job search.

2. True or False? It would be beneficial to begin your job search by networking with students who have graduated before you and are now successfully employed.

3. True or False? Poor appearance is a reason for employers not to hire a job seeker.

4. True or False? Employers like it when you know it all. They appreciate it when you do not ask questions.

5. True or False? You should never expect to receive a job from an office where you are an extern.

6. True or False? When filling out an application, it is acceptable to leave answers blank or write "see résumé."

7. True or False? You should always plan ahead and have all your information with you when picking up an application, just in case you are asked to fill it out right there.

VOCABULARY BUILDER

Misspelled Words

Find the words listed below that are misspelled; circle them, and correctly spell them in the spaces provided. Then match each correct vocabulary term to the aspect of the job-seeking process that best describes it.

accomplishment statement
application form
bullat point
carreer objective
contact tracker
cover letter
cronological résumé
functional résumé
interview
power verbs
refrences
résumé
targeted résumé

_______________ _______________ _______________

____

_______________ 1. Expresses your career goal and the position for which you are applying

_______________ 2. Résumé format used to highlight specialty areas of accomplishments and strengths

_______________ 3. A form devised by a prospective employer to collect information relative to qualifications, education, and experience in employment

_______________ 4. Individuals who have known or worked with you long enough to make an honest assessment and recommendation regarding your background history

_______________ 5. Résumé format used when focusing on a clear, specific job

_______________ 6. A statement that begins with a power verb and gives a brief description of what you did and the demonstrable results that were produced

_______________ 7. Asterisk or dot followed by a descriptive phrase

_______________ 8. A written summary data sheet or brief account of your qualifications and progress in your chosen career

_______________ 9. Action words used to describe your attributes and strengths

_______________ 10. A letter used to introduce yourself and your résumé to a prospective employer with the goal of obtaining an interview

_______________ 11. Résumé format used when you have employment experience

_______________ 12. A meeting in which you discuss employment opportunities and strengths that you can bring to the organization

_______________ 13. Form used to keep track of employment contact information, such as name of employer, name of contact person, address and telephone number, date of first contact, résumé sent, interview date, and follow-up information and dates

LEARNING REVIEW

Short Answer

1. List three types of professionals that would make excellent reference choices.

____

____

2. Identify an individual you know personally or have contact with who fits each professional reference type listed above and tell why you think they would be an excellent reference for you.

____

____

3. Identify the situations in which using a targeted résumé is advantageous by circling the number next to the statements that apply.

(1) You are just starting your career and have little experience, but you know what you want and you are clear about your capabilities.

(2) You want to use one résumé for several different applications.

(3) You are not clear about your abilities and accomplishments.

(4) You can go in several directions, and you want a different résumé for each.

(5) You are able to keep your résumé on a computer disk.

4. Identify the situations in which using a chronological résumé is advantageous by circling the number next to the statements that apply.

(1) The position is in a highly traditional field.

(2) Your job history shows real growth and development.

(3) You are changing career goals.

(4) You are looking for your first job.

(5) You are staying in the same field as prior jobs.

5. Identify the situations in which using a functional résumé is advantageous by circling the number next to the statements that apply.

(1) You have extensive specialized experience.

(2) Your most recent employers have been highly prestigious.

(3) You have had a variety of different, apparently unconnected, work experiences.

(4) You want to emphasize a management growth pattern.

(5) Much of your work has been volunteer, freelance, or temporary.

6. List four guidelines that are essential when preparing an effective cover letter.

7. List four items that are important when completing a job application.

8. Bob Thompson has an interview at Inner City Health Care for a new clinical medical assisting position. He is confident that he has prepared well for the interview. On the way to the interview, Bob reminds himself of three principles he has learned about interviewing.

   (1) ____________________ before answering questions, and try to provide the information requested in a professional manner.

   (2) ____________________ carefully so that you understand what information the interviewer is requesting.

   (3) ____________________ if you are uncertain.

9. How would you "dress for success" when preparing for your interview?

CERTIFICATION REVIEW

These questions are designed to mimic the certification examination. Select the best response.

1. Telling your friends, family, personal provider, dentist, and ophthalmologist that you are looking for a position in health care is called:

   a. networking

   b. references

   c. professionalism

   d. critiquing

2. Summarizing employment is acceptable on a résumé if it is prior to how many years ago?

   a. 1 year

   b. 5 years

   c. 10 years

   d. 15 years

3. The type of résumé that should be developed by someone who is just starting a career and has little experience is a(n):

   a. targeted résumé

   b. chronological résumé

   c. functional résumé

   d. objective résumé

4. Poise includes such things as:

   a. skill level

   b. confidence and appearance

   c. a. and b.

   d. none of the above

5. Providing a second opportunity to express your interest in an organization and a position may be done with a:

   a. cover letter

   b. recommendation letter

   c. follow-up letter

   d. strategic letter

6. Your attitude is reflected in how you react to:

   a. taking direction

   b. seeking excellence or doing just enough to get by

   c. assuming responsibility for your actions and considering your problems not to be someone else's fault

   d. all of the above

7. Some examples of transferable skills are *(circle all that apply):*

   a. leadership

   b. communication

   c. keyboarding

   d. drawing blood

8. When using someone as a reference, you should:

   a. always ask permission first before the name is printed on the reference list

   b. use your relatives

   c. verify correct spelling, title, place of employment and position, and telephone number

   d. a. and c.

9. Circle the top errors found with résumés.

   a. Typographical and grammatical errors

   b. Not mentioning jobs having transferable skills

   c. Using the same résumé for all job applications

   d. Listing your credentials

10. During the interview, it is *not* appropriate to ask:

    a. if this is a newly created position

    b. if there are opportunities for advancement

    c. about salary, sick leave, benefits, or vacation

    d. what the interviewer considers to be the most difficult task on the job

LEARNING APPLICATION

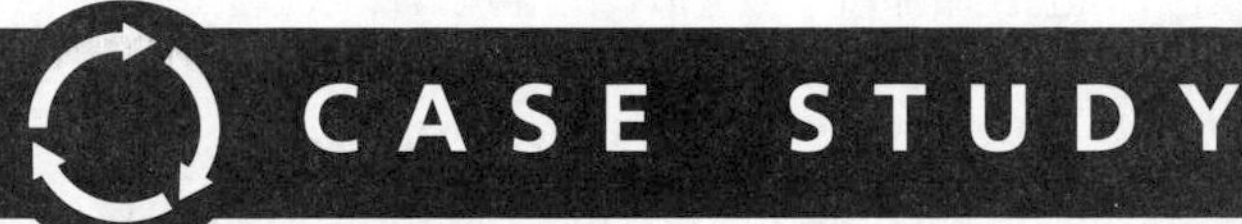

CASE STUDY REVIEW QUESTIONS

1. You are the subject of this case study. Complete the Self-Evaluation Worksheet that follows. Use your answers to help you determine the working environment you are most interested in and that best suits you. The worksheet can become a useful tool when researching prospective employers to target for your exciting first job in the medical assisting profession.

SELF-EVALUATION WORKSHEET

Respond to the following questions honestly and sincerely. They are meant to assist you in self-assessment.

1. List your strongest attributes as related to people, data, or things.

   i.e., Interpersonal skills related to people

   Accuracy related to data

   Mechanical ability related to things

   ______________________ related to ____________

   ______________________ related to ____________

   ______________________ related to ____________

2. List your three weakest attributes related to people, data, or things.

   ______________________ related to ____________

   ______________________ related to ____________

   ______________________ related to ____________

3. How do you express yourself? excellent, good, fair, poor

   Orally____________ In writing____________

4. Do you work well as a leader of a group or team? Yes _______ No_______

5. Do you prefer to work alone and on your own? Yes _______ No_______

6. Can you work under stress/pressure? Yes_______ No_______

7. Do you enjoy new ideas and situations? Yes_____ No_____

8. Are you comfortable with routines/schedules? Yes_____ No_____

9. Which work setting do you prefer?

   Single-physician setting _____ Multiphysician setting _____

   Small clinic setting _____ Large clinic setting _____

   Single-specialty setting? _____ Multispecialty setting _____

10. Are you willing to relocate? _____ Willing to travel? _____

Application Activities

1. In the Case Study, you completed a self-assessment form to help you find the type of working environment you are most interested in and best suits you. Create a contact tracker file for yourself, based on the one shown in Figure 36-2 in your textbook. Compile a list from the Yellow Pages, the Internet, want ads in your local paper, your program director, and other sources (hint: other sources are listed in the textbook).
2. Refer to Figure 36-10 in your textbook, which lists typical questions asked during an interview. Write what you would say to a potential employer in response to all of these questions. Then role play with another student, acting as interviewer and interviewee, with these questions and answers to gain confidence for an interview.
3. Recall that the interview process is a "two-way street." You, as the interviewee, should interview the employer. The text lists several example questions you might ask the interviewer during an interview. Develop a list of at least two additional questions that are important to you during the interview process.

CHAPTER POST-TEST

Perform this test without looking at your book. If an answer is "false," rewrite the sentence to make it true.

1. True or False? Positive thinking is a good thing, but it is not all that important to success in planning your career and doing your job search.

___

___

2. True or False? When beginning your job search, it would be beneficial to network with students who have graduated before you and are now successfully employed in the field.

___

___

3. True or False? Professional appearance is one reason for employers to want to hire a job seeker.

___

___

4. True or False? Employers do not expect that you will know it all. They appreciate it when you ask questions.

___

___

5. True or False? Students often receive job offers from the office where they extern.

___

___

6. True or False? When filling out an application, it is never acceptable to leave answers blank or to write "see résumé."

___

___

7. True or False? Plan ahead and have all your information with you when you pick up an application, just in case you are asked to fill it out right there.

___

___

SELF-ASSESSMENT

Imagine you are interviewing a recent graduate for a medical assisting position.

1. What questions might you ask during the interviewing process?

____

____

____

____

2. Do you think you could determine the best person for the job by meeting him or her just once? What else might you do to get to know the person better or get to know his or her work style better?

____

____

____

____

3. Did the applicant use power verbs effectively? Did they pique your interest?

____

____

____

Competency Assessment Tracking Sheet

Student Name: ____________________

Procedure Number and Title	Date Assessment Completed and Competency Achieved			
	Date/Initials	Date/Initials	Date/Initials	Date/Initials
EXAMPLE: 10-1 Medical Asepsis Hand Wash (Hand Hygiene)	**2/23/XX DF**	**3/15/XX SL**	**4/20/XX SP**	**5/1/XX JP**
4-1 Identifying Community Resources				
9-1 Control of Bleeding				
9-2 Applying an Arm Splint				
10-1 Medical Asepsis Hand Wash (Hand Hygiene)				
10-2 Removing Contaminated Gloves				
10-3 Transmission-Based Precautions: Donning a Gown, Mask, Gloves, and Cap (Isolation Technique)				
10-4 Sanitization of Instruments				
11-1 Taking a Medical History for a Paper Medical Record				
12-1 Measuring an Oral Temperature Using an Electronic Thermometer				
12-2 Measuring an Aural Temperature Using a Tympanic Thermometer				
12-3 Measuring a Temperature Using a Temporal Artery (TA) Thermometer				
12-4 Measuring a Rectal Temperature Using a Digital Thermometer				
12-5 Measuring an Axillary Temperature				
12-6 Measuring an Oral Temperature Using a Disposable Oral Strip Thermometer				
12-7 Measuring a Radial Pulse				
12-8 Taking an Apical Pulse				
12-9 Measuring the Respiration Rate				
12-10 Measuring Blood Pressure				
12-11 Measuring Height				
12-12 Measuring Adult Weight				
13-1 Assisting with a Complete Physical Examination				
14-1 Assisting with Routine Prenatal Visits				
14-2 Assisting with Pelvic Examination and Pap Test (Conventional and ThinPrep® Methods)				

Procedure Number and Title	Date Assessment Completed and Competency Achieved			
	Date/Initials	Date/Initials	Date/Initials	Date/Initials
14-3 Assisting with Insertion of an Intrauterine Device (IUD)				
14-4 Wet Prep/Wet Mount and Potassium Hydroxide (KOH) Prep				
14-5 Amplified DNA ProbeTec Test for Chlamydia and Gonorrhea				
15-1 Administration of a Vaccine				
15-2 Maintaining Immunization Records				
15-3 Measuring the Infant: Weight, Length, and Head and Chest Circumference				
15-4 Taking an Infant's Rectal Temperature with a Digital Thermometer				
15-5 Taking an Apical Pulse on an Infant				
15-6 Measuring Infant's Respiratory Rate				
15-7 Obtaining a Urine Specimen from an Infant or Young Child				
16-1 Instructing Patient in Testicular Self-Examination				
18-1 Urinary Catheterization of a Female Patient				
18-2 Urinary Catheterization of a Male Patient				
18-3 Fecal Occult Blood Test				
18-4 Performing Visual Acuity Testing Using a Snellen Chart				
18-5 Measuring Near Visual Acuity				
18-6 Testing Color Vision Using the Ishihara Plates				
18-7 Performing Eye Instillation				
18-8 Performing Eye Patch Dressing Application				
18-9 Performing Eye Irrigation				
18-10 Assisting with Audiometry				
18-11 Performing Ear Irrigation				
18-12 Performing Ear Instillation				
18-13 Assisting with Nasal Examination				
18-14 Cautery Treatment of Epistaxis				
18-15 Performing Nasal Instillation				

Procedure Number and Title	Date Assessment Completed and Competency Achieved			
	Date/Initials	Date/Initials	Date/Initials	Date/Initials
18-16 Administer Oxygen by Nasal Cannula for Minor Respiratory Distress				
18-17 Instructing Patient in Use of Metered Dose Inhaler				
18-18 Spirometry				
18-19 Pulse Oximetry				
18-20 Assisting with Plaster Cast Application				
18-21 Assisting with Cast Removal				
18-22 Assisting the Physician during a Lumbar Puncture or Cerebrospinal Fluid Aspiration				
18-23 Assisting the Provider with a Neurologic Screening Examination				
19-1 Applying Sterile Gloves				
19-2 Chemical "Cold" Sterilization of Endoscopes				
19-3 Preparing Instruments for Sterilization in Autoclave				
19-4 Sterilization of Instruments (Autoclave)				
19-5 Setting Up and Covering a Sterile Field				
19-6 Opening Sterile Packages of Instruments and Supplies and Applying Them to a Sterile Field				
19-7 Pouring a Sterile Solution into a Cup on a Sterile Field				
19-8 Assisting with Office/Ambulatory Surgery				
19-9 Dressing Change				
19-10 Wound Irrigation				
19-11 Preparation of a Patient's Skin before Surgery				
19-12 Suturing of Laceration or Incision Repair				
19-13 Sebaceous Cyst Excision				
19-14 Incision and Drainage of Localized Infection				
19-15 Aspiration of Joint Fluid				
19-16 Hemorrhoid Thrombectomy				

Procedure Number and Title	Date Assessment Completed and Competency Achieved			
	Date/Initials	Date/Initials	Date/Initials	Date/Initials
19-17 Suture/Staple Removal				
19-18 Application of Sterile Adhesive Skin Closure Strips				
21-1 Transferring Patient from Wheelchair to Examination Table				
21-2 Transferring Patient from Examination Table to Wheelchair				
21-3 Assisting the Patient to Stand and Walk				
21-4 Care of the Falling Patient				
21-5 Assisting a Patient to Ambulate with a Walker				
21-6 Teaching the Patient to Ambulate with Crutches				
21-7 Assisting a Patient to Ambulate with a Cane				
22-1 Provide Instruction for Health Maintenance and Disease Prevention				
23-1 Proper Disposal of Drugs				
24-1 Administration of Oral Medications				
24-2 Withdrawing Medication from a Vial				
24-3 Withdrawing Medication from an Ampule				
24-4 Administration of Subcutaneous, Intramuscular, and Intradermal Injections				
24-5 Administering a Subcutaneous Injection				
24-6 Administering an Intramuscular Injection				
24-7 Administering an Intradermal Injection of Purified Protein Derivative (PPD)				
24-8 Reconstituting a Powder Medication for Administration				
24-9 Z-Track Intramuscular Injection Technique				
25-1 Perform Single-Channel or Multichannel Electrocardiogram				
25-2 Holter Monitor Application (Cassette and Digital)				

Procedure Number and Title	Date Assessment Completed and Competency Achieved			
	Date/Initials	Date/Initials	Date/Initials	Date/Initials
27-1 Using the Microscope				
28-1 Palpating a Vein and Preparing a Patient for Venipuncture				
28-2 Venipuncture by Syringe				
28-3 Venipuncture by Vacuum Tube System				
28-4 Venipuncture by Butterfly Needle System				
28-5 Capillary Puncture				
28-6 Obtaining a Capillary Specimen for Transport Using a Microtainer Transport Unit				
28-7 Obtaining Blood for Blood Culture				
29-1 Hemoglobin Determination Using a CLIA Waived Hemoglobin Analyzer				
29-2 Microhematocrit Determination				
29-3 Erythrocyte Sedimentation Rate				
29-4 Prothrombin Time (Using a CLIA Waived ProTime Analyzer)				
30-1 Assessing Urine Volume, Color, and Clarity				
30-2 Using the Refractometer to Measure Specific Gravity				
30-3 Performing a Urinalysis Chemical Examination				
30-4 Preparing Slide for Microscopic Examination of Urine Sediment				
30-5 Performing a Complete Urinalysis				
30-6 Utilizing a Urine Transport System for C&S				
30-7 Instructing a Patient in the Collection of a Clean-Catch, Midstream Urine Specimen				
31-1 Procedure for Obtaining a Throat Specimen for Culture				
31-2 Wet Mount and Hanging Drop Slide Preparations				
31-3 Performing Strep Throat Testing				
31-4 Instructing a Patient on Obtaining a Fecal Specimen				

Procedure Number and Title	Date Assessment Completed and Competency Achieved			
	Date/Initials	Date/Initials	Date/Initials	Date/Initials
32-1 Pregnancy Test				
32-2 Performing Infectious Mononucleosis Test				
32-3 Obtaining Blood Specimen for Phenylketonuria (PKU) Test				
32-4 Screening Test for PKU				
32-5 Measurement of Blood Glucose Using an Automated Analyzer				
32-6 Cholesterol Testing				
33-1 Completing a Medical Incident Report				
33-2 Preparing a Meeting Agenda				
33-3 Supervising a Student Practicum				
33-4 Developing and Maintaining a Procedure Manual				
33-5 Making Travel Arrangements with a Travel Agent				
33-6 Making Travel Arrangements via the Internet				
33-7 Processing Employee Payroll				
33-8 Perform an Inventory of Equipment and Supplies				
33-9 Perform Routine Maintenance or Calibration of Administrative and Clinical Equipment				
34-1 Develop and Maintain a Policy Manual				
34-2 Prepare a Job Description				
34-3 Conduct Interviews				
34-4 Orient Personnel				

Competency Assessment Checklists

Name ________________________________ Date ____________ Score ______

COMPETENCY ASSESSMENT

Procedure 4-1 Identifying Community Resources

Task: To have a list of community resources available for patient use.

Conditions: Computer and printer, multiple resources from a variety of community services

Standards: Perform the Task within 30 minutes with a minimum score of _______ points.

Work Documentation: Electronic database or notebook of resources found

No.	Step	Points	Check #1	Check #2	Check #3
1	Determine the type of information to be in your database.				
2	Contact the sources and request any listings they may have.				
3	Search the Internet to obtain the desired resources.				
4	Develop a database on your computer so you can search easily for the resource when needed. Maintain a notebook with the resource information printed and indexed.				
Student's Total Points					
Points Possible					
Final Score (Student's Total Points/ Possible Points)					

Name ______________________ Date ____________ Score ________

WORK DOCUMENTATION

*Attach list of resources found.

Instructor's/Evaluator's Comments and Suggestions:

____

____

____

____

____

CHECK #1	
Evaluator's Signature:	Date:

CHECK #2	
Evaluator's Signature:	Date:

CHECK #3	
Evaluator's Signature:	Date:

ABHES Competency: VI.A.1.a.3.e Locate resources and information for patients and employers

CAAHEP Curriculum: IV.P.12 Develop and maintain a current list of community resources related to patients' healthcare needs; XI.P.12 Maintain a current list of community resources for emergency preparedness.

Name ______________________ **Date** __________ **Score** ______

COMPETENCY ASSESSMENT

Procedure 9-1 Control of Bleeding

Task: To control bleeding caused by an open wound.

Conditions: Sterile dressings, sterile gloves, mask, eye protection, a gown, biohazard waste container

Standards: Perform the Task within 15 minutes with a minimum score of _______ points.

Work Documentation: Simulated entry in Patient's Chart in Work Documentation area

No.	Step	Points	Check #1	Check #2	Check #3
1	Wash hands and gather equipment quickly.				
2	Apply gloves and other PPE; eye mask, gown if splashing likely.				
3	Apply pressure bandages and apply pressure for 10 minutes. If bleeding continues, elevate arm above heart. If continues, press adjacent artery against bone.				
4	Throughout procedure, demonstrate professional behavior in manner, organization and attire, including: • Recognize the effects of stress on all persons involved in emergency situations. • Demonstrate self-awareness in responding to emergency situations.				
5	Dispose of waste in biohazard container and wash hands.				
6	Document procedure.				
Student's Total Points					
Points Possible					
Final Score (Student's Total Points/ Possible Points)					

Name ______________________ **Date** ____________ **Score** ______

WORK DOCUMENTATION

Instructor's/Evaluator's Comments and Suggestions:

____

____

____

____

____

CHECK #1
Evaluator's Signature: Date:

CHECK #2
Evaluator's Signature: Date:

CHECK #3
Evaluator's Signature: Date:

ABHES Competency: VI.A.1.a(4)(f) Perform first aid and CPR; VI.A.1.a.4.e Recognize emergencies

CAAHEP Curriculum: XI.P.XI.11 Perform first aid procedures

Name ______________________________ Date ____________ Score ______

COMPETENCY ASSESSMENT

Procedure 9-2 Applying an Arm Splint

Task: To immobilize the area above and below the injured part of the arm to reduce pain and prevent further injury.

Conditions: Thin piece of rigid board and gauze roller bandage

Standards: Perform the Task within 15 minutes with a minimum score of _______ points.

Work Documentation: Simulated entry in Patient's Chart in Work Documentation area

No.	Step	Points	Check #1	Check #2	Check #3
1	Place a padded splint under the injured area. Hold the splint in place with roller gauze.				
2	Check circulation (note color and temperature of skin and nails, and check pulse).				
3	Apply sling to keep arm elevated.				
4	Throughout procedure, demonstrate professional behavior in manner, organization, and attire, including: • Recognize the effects of stress on all persons involved in emergency situations. • Demonstrate self awareness in responding to emergency situations.				
5	Wash hands.				
6	Document procedure.				
Student's Total Points					
Points Possible					
Final Score (Student's Total Points/ Possible Points)					

Name ______________________________ **Date** ____________ **Score** ______

WORK DOCUMENTATION

Instructor's/Evaluator's Comments and Suggestions:

____

____

____

____

____

CHECK #1	
Evaluator's Signature:	Date:

CHECK #2	
Evaluator's Signature:	Date:

CHECK #3	
Evaluator's Signature:	Date:

ABHES Competency: VI.A.1.a(4)(f) Perform first aid and CPR

CAAHEP Curriculum: XI.P.XI.11 Perform first aid procedures

Name ______________________________ Date ____________ Score ______

COMPETENCY ASSESSMENT

Procedure 10-1 Medical Asepsis Hand Wash (Hand Hygiene)

Task: To reduce pathogens on hands and wrists, thereby decreasing transmission of disease.

Condition: Sink with running warm water, liquid soap in dispenser, paper towels, hand lotion

Standards: Perform the Task within 3 minutes with a minimum score of _____ points.

No.	Step	Points	Check #1	Check #2	Check #3
1	Organized supplies, removed jewelry.				
2	Turned on faucet, set water temperature.				
3	Performed the procedure correctly and safely, including: • Did not touch inside of sink. • Did not lean against sink or counter. • Performed hand washing for proper amount of time. • Cleaned fingernails. • Rinsed well. • Repeated if appropriate (directed by instructor). • Dried hands well and disposed of towel without contaminating hands.				
4	Turned off faucet using barrier towel.				
5	Applied lotion.				
6	During procedure, demonstrated professional behavior in manner, organization, and attire.				
Student's Total Points					
Points Possible					
Final Score (Student's Total Points/ Possible Points)					

Name ______________________ **Date** __________ **Score** ______

Instructor's/Evaluator's Comments and Suggestions:

CHECK #1

Evaluator's Signature: Date:

CHECK #2

Evaluator's Signature: Date:

CHECK #3

Evaluator's Signature: Date:

ABHES Competency: VI.A.1.a.4.c Apply principles of aseptic techniques and infection control

CAAHEP Curriculum: III.P.4. Perform handwashing

Name ______________________________ Date ____________ Score ______

COMPETENCY ASSESSMENT

Procedure 10-2 Removing Contaminated Gloves

Task: To remove and dispose of contaminated gloves without exposing surroundings to contamination.

Condition: Biohazard waste container, contaminated gloves, hand washing equipment

Standards: Perform the Task within 3 minutes with a minimum score of _____ points.

No.	Step	Points	Check #1	Check #2	Check #3
1	Performed the procedure professionally and safely: • Held hands down and away from body, made a fist with the left hand. • Grasped the left glove with the right hand and carefully turned it inside out over left hand. • Dropped the removed glove into the right hand without contaminating the uncovered left hand. • Fisted the right hand over the left glove, turned the right hand over and carefully grasped the back inner edge of the cuff with the fingers of the left hand. • Inverted the right glove over the right hand and the left glove. • Disposed of gloves into biohazard waste container.				
2	Cleaned hands thoroughly and applied lotion.				
3	During procedure, demonstrated professional behavior in manner, organization, and attire.				
Student's Total Points					
Points Possible					
Final Score (Student's Total Points/ Possible Points)					

Name ______________________________ Date ____________ Score ______

Instructor's/Evaluator's Comments and Suggestions:

____

____

____

____

____

CHECK #1	
Evaluator's Signature:	Date:

CHECK #2	
Evaluator's Signature:	Date:

CHECK #3	
Evaluator's Signature:	Date:

ABHES Competency: VI.A.1.a.4.c Apply principles of aseptic techniques and infection control; VI.A.1.a.4.q Dispose of biohazardous materials; VI.A.1.a.4.r Practice standard precautions

CAAHEP Curriculum: III.P.2. Practice Standard Precautions

Name ______________________________ Date ____________ Score ______

COMPETENCY ASSESSMENT

Procedure 10-3 Transmission-Based Precautions: Donning a Gown, Mask, Gloves, and Cap (Isolation Technique)

Task: To provide protection from infectious diseases while in an inpatient setting.

Condition: Disposable gown, cap, mask, gloves. Hand washing equipment, biohazard waste bag, labeling pen, and writing pen

Standards: Perform the Task within 20 minutes with a minimum score of _____ points.

No.	Step	Points	Check #1	Check #2	Check #3
1	Reviewed physician orders, institutional protocol and policies, and specific isolation precautions.				
2	Organized supplies and reviewed patient's type of isolation.				
3	Removed jewelry and all unnecessary items.				
4	Performed the procedure correctly and safely: • Washed hands. • Applied barrier clothing, cap, gown, gloves, mask. • Entered patient's room with needed supplies. • Performed needed patient care, assessment, and documentation • Discarded contaminated articles into biohazard bag and labeled it. • Removed contaminated gloves, washed hands, untied waist of gown. • Removed mask, discarded properly, washed hands. • Untied neck of gown, washed hands. • Removed gown using proper technique, discarded properly. • Washed hands thoroughly, applied lotion.				
5	Demonstrated professional behavior in manner, organization, and attire.				
Student's Total Points					
Points Possible					
Final Score (Student's Total Points/ Possible Points)					

Name ______________________ **Date** __________ **Score** ______

Instructor's/Evaluator's Comments and Suggestions:

____

____

____

____

____

CHECK #1

Evaluator's Signature: Date:

CHECK #2

Evaluator's Signature: Date:

CHECK #3

Evaluator's Signature: Date:

ABHES Competency: VI.A.1.a.4.c Apply principles of aseptic techniques and infection control; VI.A.1.a.4.q Dispose of biohazardous materials; VI.A.1.a.4.r Practice standard precautions

CAAHEP Curriculum: III.P.2. Practice Standard Precautions; III.P.3. Select appropriate barrier/personal protective equipment (PPE) for potentially infectious situations

Name ______________________________ Date ____________ Score ______

COMPETENCY ASSESSMENT

Procedure 10-4 Sanitization of Instruments

Task: To properly clean instruments to remove all tissues and fluids.

Condition: Sink with running water, sanitizing agent with enzymatic action, soft brush, towels, protective plastic apron, heavy duty gloves

Standards: Perform the Task within 15 minutes with a minimum score of _____ points.

No.	Step	Points	Check #1	Check #2	Check #3
1	Organized supplies.				
2	Applied PPE.				
3	Performed the procedure correctly and safely: • Rinsed instruments in cool water. • Scrubbed each instrument well. • Rinsed in hot water. • Placed instruments on soft absorbent toweling. • Dried instruments thoroughly. • Removed gloves, washed hands.				
4	Demonstrated professional behavior in manner, organization, and attire.				
Student's Total Points					
Points Possible					
Final Score (Student's Total Points/ Possible Points)					

Name ______________________ **Date** __________ **Score** ______

Instructor's/Evaluator's Comments and Suggestions:

CHECK #1	
Evaluator's Signature:	Date:

CHECK #2	
Evaluator's Signature:	Date:

CHECK #3	
Evaluator's Signature:	Date:

ABHES Competency: VI.A.1.a.4.c Apply principles of aseptic techniques and infection control

Name ______________________________ Date ____________ Score ______

COMPETENCY ASSESSMENT

Procedure 11-1 Taking a Medical History for a Paper Medical Record

Task: To obtain and record a medical history for a new patient.

Condition: Patient history forms, clipboard, pen

Standards: Perform the Task within 25 minutes with a minimum score of _____ points.

Work Documentation: Completed patient history form

No.	Step	Points	Check #1	Check #2	Check #3
1	Introduced self to the patient, confirmed the patient's identity, and escorted her/him to the exam room.				
2	Made eye contact with the patient, established a professional and caring relationship.				
3	Performed the procedure correctly and safely: • Positioned the patient safely and comfortably, made eye contact while establishing a professional yet caring relationship. • Washed hands. • Began the interview with simple questions, spoke clearly. • Documented accurately and completely.				
4	Demonstrated professional behavior in manner, organization, and attire.				
Student's Total Points					
Points Possible					
Final Score (Student's Total Points/ Possible Points)					

Name ______________________ Date ____________ Score ______

WORK DOCUMENTATION

*Attach completed patient history form

Instructor's/Evaluator's Comments and Suggestions:

____

____

____

____

____

CHECK #1

Evaluator's Signature: Date:

CHECK #2

Evaluator's Signature: Date:

CHECK #3

Evaluator's Signature: Date:

ABHES Competency: VI.A.1.a.2.f Interview effectively; VI.A.1.a.2.g Use appropriate medical terminology; VI.A.1.a.4.a Interview and record patient history

CAAHEP Curriculum: I.P.6. Perform patient screening using established protocols; IV.P.1. Use reflection, restatement and clarification techniques to obtain a patient history; IV.P.3. Use medical terminology, pronouncing medical terms correctly, to communicate information, patient history, data and observations; IV.P.8. Document patient care

Name ______________________ Date __________ Score ______

COMPETENCY ASSESSMENT

Procedure 12-1 Measuring an Oral Temperature Using an Electronic Thermometer

Task: Obtain an accurate oral temperature.

Condition: Electronic thermometer, probe cover, biohazard waste container, patient chart

Standards: Perform the Task within 3 minutes with a minimum score of _____ points.

Work Documentation: Patient chart entry

No.	Step	Points	Check #1	Check #2	Check #3
1	Organized supplies and room.				
2	Greeted the patient correctly and appropriately.				
3	Washed hands and used proper PPE.				
4	Performed the procedure correctly and safely: • Ensured the thermometer was calibrated. • Placed thermometer gently and correctly. • Ensured patient comfort. • Removed thermometer gently when it beeped.				
5	Obtained accurate temperature.				
6	Demonstrated professional behavior in manner, organization, and attire, including: • Communicated appropriately and comfortably with the patient.				
7	Cleaned/disposed of supplies and equipment appropriately and washed hands.				
8	Documented correctly.				
Student's Total Points					
Points Possible					
Final Score (Student's Total Points/ Possible Points)					

Name ______________________ **Date** __________ **Score** ______

WORK DOCUMENTATION

Instructor's/Evaluator's Comments and Suggestions:

CHECK #1
Evaluator's Signature: Date:

CHECK #2
Evaluator's Signature: Date:

CHECK #3
Evaluator's Signature: Date:

ABHES Competency: VI.A.1.a.4.d Take vital signs

CAAHEP Curriculum: I.P.1 Obtain vital signs

Name ______________________ Date __________ Score ______

COMPETENCY ASSESSMENT

Procedure 12-2 Measuring an Aural Temperature Using a Tympanic Thermometer

Task: Obtain an accurate aural temperature.

Condition: Tympanic thermometer, probe cover, biohazard waste container, patient chart

Standards: Perform the Task within 3 minutes with a minimum score of _____ points.

Work Documentation: Patient chart entry

No.	Step	Points	Check #1	Check #2	Check #3
1	Organized supplies and room.				
2	Greeted the patient correctly and appropriately.				
3	Washed hands and used proper PPE.				
4	Performed the procedure correctly and safely: • Ensured the thermometer was calibrated. • Placed thermometer gently and correctly. • Ensured patient comfort. • Removed thermometer gently when it beeped.				
5	Obtained accurate temperature.				
6	Demonstrated professional behavior in manner, organization, and attire, including: • Communicated appropriately and comfortably with the patient.				
7	Cleaned/disposed of supplies and equipment appropriately and washed hands.				
8	Documented correctly.				
Student's Total Points					
Points Possible					
Final Score (Student's Total Points/ Possible Points)					

Name ______________________ **Date** __________ **Score** ______

WORK DOCUMENTATION

Instructor's/Evaluator's Comments and Suggestions:

____

____

____

____

____

CHECK #1	
Evaluator's Signature:	Date:

CHECK #2	
Evaluator's Signature:	Date:

CHECK #3	
Evaluator's Signature:	Date:

ABHES Competency: VI.A.1.a.4.d Take vital signs

CAAHEP Curriculum: I.P.1 Obtain vital signs

Name ______________________ Date __________ Score ______

COMPETENCY ASSESSMENT

Procedure 12-3 Measuring a Temperature Using a Temporal Artery (TA) Thermometer

Task: Obtain an accurate temporal artery temperature.

Condition: Temporal artery thermometer, probe cap or cover, alcohol wipes, patient chart

Standards: Perform the Task within 3 minutes with a minimum score of _____ points.

Work Documentation: Patient chart entry

No.	Step	Points	Check #1	Check #2	Check #3
1	Organized supplies and room.				
2	Greeted the patient correctly and appropriately.				
3	Washed hands and used proper PPE.				
4	Performed the procedure correctly and safely: • Ensured the thermometer was calibrated. • Cleared patient's forehead of perspiration, hair. • Placed thermometer gently and correctly. • Slid thermometer gently and correctly over the forehead. • Ensured patient comfort.				
5	Obtained accurate temperature.				
6	Demonstrated professional behavior in manner, organization, and attire, including: • Communicated appropriately and comfortably with the patient.				
7	Cleaned/disposed of supplies and equipment appropriately and washed hands.				
8	Documented correctly.				
Student's Total Points					
Points Possible					
Final Score (Student's Total Points/ Possible Points)					

Name ______________________________ **Date** ____________ **Score** ______

WORK DOCUMENTATION

Instructor's/Evaluator's Comments and Suggestions:

____

____

____

____

____

CHECK #1
Evaluator's Signature: Date:

CHECK #2
Evaluator's Signature: Date:

CHECK #3
Evaluator's Signature: Date:

ABHES Competency: VI.A.1.a.4.d Take vital signs

CAAHEP Curriculum: I.P.1 Obtain vital signs

Name ______________________________ Date __________ Score ______

COMPETENCY ASSESSMENT

Procedure 12-4 Measuring a Rectal Temperature Using a Digital Thermometer

Task: Obtain an accurate rectal temperature.

Conditions: Digital rectal thermometer, probe cover, lubricating jelly, biohazard waste container, patient chart

Standards: Perform the Task within 3 minutes with a minimum score of _____ points.

Work Documentation: Patient chart entry

No.	Step	Points	Check #1	Check #2	Check #3
1	Organized supplies and room.				
2	Greeted the patient correctly and appropriately.				
3	Washed hands and used proper PPE.				
4	Performed the procedure correctly and safely: • Ensured the thermometer was calibrated. • Placed thermometer gently and correctly. • Ensured patient comfort. • Removed thermometer gently when it beeped.				
5	Obtained accurate temperature.				
6	Demonstrated professional behavior in manner, organization, and attire, including: • Communicated appropriately and comfortably with the patient.				
7	Cleaned/disposed of supplies and equipment appropriately and washed hands.				
8	Documented correctly.				
Student's Total Points					
Points Possible					
Final Score (Student's Total Points/ Possible Points)					

Name ______________________ Date __________ Score ______

WORK DOCUMENTATION

Instructor's/Evaluator's Comments and Suggestions:

____

____

____

____

____

CHECK #1	
Evaluator's Signature:	Date:

CHECK #2	
Evaluator's Signature:	Date:

CHECK #3	
Evaluator's Signature:	Date:

ABHES Competency: VI.A.1.a.4.d Take vital signs

CAAHEP Curriculum: I.P.1 Obtain vital signs

Name ______________________________ Date ____________ Score ______

COMPETENCY ASSESSMENT

Procedure 12-5 Measuring an Axillary Temperature

Task: Obtain an accurate axillary temperature.

Conditions: Digital thermometer, probe cover, tissues, biohazard waste container, patient chart

Standards: Perform the Task within 3 minutes with a minimum score of _____ points.

Work Documentation: Patient chart entry

No.	Step	Points	Check #1	Check #2	Check #3
1	Organized supplies and room.				
2	Greeted the patient correctly and appropriately.				
3	Washed hands and used proper PPE.				
4	Performed the procedure correctly and safely: • Ensured the thermometer was calibrated. • Dried the axillary space if needed. • Placed thermometer gently and correctly. • Ensured patient comfort. • Removed thermometer gently when it beeped.				
5	Obtained accurate temperature.				
6	Demonstrated professional behavior in manner, organization, and attire, including: • Communicated appropriately and comfortably with the patient.				
7	Cleaned/disposed of supplies and equipment appropriately and washed hands.				
8	Documented correctly.				
Student's Total Points					
Points Possible					
Final Score (Student's Total Points/ Possible Points)					

Name ______________________________ **Date** ____________ **Score** ______

WORK DOCUMENTATION

Instructor's/Evaluator's Comments and Suggestions:

____

____

____

____

____

CHECK #1

Evaluator's Signature: Date:

CHECK #2

Evaluator's Signature: Date:

CHECK #3

Evaluator's Signature: Date:

ABHES Competency: VI.A.1.a.4.d Take vital signs

CAAHEP Curriculum: I.P.1 Obtain vital signs

Name ______________________________ Date ____________ Score _______

COMPETENCY ASSESSMENT

Procedure 12-6 Measuring an Oral Temperature Using a Disposable Oral Strip Thermometer

Task: Obtain an accurate oral temperature.

Conditions: Disposable oral strip thermometer, biohazard waste container, patient chart

Standards: Perform the Task within 3 minutes with a minimum score of _____ points.

Work Documentation: Patient chart entry

No.	Step	Points	Check #1	Check #2	Check #3
1	Organized supplies and room.				
2	Greeted the patient correctly and appropriately.				
3	Washed hands and used proper PPE.				
4	Performed the procedure correctly and safely: • Checked the package expiration date. • Placed thermometer gently and correctly. • Ensured patient comfort. • Removed thermometer gently at the appropriate time.				
5	Obtained accurate temperature.				
6	Demonstrated professional behavior in manner, organization, and attire, including: • Communicated appropriately and comfortably with the patient.				
7	Cleaned/disposed of supplies and equipment appropriately and washed hands.				
8	Documented correctly.				
Student's Total Points					
Points Possible					
Final Score (Student's Total Points/ Possible Points)					

Name ______________________________ **Date** ____________ **Score** ______

WORK DOCUMENTATION

Instructor's/Evaluator's Comments and Suggestions:

____

____

____

____

____

CHECK #1	
Evaluator's Signature:	Date:

CHECK #2	
Evaluator's Signature:	Date:

CHECK #3	
Evaluator's Signature:	Date:

ABHES Competency: VI.A.1.a.4.d Take vital signs

CAAHEP Curriculum: I.P.1 Obtain vital signs

Name ______________________ Date __________ Score ______

COMPETENCY ASSESSMENT

Procedure 12-7 Measuring a Radial Pulse

Task: Obtain an accurate radial pulse.

Conditions: Watch or clock with a second hand, patient chart

Standards: Perform the Task within 3 minutes with a minimum score of _____ points.

Work Documentation: Patient chart entry

No.	Step	Points	Check #1	Check #2	Check #3
1	Organized supplies and room and washed hands.				
2	Greeted the patient correctly and appropriately.				
3	Performed the procedure correctly and safely: • Counted the pulse for 30 seconds or a full minute if irregularities noted. • Assessed the pulse for irregularities in rate, rhythm, force/volume. • Ensured patient comfort and safety.				
4	Obtained accurate pulse rate.				
5	Demonstrated professional behavior in manner, organization, and attire, including: • Communicated appropriately and comfortably with the patient.				
6	Washed hands.				
7	Documented correctly.				
Student's Total Points					
Points Possible					
Final Score (Student's Total Points/ Possible Points)					

Name ______________________ Date ____________ Score ______

WORK DOCUMENTATION

Instructor's/Evaluator's Comments and Suggestions:

____

____

____

____

____

CHECK #1
Evaluator's Signature: Date:

CHECK #2
Evaluator's Signature: Date:

CHECK #3
Evaluator's Signature: Date:

ABHES Competency: VI.A.1.a.4.d Take vital signs

CAAHEP Curriculum: I.P.1 Obtain vital signs

Name ______________________________ Date ____________ Score ______

COMPETENCY ASSESSMENT

Procedure 12-8 Taking an Apical Pulse

Task: Obtain an accurate apical pulse rate.

Conditions: Watch or clock with a second hand, patient chart

Standards: Perform the Task within 3 minutes with a minimum score of _____ points.

Work Documentation: Patient chart entry

No.	Step	Points	Check #1	Check #2	Check #3
1	Organized supplies and room and washed hands.				
2	Greeted the patient correctly and appropriately.				
3	Performed the procedure correctly and safely: • Prepared patient properly, assisting if needed. • Draped patient appropriately. • Determined correct location of apical pulse site. • Counted the pulse rate for respirations for full minute. • Assessed the pulse for irregularities in rate, rhythm, and sounds. • Assisted patient while ensuring his/her comfort and safety.				
4	Obtained accurate pulse rate.				
5	Demonstrated professional behavior in manner, organization, and attire, including: • Communicated appropriately and comfortably with the patient.				
6	Washed hands.				
7	Documented correctly.				
Student's Total Points					
Points Possible					
Final Score (Student's Total Points/ Possible Points)					

Name ______________________________ Date ____________ Score ______

WORK DOCUMENTATION

Instructor's/Evaluator's Comments and Suggestions:

____

____

____

____

____

CHECK #1	
Evaluator's Signature:	Date:

CHECK #2	
Evaluator's Signature:	Date:

CHECK #3	
Evaluator's Signature:	Date:

ABHES Competency: VI.A.1.a.4.d Take vital signs

CAAHEP Curriculum: I.P.1 Obtain vital signs

Name ______________________________ Date __________ Score ______

COMPETENCY ASSESSMENT

Procedure 12-9 Measuring the Respiration Rate

Task: Obtain an accurate respiratory rate.

Conditions: Watch or clock with a second hand, patient chart

Standards: Perform the Task within 3 minutes with a minimum score of ____ points.

Work Documentation: Patient chart entry

No.	Step	Points	Check #1	Check #2	Check #3
1	Organized supplies and room and washed hands.				
2	Greeted the patient correctly and appropriately.				
3	Performed the procedure correctly and safely: • Counted the respirations for 30 seconds or a full minute if irregularities noted. • Assessed the breathing for irregularities in rate, rhythm, and breath sounds. • Ensured patient comfort and safety.				
4	Obtained accurate respiratory rate.				
5	Demonstrated professional behavior in manner, organization, and attire, including: • Communicated appropriately and comfortably with the patient.				
6	Washed hands.				
7	Documented correctly.				
Student's Total Points					
Points Possible					
Final Score (Student's Total Points/ Possible Points)					

Name ______________________ **Date** __________ **Score** ______

WORK DOCUMENTATION

Instructor's/Evaluator's Comments and Suggestions:

CHECK #1	
Evaluator's Signature:	Date:

CHECK #2	
Evaluator's Signature:	Date:

CHECK #3	
Evaluator's Signature:	Date:

ABHES Competency: VI.A.1.a.4.d Take vital signs

CAAHEP Curriculum: I.P.1 Obtain vital signs

Name ______________________________ Date ____________ Score ______

COMPETENCY ASSESSMENT

Procedure 12-10 Measuring Blood Pressure

Task: Obtain an accurate blood pressure.

Conditions: Stethoscope, sphygmomanometer/BP cuff, patient chart

Standards: Perform the Task within 3 minutes with a minimum score of _____ points.

Work Documentation: Patient chart entry

No.	Step	Points	Check #1	Check #2	Check #3
1	Organized supplies and room and washed hands.				
2	Greeted the patient correctly and appropriately.				
3	Performed the procedure correctly and safely using proper body mechanics: • Positioned the patient properly. • Exposed arm appropriately. • Determined proper cuff size. • Positioned cuff correctly. • Held patient arm at proper level in relaxed position. • Positioned stethoscope ear buds at proper angle, positioned diaphragm correctly. • Released pressure at appropriate speed.				
4	Obtained accurate blood pressure reading.				
5	Demonstrated professional behavior in manner, organization, and attire, including: • Communicated appropriately and comfortably with the patient.				
6	Washed hands.				
7	Documented correctly.				
Student's Total Points					
Points Possible					
Final Score (Student's Total Points/ Possible Points)					

Name ______________________ **Date** __________ **Score** ______

WORK DOCUMENTATION

Instructor's/Evaluator's Comments and Suggestions:

____

____

____

____

____

CHECK #1	
Evaluator's Signature:	Date:

CHECK #2	
Evaluator's Signature:	Date:

CHECK #3	
Evaluator's Signature:	Date:

ABHES Competency: VI.A.1.a.4.d Take vital signs

CAAHEP Curriculum: I.P.1 Obtain vital signs

Name ______________________________ Date __________ Score _______

COMPETENCY ASSESSMENT

Procedure 12-11 Measuring Height

Task: Obtain an accurate patient height.

Conditions: Height scale, patient chart

Standards: Perform the Task within 3 minutes with a minimum score of _____ points.

Work Documentation: Patient chart entry

No.	Step	Points	Check #1	Check #2	Check #3
1	Prepared scale and area around scale: • Arranged for a place for patient to sit to remove shoes and hang coat. • Ensured that height scale was properly calibrated and functioning.				
2	Washed hands.				
3	Greeted the patient correctly and appropriately.				
4	Performed the procedure correctly and safely: • Assisted patient with removal of coat and shoes as needed. • Assisted patient in storing coat, shoes, and other property. • Positioned patient correctly and safely for proper height measurement. • Measured properly. • Returned height scale to original position.				
5	Obtained accurate height measurement.				
6	Demonstrated professional behavior in manner, organization, and attire, including: • Communicated appropriately and comfortably with the patient.				
7	Washed hands.				
8	Documented correctly.				
Student's Total Points					
Points Possible					
Final Score (Student's Total Points/ Possible Points)					

Name ______________________________ **Date** ____________ **Score** ________

WORK DOCUMENTATION

Instructor's/Evaluator's Comments and Suggestions:

____

____

____

____

____

CHECK #1	
Evaluator's Signature:	Date:

CHECK #2	
Evaluator's Signature:	Date:

CHECK #3	
Evaluator's Signature:	Date:

ABHES Competency: VI.A.1.a.4.d Take vital signs

CAAHEP Curriculum: I.P.1 Obtain vital signs

Name ______________________ Date __________ Score ______

COMPETENCY ASSESSMENT

Procedure 12-12 Measuring Adult Weight

Task: Obtain an accurate patient weight.

Conditions: Weight scale, patient chart

Standards: Perform the Task within 3 minutes with a minimum score of _____ points.

Work Documentation: Patient chart entry

No.	Step	Points	Check #1	Check #2	Check #3
1	Prepared scale and area around scale: • Arranged for a place for patient to sit to remove shoes and hang coat. • Ensured that height scale was properly calibrated and functioning.				
2	Washed hands.				
3	Greeted the patient correctly and appropriately.				
4	Performed the procedure correctly and safely: • Assisted patient with removal of coat and shoes as needed. • Assisted patient in storing coat, shoes, and other property. • Positioned patient correctly and safely for proper weight measurement. • Measured weight properly. • Returned weight balance to original position.				
5	Obtained accurate weight measurement.				
6	Demonstrated professional behavior in manner, organization, and attire, including: • Communicated appropriately and comfortably with the patient.				
7	Washed hands.				
8	Documented correctly.				
Student's Total Points					
Points Possible					
Final Score (Student's Total Points/ Possible Points)					

Name ______________________ **Date** __________ **Score** ______

WORK DOCUMENTATION

Instructor's/Evaluator's Comments and Suggestions:

____

____

____

____

____

CHECK #1

Evaluator's Signature: Date:

CHECK #2

Evaluator's Signature: Date:

CHECK #3

Evaluator's Signature: Date:

ABHES Competency: VI.A.1.a.4.d Take vital signs

CAAHEP Curriculum: I.P.1 Obtain vital signs

Name ______________________________ Date ____________ Score ______

COMPETENCY ASSESSMENT

Procedure 13-1 Assisting with a Complete Physical Examination

Task: To assist the physician with a complete examination.

Conditions: Scale for height and weight, patient gown, drape, thermometer, stethoscope, sphygmomanometer, alcohol wipes, examination light, otoscope, ophthalmoscope, penlight, nasal speculum, tongue depressor, percussion hammer, tape measure, cotton balls, safety pin or sensory wheel, gloves, tissues, lubricant, emesis basin, gauze sponges, specimen bottle, slides and requisition form, biohazard waste container, and specific test kits as needed

Standards: Perform the Task within 25 minutes with a minimum score of _____ points.

Work Documentation: Patient chart entry

No.	Step	Points	Check #1	Check #2	Check #3
1	Washed hands, organized equipment and exam room.				
2	Introduced self to the patient, confirmed the patient's identity. Made eye contact with the patient.				
3	Performed the procedure correctly and safely: • Positioned the patient safely and comfortably. • Washed hands in front of the patient. • Interviewed the patient for current medications, tetanus status, update of medical history, determination of chief complaint. • Obtained and recorded vital signs. • Obtained lab work if previously ordered. • Performed diagnostic tests if previously ordered (EKG or spirometry). • Assisted the patient to prepare for examination. • Assisted the physician during and after the examination as needed. • Escorted the patient to the next phase (such as to the front desk for rescheduling, to the laboratory for testing).				
4	Demonstrated professional behavior in manner, organization, and attire.				
5	Washed hands and cleaned, sanitized, and disinfected the exam room for the next patient.				
6	Documented accurately and completely.				
Student's Total Points					
Points Possible					
Final Score (Student's Total Points/ Possible Points)					

Name ______________________ **Date** ____________ **Score** _______

WORK DOCUMENTATION

Instructor's/Evaluator's Comments and Suggestions:

CHECK #1	
Evaluator's Signature:	Date:

CHECK #2	
Evaluator's Signature:	Date:

CHECK #3	
Evaluator's Signature:	Date:

ABHES Competency: VI.A.1.a.4.b Prepare patients for procedures; VI.A.1.a.4.d Take vital signs; VI.A.1.a.4.g Prepare and maintain examination and treatment area; VI.A.1.a.4.h Prepare patient for and assist physician with routine and specialty examinations and treatments and minor office surgeries

CAAHEP Curriculum: I.P.1 Obtain vital signs; I.P.10 Assist physician with patient care; IV.P.6 Prepare a patient for procedures and/or treatments

Name ______________________ Date __________ Score ______

COMPETENCY ASSESSMENT

Procedure 14-1 Assisting with Routine Prenatal Visits

Task: To assist in routine examination to monitor the progress of a pregnancy.

Conditions: Disposable gloves, patient gown, scale, tape measure, sphygmomanometer, stethoscope, Doppler fetoscope and accessories, urine specimen container, urinalysis supplies, thermometer, patient chart

Standards: Perform the Task within 10 minutes with a minimum score of _____ points.

Work Documentation: Patient chart entry

No.	Step	Points	Check #1	Check #2	Check #3
1	Organized supplies and room.				
2	Greeted the patient correctly and appropriately.				
3	Washed hands and used proper PPE.				
4	Performed the procedure correctly and safely: • Obtained accurate weight. • Obtained accurate blood pressure and pulse. • Performed chemical examination of urine accurately and safely. • Assisted the provider as needed. • Assisted the patient as needed.				
5	Demonstrated professional behavior in manner, organization, and attire, including: • Communicating appropriately and comfortably with the patient.				
6	Cleaned/disposed of supplies and equipment appropriately and washed hands.				
7	Documented correctly.				
Student's Total Points					
Points Possible					
Final Score (Student's Total Points/ Possible Points)					

Name ______________________ Date __________ Score ______

WORK DOCUMENTATION

Instructor's/Evaluator's Comments and Suggestions:

____

____

____

____

____

CHECK #1

Evaluator's Signature: Date:

CHECK #2

Evaluator's Signature: Date:

CHECK #3

Evaluator's Signature: Date:

ABHES Competency: VI.A.1.a.4.b Prepare patients for procedures; VI.A.1.a.4.d Take vital signs; VI.A.1.a.4.h Prepare patient for and assist physician with routine and specialty examinations and treatments and minor office surgeries

CAAHEP Curriculum: I.P.1 Obtain vital signs; I.P.10 Assist physician with patient care; IV.P.6 Prepare a patient for procedures and/or treatments

Name ______________________________ Date ____________ Score ______

COMPETENCY ASSESSMENT

Procedure 14-2 Assisting with Pelvic Examination and Pap Test (Conventional and ThinPrep® Methods)

Task: To assist the provider in collection of cervical cells for laboratory analysis for early detection of abnormal cells of the cervix, including cancer, to assess the health of the patient's reproductive organs, to detect disease, leading to diagnosis and treatment.

Conditions: Patient chart, patient gown, patient drape, disposable gloves, tissues, lubricant, 4 × 4, vaginal speculum, tissues, urine cup and testing supplies, warm water or warming light, light for viewing, adjustable stool for provider, supplies for Pap test according to method used (see Procedure 14-2)

Standards: Perform the Task within 25 minutes with a minimum score of _____ points.

Work Documentation: Patient chart entry, lab requisition

No.	Step	Points	Check #1	Check #2	Check #3
1	Organized supplies and room.				
2	Prepared patient for pelvic examination: • Greeted patient correctly and appropriately. • Had patient empty bladder, saving the specimen for testing if needed. • Instructed patient to undress and put on a gown. • Explained procedure to patient. • Asked patient to sit at end of table. • Draped patient for privacy.				
3	Labeled the Pap bottles and completed the requisition as required for method used.				
4	Assisted the physician as needed through examination: • Assisted patient into lithotomy position safely and correctly, and draped patient. • Applied gloves. • Warmed the speculum. • Handed supplies to the physician as needed. • Prepared the specimen for the laboratory properly. • Disposed of waste into proper containers. • Removed gloves, washed hands.				

No.	Step	Points	Check #1	Check #2	Check #3
5	Assisted the patient as needed after the examination: • Helped her to a sitting position, using safe and correct body mechanics. • Helped her dress as needed. • Answered any questions she had. • Informed her of when the results would be available. • Scheduled her next regular examination or set up a reminder at a later date.				
6	Demonstrated professional behavior in manner, organization, and attire, including: • Communicated appropriately and comfortably with the patient throughout.				
7	Prepared the specimen for transport to the laboratory and completed the requisition properly.				
8	Documented correctly.				
9	Cleaned and prepared room for next patient; took instruments to the cleaning area for sanitization and sterilization.				
Student's Total Points					
Points Possible					
Final Score (Student's Total Points/ Possible Points)					

Name ______________________ Date __________ Score ______

WORK DOCUMENTATION

*Also attach lab requisition.

Instructor's/Evaluator's Comments and Suggestions:

CHECK #1	
Evaluator's Signature:	Date:

CHECK #2	
Evaluator's Signature:	Date:

CHECK #3	
Evaluator's Signature:	Date:

ABHES Competency: VI.A.1.a.4.b Prepare patients for procedures; VI.A.1.a.4.h Prepare patient for and assist physician with routine and specialty examinations and treatments and minor office surgeries

CAAHEP Curriculum: I.P.10 Assist physician with patient care; IV.P.6 Prepare a patient for procedures and/or treatments

Name ______________________ Date __________ Score ______

COMPETENCY ASSESSMENT

Procedure 14-3 Assisting with Insertion of an Intrauterine Device (IUD)

Task: To assist the provider with the insertion of an intrauterine device.

Condition: Nonsterile gloves, sterile gloves, vaginal speculum, light source and stool for provider, drape and gown, tissue, lubricant, prepackaged IUD, biohazard waste container, local anesthetic, syringe and needle, antiseptic such as Betadine® solution or swabs, emesis basin for used items such as speculum

Standards: Perform the Task within 25 minutes with a minimum score of _____ points.

Work Documentation: Patient chart entry

No.	Step	Points	Check #1	Check #2	Check #3
1	Washed hands and organized supplies and room, including drawing up anesthetic into syringe as directed by the provider.				
2	Prepared patient for pelvic examination.				
3	Assisted the provider as needed through procedure: • Applied gloves. • Warmed the speculum. • Handed supplies to the physician as needed. • Prepared the specimen for the laboratory properly. • Disposed of waste into proper containers. • Removed gloves, washed hands.				
4	Assisted the patient as needed after the procedure: • Checked vital signs. • Helped her to a sitting position, using safe and correct body mechanics. • Helped her dress as needed. • Answered any questions she had. • Scheduled a follow-up appointment.				
5	Demonstrated professional behavior in manner, organization, and attire, including: • Communicated appropriately and comfortably with the patient throughout.				
6	Documented correctly.				
7	Cleaned and prepared room for next patient; took instruments to the cleaning area for sanitization and sterilization.				
Student's Total Points					
Points Possible					
Final Score (Student's Total Points/ Possible Points)					

Name ______________________________ Date ____________ Score _______

WORK DOCUMENTATION

Instructor's/Evaluator's Comments and Suggestions:

____

____

____

____

____

CHECK #1

Evaluator's Signature: Date:

CHECK #2

Evaluator's Signature: Date:

CHECK #3

Evaluator's Signature: Date:

ABHES Competency: VI.A.1.a.4.b Prepare patients for procedures; VI.A.1.a.4.h Prepare patient for and assist physician with routine and specialty examinations and treatments and minor office surgeries

CAAHEP Curriculum: I.P.10 Assist physician with patient care; IV.P.6 Prepare a patient for procedures and/or treatments

Name ______________________________ Date ____________ Score ______

COMPETENCY ASSESSMENT

Procedure 14-4 Wet Prep/Wet Mount and Potassium Hydroxide (KOH) Prep

Task: To test the vaginal area for the determination and diagnosis of vaginitis. The wet prep mount test for yeast, bacteria, and trichomonas; the KOH prep tests for fungi.

Conditions: Patient chart, patient gown, patient drape, urine cup, disposable gloves, tissues, lubricant, 4 × 4, vaginal speculum and other supplies as needed for the vaginal examination. For wet prep: Cotton-tipped applicators, small test tubes, normal saline (0.5 mL, or a few drops), two microscope slides and cover slips. For KOH: 10% potassium hydrochloride solution (0.5 mL or a few drops), two microscope slides and cover slips, microscope

Standards: Perform the Task within 25 minutes with a minimum score of _____ points.

Work Documentation: Patient chart entry, lab report

No.	Step	Points	Check #1	Check #2	Check #3
1	Organized supplies and room.				
2	Prepared patient for pelvic examination.				
3	Assisted the physician as needed through examination.				
4	Prepared the specimen for the laboratory properly: • Placed several drops of normal saline in small test tube. • After physician obtained vaginal discharge sample, rinsed the swab in the saline solution, pressing the cotton tip against the inside of the tube to express the specimen. • Disposed of the applicator into sharps container. • Applied a drop of sample/solution onto a microscope slide and covered with cover slip.				
5	Assisted the patient as needed after the examination: • Helped her to a sitting position, using safe and correct body mechanics. • Helped her dress as needed. • Informed her that you and the provider would return when lab testing was finished.				
6	Removed gloves and washed hands.				

No.	Step	Points	Check #1	Check #2	Check #3
7	Took sample to laboratory, set up for physician to perform the microscopic examination.				
8	While the physician was examining the slide, prepared the sample for KOH examination: • Applied a few drops of KOH into the remaining solution in the test tube. • Mixed well. • Applied a drop onto a fresh slide, covered with a cover slip. • Set up for the provider to perform the microscopic examination.				
9	After the microscopy was performed, cleaned and disinfected the laboratory, disposing of supplies into proper receptacles.				
10	Went back to assist patient as needed.				
11	Demonstrated professional behavior in manner, organization, and attire, including: • Communicated appropriately and comfortably with the patient throughout.				
12	Documented correctly.				
13	Cleaned and prepared room for next patient; took instruments to the cleaning area for sanitization and sterilization.				
Student's Total Points					
Points Possible					
Final Score (Student's Total Points/ Possible Points)					

Name ______________________________ Date ____________ Score ______

WORK DOCUMENTATION

*Also attach lab report.

Instructor's/Evaluator's Comments and Suggestions:

____

____

____

____

____

CHECK #1	
Evaluator's Signature:	Date:

CHECK #2	
Evaluator's Signature:	Date:

CHECK #3	
Evaluator's Signature:	Date:

ABHES Competency: VI.A.1.a.4.b Prepare patients for procedures; VI.A.1.a.4.h Prepare patient for and assist physician with routine and specialty examinations and treatments and minor office surgeries

CAAHEP Curriculum: I.P.10 Assist physician with patient care; IV.P.6 Prepare a patient for procedures and/or treatments

Name ____________________ Date __________ Score ______

COMPETENCY ASSESSMENT

Procedure 14-5 Amplified DNA ProbeTec Test for Chlamydia and Gonorrhea

Task: To test the vaginal area for diagnosis of chlamydia and gonorrhea and to use as a screening for pregnant women.

Conditions: Patient chart, patient gown, patient drape, urine cup, disposable gloves, tissues, lubricant, 4 × 4, vaginal speculum and other supplies as needed for the vaginal examination; Amplified DNA ProbeTec Kit (pink), laboratory requisition, biohazard transport bag

Standards: Perform the Task within 25 minutes with a minimum score of _____ points.

Work Documentation: Patient chart entry, lab requisition

No.	Step	Points	Check #1	Check #2	Check #3
1	Organized supplies and room.				
2	Prepared patient for pelvic examination.				
3	Assisted the physician as needed through examination: • First handed the large swab to provider. • Discarded it into biohazard. • Handed the Mini-tip Culturette Swab to provider.				
4	Prepared the specimen for the laboratory properly: • After the physician obtained a sample of the vaginal secretion on the mini-tip swab, immediately placed the swab into the transport tube and recapped it (per ProbeTec Wet Transport tube directions: broke off the tip of the swab into the liquid and recapped). • Placed specimen into biohazard specimen transport bag.				
5	Removed gloves and washed hands.				
6	Assisted the patient as needed after the examination: • Helped her to a sitting position, using safe and correct body mechanics. • Helped her dress as needed.				
7	Completed lab requisition, placed it into the outer pocket of the transport bag.				

No.	Step	Points	Check #1	Check #2	Check #3
8	Demonstrated professional behavior in manner, organization, and attire, including: • Communicated appropriately and comfortably with the patient throughout.				
9	Documented correctly.				
10	Cleaned and prepared room for next patient; took instruments to the cleaning area for sanitization and sterilization.				
Student's Total Points					
Points Possible					
Final Score (Student's Total Points/ Possible Points)					

Name ______________________ Date __________ Score ______

WORK DOCUMENTATION

*Also attach lab requisition.

Instructor's/Evaluator's Comments and Suggestions:

____

____

____

____

____

CHECK #1

Evaluator's Signature: Date:

CHECK #2

Evaluator's Signature: Date:

CHECK #3

Evaluator's Signature: Date:

ABHES Competency: VI.A.1.a.4.b Prepare patients for procedures; VI.A.1.a.4.h Prepare patient for and assist physician with routine and specialty examinations and treatments and minor office surgeries

CAAHEP Curriculum: I.P.10 Assist physician with patient care; IV.P.6 Prepare a patient for procedures and/or treatments

Name ______________________________ Date ____________ Score ______

COMPETENCY ASSESSMENT

Procedure 15-1 Administration of a Vaccine

Task: To administer a vaccine.

Conditions: Vaccination order, vaccine, child's vaccination record, patient chart, pen or electronic chart, current VIS (Vaccine Information Statement); if administering by injection: syringe/needle as appropriate, alcohol wipe, sharps container

Standards: Perform the Task within 15 minutes with a minimum score of _____ points.

Work Documentation: Patient chart entry, vaccine administration record

No.	Step	Points	Check #1	Check #2	Check #3
1	Gave the parent the most recent copy of the Vaccine Information Statement (VIS).				
2	Followed the proper steps for selecting and drawing up medication, including checking the order with the medication three times and checking expiration date.				
3	Administered the medication properly: • Used correct route. • If injecting, used proper technique and site.				
4	After administering the vaccine, documented the procedure in the patient's medical chart and in his/her vaccine record: • Used the medication note and the vaccine vial to fill out the vaccine record. • Noted the type of vaccine, the date given, dose, site, route, vaccine lot number, and manufacturer. • Documented which VIS was given to the patient.				
5	Filed the clinic copy and gave the parent the patient copy.				
6	Demonstrated professional behavior in manner, organization, and attire.				
Student's Total Points					
Points Possible					
Final Score (Student's Total Points/ Possible Points)					

Name ______________________________ Date ____________ Score ______

WORK DOCUMENTATION

*Also attach vaccination administration record.

Instructor's/Evaluator's Comments and Suggestions:

____

____

____

____

____

CHECK #1

Evaluator's Signature: Date:

CHECK #2

Evaluator's Signature: Date:

CHECK #3

Evaluator's Signature: Date:

ABHES Competency: VI.A.1.a.4.m Prepare and administer oral and parenteral medications as directed by physician; VI.A.1.a.4.n Maintain medication and immunization records

CAAHEP Curriculum: I.P.7 Select proper sites for administering parenteral medication; I.P.9 Administer parenteral (excluding IV) medications; IV.P.8 Document patient care

Name ______________________________ Date ____________ Score ______

COMPETENCY ASSESSMENT

Procedure 15-2 Maintaining Immunization Records

Task: To establish and maintain a record of childhood immunizations.

Conditions: Medication order, vial of vaccination administered, child's vaccination record, patient chart, pen or electronic chart

Standards: Perform the Task within 15 minutes with a minimum score of _____ points.

Work Documentation: Patient chart entry, vaccine administration record

No.	Step	Points	Check #1	Check #2	Check #3
1	Gave the parent the most recent copy of the Vaccine Information Statement (VIS).				
2	After administering the vaccine, documented the procedure in the patient's medical chart and in his/her vaccine record: • Used the medication note and the vaccine vial to fill out the vaccine record. • Noted the type of vaccine, the date given, dose, site, route, vaccine lot number, and manufacturer. • Documented which VIS was given to the patient.				
3	Filed the clinic copy and gave the parent the patient copy.				
4	Demonstrated professional behavior in manner, organization, and attire.				
Student's Total Points					
Points Possible					
Final Score (Student's Total Points/ Possible Points)					

Name ______________________________ Date ____________ Score ______

WORK DOCUMENTATION

*Also attach vaccine administration record.

Instructor's/Evaluator's Comments and Suggestions:

____

____

____

____

____

CHECK #1

Evaluator's Signature: Date:

CHECK #2

Evaluator's Signature: Date:

CHECK #3

Evaluator's Signature: Date:

ABHES Competency: VI.A.1.a.4.m Prepare and administer oral and parenteral medications as directed by physician; VI.A.1.a.4.n Maintain medication and immunization records

CAAHEP Curriculum: I.P.7 Select proper sites for administering parenteral medication; I.P.9 Administer parenteral (excluding IV) medications; IV.P.8 Document patient care

Name ______________________________ Date __________ Score ______

COMPETENCY ASSESSMENT

Procedure 15-3 Measuring the Infant: Weight, Length, and Head and Chest Circumference

Task: To obtain an accurate measurement of an infant's weight, length, and head and chest circumferences.

Conditions: Patient chart including a growth grid, infant scale with protector, measuring tape or calibrated measuring mat, patient drape or blanket

Standards: Perform the Task within 30 minutes with a minimum score of _____ points.

Work Documentation: Patient chart entry, growth chart

No.	Step	Points	Check #1	Check #2	Check #3
1	Assembled equipment and arranged the room.				
2	Identified patient and explained the procedure to the parents; washed hands.				
3	Correctly weighed the infant: • Undressed the infant and/or assisted the parents as needed. • Placed protective sheet on scale and calibrated scale. • Gently placed infant on scale and ensured patient safety while on scale. • Adjusted the scale until weight was determined, while infant was lying still. • Noted infant's weight. • Returned scale weights to original position. • Removed protective sheet, disposed of it properly, and disinfected the scale. • Assisted parents to re-dress infant as needed.				
4	Correctly measured infant's length: If using a calibrated measuring mat: • Placed the infant on the mat with head touching the headboard. • Adjusted the foot board so the infant's heel and foot were flat against it and infant was lying straight; noted the length.				

No.	Step	Points	Check #1	Check #2	Check #3
	If using tape measure on examination table: • Laid the infant on the examination table, noted head position on the table paper. • Straightened the infant gently and marked the heel position on the table paper. • Lifted infant carefully and gave to parent. • Measured the distance between the head and heel marks, and noted the length.				
5	Correctly measured the head circumference: • Placed measuring tape around the largest part of the head, keeping the tape straight. • Noted head circumference in centimeters.				
6	Correctly measured the chest circumference: • Placed the measuring tape around the infant's chest, under the arms, just above the nipples, keeping the tape straight. • Noted chest circumference in centimeters.				
7	Correctly documented all measurements in the patient's record and on the growth chart.				
8	Demonstrated professional behavior in manner, organization, and attire, including communicating professionally with the patient and parents.				
Student's Total Points					
Points Possible					
Final Score (Student's Total Points/ Possible Points)					

Name ______________________ **Date** __________ **Score** ______

WORK DOCUMENTATION

*Also attach growth chart.

Instructor's/Evaluator's Comments and Suggestions:

____

____

____

____

____

CHECK #1

Evaluator's Signature: Date:

CHECK #2

Evaluator's Signature: Date:

CHECK #3

Evaluator's Signature: Date:

CAAHEP Curriculum: II.P.3 Maintain growth charts; IV.P.8 Document patient care

Name ______________________________ **Date** ____________ **Score** ______

COMPETENCY ASSESSMENT

Procedure 15-4 Taking an Infant's Rectal Temperature with a Digital Thermometer

Task: To obtain an accurate rectal temperature.

Conditions: Digital thermometer and probe cover, lubricating jelly, 4 × 4 gauze square, spare diaper, gloves, patient chart, pen or electronic chart

Standards: Perform the Task within 15 minutes with a minimum score of _____ points.

Work Documentation: Patient chart entry

No.	Step	Points	Check #1	Check #2	Check #3
1	Assembled equipment and supplies.				
2	Identified patient and explained the procedure to the parents.				
3	Used proper technique to obtain rectal temperature: • Removed the infant's diaper or assisted the parents as needed. • Applied gloves. • Positioned infant properly and safely. • Attached the probe cover to thermometer. • Lubricated the tip. • Inserted thermometer properly (0.5 inch). • Restrained infant as needed for safety. • When thermometer beeped, removed it and noted temperature. • Discarded probe cover into biohazard waste, removed gloves, washed hands. • Assisted parents in dressing the infant as needed.				
4	Disinfected thermometer and area.				
5	Correctly documented temperature.				
6	Demonstrated professional behavior in manner, organization, and attire, including communicating clearly with parents.				
Student's Total Points					
Points Possible					
Final Score (Student's Total Points/ Possible Points)					

Name ______________________________ **Date** ____________ **Score** ______

WORK DOCUMENTATION

Instructor's/Evaluator's Comments and Suggestions:

____

____

____

____

____

CHECK #1

Evaluator's Signature: Date:

CHECK #2

Evaluator's Signature: Date:

CHECK #3

Evaluator's Signature: Date:

ABHES Competency: VI.A.1.a.4.d Take vital signs

CAAHEP Curriculum: I.P.1 Obtain vital signs

Name ______________________________ Date ____________ Score ________

COMPETENCY ASSESSMENT

Procedure 15-5 Taking an Apical Pulse on an Infant

Task: To obtain an accurate apical pulse rate of an infant.

Conditions: Stethoscope, watch with second hand, alcohol wipes, patient drape, patient chart, pen or electronic chart

Standards: Perform the Task within 15 minutes with a minimum score of _____ points.

Work Documentation: Patient chart entry

No.	Step	Points	Check #1	Check #2	Check #3
1	Assembled equipment and supplies.				
2	Identified patient and explained the procedure to the parents; washed hands.				
3	Prepared the infant for the procedure: • Undressed the infant and/or assisted the parent(s) as needed. • Provided a drape sheet for comfort if appropriate. • Positioned the patient in supine position.				
4	Took the apical pulse rate: • Located the 5th intercostal space at the midclavicular line on the left side of the chest. • Placed the warmed stethoscope bell on the space and listened for the heartbeat. • Counted the pulse for one full minute. • Noted the rate.				
5	Correctly documented apical pulse rate.				
6	Demonstrated professional behavior in manner, organization, and attire, including communicating clearly with parents.				
Student's Total Points					
Points Possible					
Final Score (Student's Total Points/ Possible Points)					

Name ______________________________ Date ____________ Score ______

WORK DOCUMENTATION

Instructor's/Evaluator's Comments and Suggestions:

____

____

____

____

____

CHECK #1

Evaluator's Signature: Date:

CHECK #2

Evaluator's Signature: Date:

CHECK #3

Evaluator's Signature: Date:

ABHES Competency: VI.A.1.a.4.d Take vital signs

CAAHEP Curriculum: I.P.1 Obtain vital signs

Name ______________________________ Date ____________ Score ______

COMPETENCY ASSESSMENT

Procedure 15-6 Measuring Infant's Respiratory Rate

Task: To obtain an accurate respiratory rate of an infant.

Conditions: Watch with second hand, patient chart, pen or electronic chart

Standards: Perform the Task within 15 minutes with a minimum score of _____ points.

Work Documentation: Patient chart entry

No.	Step	Points	Check #1	Check #2	Check #3
1	Assembled equipment and supplies.				
2	Identified patient and explained the procedure to the parents; washed hands.				
3	Took the respiratory rate: • Positioned the patient in supine position. • Placed hand on infant's chest to feel the respirations. • Counted the respirations for one full minute. • Noted the rate, depth, rhythm, and breath sounds. • Returned infant to parents.				
4	Correctly documented the respiration rate.				
5	Demonstrated professional behavior in manner, organization, and attire, including communicating clearly with parents.				
Student's Total Points					
Points Possible					
Final Score (Student's Total Points/ Possible Points)					

Name ______________________ **Date** __________ **Score** ______

WORK DOCUMENTATION

Instructor's/Evaluator's Comments and Suggestions:

CHECK #1	
Evaluator's Signature:	Date:

CHECK #2	
Evaluator's Signature:	Date:

CHECK #3	
Evaluator's Signature:	Date:

ABHES Competency: VI.A.1.a.4.d Take vital signs

CAAHEP Curriculum: I.P.1 Obtain vital signs

Name ______________________________ Date ____________ Score ______

COMPETENCY ASSESSMENT

Procedure 15-7 Obtaining a Urine Specimen from an Infant or Young Child

Task: To obtain a specimen of urine from an infant or young child.

Conditions: Urine collection bag, laboratory request form, urine cup, urinalysis supplies, gloves, cleansing cloth, drying pad, patient chart, pen or electronic chart

Standards: Perform the Task within 15 minutes with a minimum score of _____ points.

Work Documentation: Patient chart entry, urinalysis report form, lab requisition

No.	Step	Points	Check #1	Check #2	Check #3
1	Assembled equipment and supplies.				
2	Identified patient and explained the procedure to the parents; washed hands.				
3	Prepared the patient for the procedure: • Positioned patient in supine position. • Removed diaper or assisted parent(s) as needed.				
4	Obtained the urine specimen: • Applied the bag to the patient properly. • Replaced the diaper. • Checked frequently or instructed parents • When specimen was collected, carefully removed bag and returned infant to parents. • Transported specimen to urine cup. • Prepared for transport or test in POL.				
5	Correctly documented the procedure.				
6	Demonstrated professional behavior in manner, organization, and attire, including communicating clearly with parents.				
Student's Total Points					
Points Possible					
Final Score (Student's Total Points/ Possible Points)					

Name ______________________________ **Date** __________ **Score** ______

WORK DOCUMENTATION

*Also attach urinalysis report form and lab requisition.

Instructor's/Evaluator's Comments and Suggestions:

CHECK #1

Evaluator's Signature: Date:

CHECK #2

Evaluator's Signature: Date:

CHECK #3

Evaluator's Signature: Date:

ABHES Competency: VI.A.1.a.4.j Collect and process specimens

CAAHEP Curriculum: III.P.7 Obtain specimens for microbiological testing

Name ________________________ Date ____________ Score ______

COMPETENCY ASSESSMENT

Procedure 16-1 Instructing Patient in Testicular Self-Examination

Task: To provide the patient with the correct procedure for performing monthly testicular self-examination.

Conditions: Patient chart, testicular model, testicular self-examination brochure and/or DVD

Standards: Perform the Task within 15 minutes with a minimum score of _____ points.

Work Documentation: Patient chart entry

No.	Step	Points	Check #1	Check #2	Check #3
1	Organized supplies and room.				
2	Identified and greeted patient appropriately.				
3	Performed the instruction correctly and professionally: • Using a DVD and/or patient brochure, instructed the patient on the proper method to perform the self-examination. • Discussed ideal positioning, frequency, and method to follow while examining the testicles, as well as what the patient is to be aware of during the self-examination. • Answered any questions from the patient. • Provided additional educational resources as approved by the provider.				
4	Instructed patient to notify the provider immediately if any abnormalities are found.				
5	Demonstrated professional behavior in manner, organization, and attire, including communicating clearly and comfortably with patient.				
6	Washed hands.				
7	Correctly documented the procedure.				
Student's Total Points					
Points Possible					
Final Score (Student's Total Points/ Possible Points)					

Name ______________________________ Date ____________ Score ______

WORK DOCUMENTATION

Instructor's/Evaluator's Comments and Suggestions:

____

____

____

____

____

CHECK #1

Evaluator's Signature: Date:

CHECK #2

Evaluator's Signature: Date:

CHECK #3

Evaluator's Signature: Date:

ABHES Competency: VI.A.1.a.2.m Adaptation for individualized needs; VI.A.1.a.7.c Teach patients methods of health promotion and disease prevention

CAAHEP Curriculum: IV.P.5 Instruct patients according to their needs to promote health maintenance and disease prevention; IV.P.9 Document patient education

Name ______________________ Date __________ Score ______

COMPETENCY ASSESSMENT

Procedure 18-1 Urinary Catheterization of a Female Patient

Task: To obtain a sterile urine specimen for analysis, to measure post-void residual, or to relieve urinary retention.

Conditions: Catheter kit containing needed supplies, sterile gloves, antiseptic cleansing solution, waxed bag or nearby biohazard bag, lubricant, sterile cotton balls, sterile forceps and Betadine® or Betadine® swabs, sterile urine cup, sterile 2 × 2 gauze, sterile absorbent pad, sterile fenestrated drape, tissue, sterile catheter as ordered, laboratory requisition, biohazard specimen transfer bag if needed

Standards: Perform the Task within 20 minutes with a minimum score of _____ points.

Work Documentation: Patient chart entry

No.	Step	Points	Check #1	Check #2	Check #3
1	Organized supplies and room.				
2	Identified and greeted patient appropriately; washed hands.				
3	Prepared the patient for the procedure: • Directed the patient to undress from the waist down and provided a drape. • Helped the patient onto the examination table. • Positioned the patient on back with feet together and knees apart.				
4	Set up the catheter tray, using sterile technique: • Opened the catheter kit using sterile technique on Mayo tray. • Placed the non-fenestrated drape under the patient's buttocks. • Emptied the kit onto the sterile field. • Placed the container into position without compromising sterility. • Applied sterile gloves. • Prepared Betadine cleansers and lubricant within sterile field.				

No.	Step	Points	Check #1	Check #2	Check #3
5	Performed catheterization properly without compromising sterility: • Placed fenestrated drape over patient's genitalia to create a sterile field. • Used nondominant hand to hold labia apart. • Cleansed area with three Betadine wipes using sterile dominant hand. • Dipped catheter tip into lubricant, placed other end into the container between patient's legs, and gently inserted the lubricated tip into the urethra. • Inserted catheter about 4 inches or until urine flowed. • When urine ceased, removed the catheter gently and slowly.				
6	Cared for the patient and the urine sample after catheterization: • Moved the urine container to the tray. • Transferred the urine to a capped sterile urine cup. • Disposed of contents of tray into biohazard bag. • Removed gloves, washed hands. • Assisted the patient to sit up and get dressed as needed.				
7	Demonstrated professional behavior in manner, organization, and attire, including communicating clearly and comfortably with patient.				
8	Correctly documented the procedure.				
Student's Total Points					
Points Possible					
Final Score (Student's Total Points/ Possible Points)					

Name ______________________ **Date** __________ **Score** ______

WORK DOCUMENTATION

Instructor's/Evaluator's Comments and Suggestions:

CHECK #1	
Evaluator's Signature:	Date:

CHECK #2	
Evaluator's Signature:	Date:

CHECK #3	
Evaluator's Signature:	Date:

ABHES Competency: VI.A.1.a.4.h Prepare patient for and assist physician with routine and specialty examinations and treatments and minor office surgeries

Name ______________________________ Date ____________ Score ______

COMPETENCY ASSESSMENT

Procedure 18-2 Urinary Catheterization of a Male Patient

Task: To obtain a sterile urine specimen for analysis, to measure post-void residual, or to relieve urinary retention.

Conditions: Catheter kit containing needed supplies, sterile gloves, antiseptic cleansing solution, waxed bag or nearby biohazard bag, lubricant, sterile cotton balls, sterile forceps and Betadine® or Betadine® swabs, sterile urine cup, sterile 2×2 gauze, sterile absorbent pad, sterile fenestrated drape, tissue, sterile catheter as ordered, laboratory requisition, biohazard specimen transfer bag if needed

Standards: Perform the Task within 15 minutes with a minimum score of _____ points.

Work Documentation: Patient chart entry

No.	Step	Points	Check #1	Check #2	Check #3
1	Organized supplies and room.				
2	Identified and greeted patient appropriately; washed hands.				
3	Prepared the patient for the procedure: • Directed the patient to undress from the waist down and provided a drape. • Helped the patient onto the examination table. • Positioned the patient on his back with legs straight.				
4	Set up the catheter tray, using sterile technique: • Opened the catheter kit using sterile technique on Mayo tray. • Placed the non-fenestrated drape on the patient's thighs. • Emptied the kit onto the sterile field. • Placed the container into position without compromising sterility. • Applied sterile gloves. • Prepared Betadine cleansers and lubricant within sterile field.				

No.	Step	Points	Check #1	Check #2	Check #3
5	Performed catheterization properly without compromising sterility: • Placed non-fenestrated drape over patient's thighs and fenestrated drape over penis to create a sterile field. • Used nondominant hand to hold penis taut, pulled back foreskin if necessary. • Cleansed area with three Betadine wipes using sterile dominant hand. • Dipped catheter tip into lubricant, placed other end into the container between patient's legs, and gently inserted the lubricated tip into the urethra. • Inserted catheter about 6 inches or until urine flowed. • When urine ceased, removed the catheter gently and slowly.				
6	Cared for the patient and the urine sample after catheterization: • Moved the urine container to the tray. • Transferred the urine to a capped sterile urine cup. • Disposed of contents of tray into biohazard bag. • Removed gloves, washed hands. • Assisted the patient to sit up and get dressed as needed.				
7	Demonstrated professional behavior in manner, organization, and attire, including communicating clearly and comfortably with patient.				
8	Correctly documented the procedure.				
Student's Total Points					
Points Possible					
Final Score (Student's Total Points/ Possible Points)					

Name ______________________ Date ____________ Score ______

WORK DOCUMENTATION

Instructor's/Evaluator's Comments and Suggestions:

CHECK #1

Evaluator's Signature: Date:

CHECK #2

Evaluator's Signature: Date:

CHECK #3

Evaluator's Signature: Date:

ABHES Competency: VI.A.1.a.4.h Prepare patient for and assist physician with routine and specialty examinations and treatments and minor office surgeries

Name ______________________________ Date __________ Score ______

COMPETENCY ASSESSMENT

Procedure 18-3 Fecal Occult Blood Test

Task: To teach the patient how to properly obtain a fecal specimen and then return it to the office for testing. To test feces for occult blood in the provider's office laboratory (POL).

Conditions: *Obtaining the specimen:* An occult slide test kit containing three slides, six applicators, envelope, and instructions. *Testing the specimen:* Prepared slides from the patient, occult blood developer from same manufacturer, gloves, biohazard waste container

Standards: Perform the Task within 15 minutes with a minimum score of _____ points.

Work Documentation: Two patient chart entries

No.	Step	Points	Check #1	Check #2	Check #3
1	Organized supplies and room.				
2	Identified and greeted patient appropriately; washed hands.				
3	Explained the procedure to the patient. Directed the patient to: • Follow the instructions on the slides. • Keep slides away from moisture, heat, and direct sunlight. • Label slide prior to obtaining the specimen. • Take a specimen each day for three days or three separate bowel movements. • Return the specimen to the office for testing. • Ingest no red meat, vitamin C, or aspirin products for three days prior to testing.				
4	Provided the patient with a biohazard envelope for the completed slides.				
5	Correctly documented the procedure.				
6	Demonstrated professional behavior in manner, organization, and attire, including communicating clearly and comfortably with patient.				

No.	Step	Points	Check #1	Check #2	Check #3
7	Tested for occult fecal blood by developing the slides: • Applied gloves. • Checked the dates and name on the slides. • Checked expiration date and label for the developing reagent. • Opened the back of each slide and, following instructions, applied drops of reagent onto the specimens and the controls. • Read the slides immediately for any evidence of blue color.				
8	Disposed of slides into biohazard waste container.				
9	Disinfected area, removed gloves, washed hands.				
10	Correctly documented the procedure.				
Student's Total Points					
Points Possible					
Final Score (Student's Total Points/ Possible Points)					

Name ______________________ Date __________ Score ______

WORK DOCUMENTATION

Instructor's/Evaluator's Comments and Suggestions:

____

____

____

____

____

CHECK #1

Evaluator's Signature: Date:

CHECK #2

Evaluator's Signature: Date:

CHECK #3

Evaluator's Signature: Date:

ABHES Competency: VI.A.1.a.4.j Collect and process specimens; VI.A.1.a.4.l Screen and follow up patient test results; VI.A.1.a.4.x Instruct patient in the collection of fecal specimen

CAAHEP Curriculum: I.P.6 Screen test results; IV.P.9 Document patient education

Name ______________________________ Date __________ Score ______

COMPETENCY ASSESSMENT

Procedure 18-4 Performing Visual Acuity Testing Using a Snellen Chart

Task: To perform a visual screening test to determine a patient's distance visual acuity.

Conditions: Snellen eye chart (appropriate for age and language ability) placed at eye level without glare on it, occluder, pointer, disinfectant wipes

Standards: Perform the Task within 15 minutes with a minimum score of _____ points.

Work Documentation: Patient chart entry

No.	Step	Points	Check #1	Check #2	Check #3
1	Organized supplies and area for testing, ensured good lighting with no glare at a distance of 20 feet.				
2	Identified and greeted patient appropriately; washed hands.				
3	Explained the procedure to the patient.				
4	Performed the procedure, directing the patient to: • Stand back at 20 feet, cover one eye with the occluder, and read the chart as directed. • Cover the other eye and read the chart again as directed. • Point to each line on the chart, starting large and going smaller while noting the patient's accuracy, reactions, and comfort. • Perform the same test with both eyes.				
5	Demonstrated professional behavior in manner, organization, and attire, including communicating clearly and comfortably with patient.				
6	Disinfected the occluder, washed hands.				
7	Correctly documented the procedure.				
Student's Total Points					
Points Possible					
Final Score (Student's Total Points/ Possible Points)					

Name ______________________________ **Date** ____________ **Score** ______

WORK DOCUMENTATION

Instructor's/Evaluator's Comments and Suggestions:

____

____

____

____

____

CHECK #1

Evaluator's Signature: Date:

CHECK #2

Evaluator's Signature: Date:

CHECK #3

Evaluator's Signature: Date:

ABHES Competency: VI.A.1.a.4.h Prepare patient for and assist physician with routine and specialty examinations and treatments and minor office surgeries

Name ______________________________ Date ____________ Score ______

COMPETENCY ASSESSMENT

Procedure 18-5 Measuring Near Visual Acuity

Task: To measure the near vision of a patient.

Conditions: Visual acuity eye chart, occluder, disinfectant wipes

Standards: Perform the Task within 15 minutes with a minimum score of _____ points.

Work Documentation: Patient chart entry

No.	Step	Points	Check #1	Check #2	Check #3
1	Organized supplies and area for testing, ensured good lighting with no glare.				
2	Identified and greeted patient appropriately; washed hands.				
3	Explained the procedure to the patient.				
4	Performed the procedure: • Instructed patient to cover one eye with occluder and hold vision card 14 inches from bridge of nose. • Instructed patient to read the paragraphs on the card. • Noted the acuity measurement number. • Instructed the patient to cover the other eye and read the chart again as before. • Noted the number for the second eye. • Performed the same test with both eyes and noted the number.				
5	Demonstrated professional behavior in manner, organization, and attire, including communicating clearly and comfortably with patient.				
6	Disinfected the occluder, washed hands.				
7	Correctly documented the procedure.				
Student's Total Points					
Points Possible					
Final Score (Student's Total Points/ Possible Points)					

Name ______________________ **Date** __________ **Score** _____

WORK DOCUMENTATION

Instructor's/Evaluator's Comments and Suggestions:

____

____

____

____

____

CHECK #1	
Evaluator's Signature:	Date:

CHECK #2	
Evaluator's Signature:	Date:

CHECK #3	
Evaluator's Signature:	Date:

ABHES Competency: VI.A.1.a.4.h Prepare patient for and assist physician with routine and specialty examinations and treatments and minor office surgeries

Name ____________________ Date __________ Score ______

COMPETENCY ASSESSMENT

Procedure 18-6 Testing Color Vision Using the Ishihara Plates

Task: To assess a patient's ability to distinguish between the colors red and green.

Conditions: Ishihara color plates

Standards: Perform the Task within 15 minutes with a minimum score of _____ points.

Work Documentation: Patient chart entry

No.	Step	Points	Check #1	Check #2	Check #3
1	Organized supplies and area for testing, ensured good lighting with no glare.				
2	Identified and greeted patient appropriately; washed hands.				
3	Explained the procedure to the patient.				
4	Tested the patient's color vision: • Held each plate 30 inches and directly within the patient's line of vision. • Recorded the number the patient saw on each plate. • Assessed the accuracy and noted the correctly read plates.				
5	Demonstrated professional behavior in manner, organization, and attire, including communicating clearly and comfortably with patient.				
6	Disinfected the occluder, washed hands.				
7	Correctly documented the procedure.				
Student's Total Points					
Points Possible					
Final Score (Student's Total Points/ Possible Points)					

Name ______________________________ Date ____________ Score ______

WORK DOCUMENTATION

Instructor's/Evaluator's Comments and Suggestions:

____

____

____

____

____

CHECK #1	
Evaluator's Signature:	Date:

CHECK #2	
Evaluator's Signature:	Date:

CHECK #3	
Evaluator's Signature:	Date:

ABHES Competency: VI.A.1.a.4.h Prepare patient for and assist physician with routine and specialty examinations and treatments and minor office surgeries

Name ______________________________ Date ____________ Score ______

COMPETENCY ASSESSMENT

Procedure 18-7 Performing Eye Instillation

Task: To treat eye infections, soothe irritations, anesthetize the eye, or dilate the pupils.

Conditions: Sterile eye dropper, sterile ophthalmic medication as ordered by the physician, sterile cotton balls, sterile gloves, tissue or gauze

Standards: Perform the Task within 10 minutes with a minimum score of _____ points.

Work Documentation: Patient chart entry

No.	Step	Points	Check #1	Check #2	Check #3
1	Organized supplies and room. Selected the ordered medication properly, checked order, dose, and expiration date.				
2	Identified and greeted patient appropriately; washed hands.				
3	Set the sterile field.				
4	Checked the medication order carefully again, including the order, the dose, and the expiration date.				
5	Explained the procedure to the patient, including that medication may blur vision temporarily.				
6	Instilled the eye medication: • Positioned the patient properly. • Applied gloves. • Instructed the patient to look up at a fixed spot and exposed the lower conjunctiva by using the gauze. • Applied the amount of medication ordered without touching the applicator to the eye or surrounding area. • Instructed the patient to close the eye and roll the eyeball gently to distribute the medication. • Blotted the excess medication or tears from the skin with tissue without rubbing or wiping the eye.				
7	Disposed of all supplies according to OSHA regulations; removed gloves, washed hands.				

No.	Step	Points	Check #1	Check #2	Check #3
8	Demonstrated professional behavior in manner, organization, and attire, including communicating clearly and comfortably with patient.				
9	Correctly documented the procedure.				
Student's Total Points					
Points Possible					
Final Score (Student's Total Points/ Possible Points)					

Name ______________________ Date __________ Score ______

WORK DOCUMENTATION

Instructor's/Evaluator's Comments and Suggestions:

____

____

____

____

____

CHECK #1	
Evaluator's Signature:	Date:

CHECK #2	
Evaluator's Signature:	Date:

CHECK #3	
Evaluator's Signature:	Date:

ABHES Competency: VI.A.1.a.4.h Prepare patient for and assist physician with routine and specialty examinations and treatments and minor office surgeries

CAAHEP Curriculum: I.P.10 Assisting physician with patient care

Name ______________________________ Date ____________ Score ______

COMPETENCY ASSESSMENT

Procedure 18-8 Performing Eye Patch Dressing Application

Task: To apply a sterile eye patch.

Conditions: Sterile eye patch(es) (some physicians request double layer), tape

Standards: Perform the Task within 10 minutes with a minimum score of _____ points

Work Documentation: Patient chart entry

No.	Step	Points	Check #1	Check #2	Check #3
1	Organized supplies and room.				
2	Identified and greeted patient appropriately; washed hands.				
3	Prepared the patient for procedure: • Explained the procedure. • Determined if patient had a ride home. • Positioned the patient in supine position. • Instructed patient to close both eyes during procedure.				
4	Performed the dressing application: • Opened eye patch using sterile technique. • Applied the eye patch, keeping inside sterile. • Correctly secured patch(es) in place with tape.				
5	Washed hands.				
6	Demonstrated professional behavior in manner, organization, and attire, including communicating clearly and comfortably with patient.				
7	Correctly documented the procedure.				
Student's Total Points					
Points Possible					
Final Score (Student's Total Points/ Possible Points)					

Name ______________________________ Date ____________ Score ______

WORK DOCUMENTATION

Instructor's/Evaluator's Comments and Suggestions:

____

____

____

____

____

CHECK #1

Evaluator's Signature: Date:

CHECK #2

Evaluator's Signature: Date:

CHECK #3

Evaluator's Signature: Date:

ABHES Competency: VI.A.1.a.4.h Prepare patient for and assist physician with routine and specialty examinations and treatments and minor office surgeries

CAAHEP Curriculum: I.P.10 Assisting physician with patient care

Name ______________________________ Date ____________ Score ______

COMPETENCY ASSESSMENT

Procedure 18-9 Performing Eye Irrigation

Task: To irrigate the patient's eye to remove foreign debris, cleanse discharge, remove chemicals, or apply antiseptic.

Conditions: Sterile irrigation solution as ordered by provider, sterile bulb syringe (rubber), kidney-shaped basin to catch irrigation solution, sterile cotton balls, sterile gloves, biohazard waste container, towel, pillow

Standards: Perform the Task within 15 minutes with a minimum score of _____ points.

Work Documentation: Patient chart entry

No.	Step	Points	Check #1	Check #2	Check #3
1	Organized supplies and room. Selected and prepared the irrigation solution carefully including the amount or dose and expiration date.				
2	Identified and greeted patient appropriately; washed hands.				
3	Prepared the patient for the procedure: • Explained the procedure. • Positioned patient in supine position with towel on shoulder and basin beside affected eye. • Tilted the patient's head toward the affected eye and instructed the patient to stare at a fixed spot during the irrigation.				
4	Checked the solution/medication order carefully again, including the order, amount or dose, and the expiration date.				
5	Performed the irrigation: • Applied sterile gloves. • Correctly cleansed the eyelids and eyelashes of affected eye with cotton balls moistened with irrigation solution, from inner to outer canthus. • Exposed the lower conjunctiva by separating the eyelid with index finger and thumb. • Irrigated the affected eye with sterile solution by resting the bulb on the bridge of the nose. Allowed solution to flow from inner to outer canthus. Did not touch the eye or surrounding area with the tip of the bulb. • After irrigation, dried the eyelid and eyelashes with sterile cotton balls.				

No.	Step	Points	Check #1	Check #2	Check #3
6	Discarded supplies according to OSHA standards; removed gloves and washed hands.				
7	Demonstrated professional behavior in manner, organization, and attire, including communicating clearly and comfortably with patient.				
8	Correctly documented the procedure.				
Student's Total Points					
Points Possible					
Final Score (Student's Total Points/ Possible Points)					

Name ______________________ **Date** __________ **Score** ______

WORK DOCUMENTATION

Instructor's/Evaluator's Comments and Suggestions:

____

____

____

____

____

CHECK #1

Evaluator's Signature: Date:

CHECK #2

Evaluator's Signature: Date:

CHECK #3

Evaluator's Signature: Date:

ABHES Competency: VI.A.1.a.4.h Prepare patient for and assist physician with routine and specialty examinations and treatments and minor office surgeries

CAAHEP Curriculum: I.P.10 Assisting physician with patient care

Name ______________________________ Date ____________ Score ______

COMPETENCY ASSESSMENT

Procedure 18-10 Assisting with Audiometry

Task: To assist in testing a patient for hearing loss.

Conditions: Audiometer with headphones, quiet room

Standards: Perform the Task within 20 minutes with a minimum score of _____ points.

Work Documentation: Patient chart entry

No.	Step	Points	Check #1	Check #2	Check #3
1	Organized supplies and area for testing.				
2	Identified and greeted patient appropriately; washed hands.				
3	Prepared the patient for the procedure: • Explained the procedure. • Positioned patient in sitting position. • Instructed patient to put on headphones.				
4	Performed the audiometry test: • Checked one ear first, then the other. • Plotted the graph as the patient indicated a sound was heard.				
5	Gave the results to the provider.				
6	Cleaned and stored equipment properly; washed hands.				
7	Demonstrated professional behavior in manner, organization, and attire, including communicating clearly and comfortably with patient.				
8	Correctly documented the procedure.				
Student's Total Points					
Points Possible					
Final Score (Student's Total Points/ Possible Points)					

Name ______________________ **Date** __________ **Score** ______

WORK DOCUMENTATION

Instructor's/Evaluator's Comments and Suggestions:

____

____

____

____

____

CHECK #1

Evaluator's Signature: Date:

CHECK #2

Evaluator's Signature: Date:

CHECK #3

Evaluator's Signature: Date:

ABHES Competency: VI.A.1.a.4.h Prepare patient for and assist physician with routine and specialty examinations and treatments and minor office surgeries

CAAHEP Curriculum: I.P.10 Assisting physician with patient care

Name ______________________ Date __________ Score ______

COMPETENCY ASSESSMENT

Procedure 18-11 Performing Ear Irrigation

Task: To remove impacted cerumen, discharge, or foreign materials from the patient's ear canal as directed by the provider.

Conditions: Irrigation solution as ordered by the provider warmed to 98.6°F to 103°F, ear syringe or bulb or ear irrigation equipment, kidney-shaped basin or ear irrigation basin, larger basin for warmed solution, towel, cotton balls, tissues, otoscope

Standards: Perform the Task within 25 minutes with a minimum score of _____ points.

Work Documentation: Patient chart entry

No.	Step	Points	Check #1	Check #2	Check #3
1	Organized supplies and room. Selected and prepared irrigation solution properly.				
2	Identified and greeted patient appropriately; washed hands.				
3	Prepared the patient for the procedure: • Explained the procedure and that slight discomfort or dizziness may be experienced. • Determined that provider has examined ear. • Positioned patient in sitting position with towel on shoulder and basin against neck. • Cleansed outer ear with moistened cotton ball.				
4	Checked the irrigation solution again for correctness and proper temperature.				
5	Prepared the solution in the syringe.				
6	Performed the irrigation correctly and safely: • Straightened external auditory canal as appropriate for patient's age. • Gently inserted the syringe tip into the ear canal at the appropriate depth. • Directed the flow upward and toward the roof of the canal. • Periodically checked with the patient for discomfort or pain. • Repeated the irrigation until ear canal was clear or solution was finished. • Noted the results by examining the ear with the otoscope. • Dried the outer ear.				

No.	Step	Points	Check #1	Check #2	Check #3
7	Discarded supplies according to OSHA standards; removed gloves and washed hands.				
8	Demonstrated professional behavior in manner, organization, and attire, including communicating clearly and comfortably with patient.				
9	Correctly documented the procedure.				
Student's Total Points					
Points Possible					
Final Score (Student's Total Points/ Possible Points)					

Name ______________________________ Date ____________ Score ______

WORK DOCUMENTATION

Instructor's/Evaluator's Comments and Suggestions:

CHECK #1	
Evaluator's Signature:	Date:

CHECK #2	
Evaluator's Signature:	Date:

CHECK #3	
Evaluator's Signature:	Date:

ABHES Competency: VI.A.1.a.4.h Prepare patient for and assist physician with routine and specialty examinations and treatments and minor office surgeries

CAAHEP Curriculum: I.P.10 Assisting physician with patient care

Name ______________________________ Date ____________ Score ______

COMPETENCY ASSESSMENT

Procedure 18-12 Performing Ear Instillation

Task: To soften impacted cerumen, treat infection with antibiotics, or relieve pain.

Conditions: Otic medication as prescribed by the provider, sterile ear dropper, cotton balls, gloves

Standards: Perform the Task within 15 minutes with a minimum score of _____ points.

Work Documentation: Patient chart entry

No.	Step	Points	Check #1	Check #2	Check #3
1	Organized supplies and room. Selected medication as ordered and carefully checked dose and expiration date.				
2	Identified and greeted patient appropriately; washed hands.				
3	Prepared the patient for the procedure: • Explained the procedure and that slight discomfort or dizziness may be experienced. • Determined that provider has examined ear. • Positioned patient in sitting position with towel on shoulder and basin against neck.				
4	Checked the medication order again, including the dose and expiration date.				
5	Drew up the prescribed medication.				
6	Performed the irrigation correctly and safely: • Straightened external auditory canal as appropriate for patient's age. • Instilled prescribed dose into the ear. • Instructed patient to maintain position for 5 minutes to retain medication. • When instructed by provider, inserted moistened cotton ball into external canal for 15 minutes.				
7	Discarded supplies according to OSHA standards; removed gloves and washed hands.				

No.	Step	Points	Check #1	Check #2	Check #3
8	Demonstrated professional behavior in manner, organization, and attire, including communicating clearly and comfortably with patient.				
9	Correctly documented the procedure.				
Student's Total Points					
Points Possible					
Final Score (Student's Total Points/ Possible Points)					

Name ______________________ Date __________ Score ______

WORK DOCUMENTATION

Instructor's/Evaluator's Comments and Suggestions:

____

____

____

____

____

CHECK #1	
Evaluator's Signature:	Date:

CHECK #2	
Evaluator's Signature:	Date:

CHECK #3	
Evaluator's Signature:	Date:

ABHES Competency: VI.A.1.a.4.h Prepare patient for and assist physician with routine and specialty examinations and treatments and minor office surgeries

CAAHEP Curriculum: I.P.10 Assisting physician with patient care

Name ______________________________ Date __________ Score ______

COMPETENCY ASSESSMENT

Procedure 18-13 Assisting with Nasal Examination

Task: To assist the provider with the nasal examination when looking for polyps, engorged superficial blood vessels, and to assist in the possible removal of a foreign object.

Conditions: Nasal speculum, hands-free light source, gloves, kidney basin, bayonet forceps, patient drape

Standards: Perform the Task within 15 minutes with a minimum score of _____ points.

Work Documentation: Patient chart entry

No.	Step	Points	Check #1	Check #2	Check #3
1	Organized supplies and room.				
2	Identified and greeted patient appropriately; washed hands and applied gloves.				
3	Prepared the patient for the procedure: • Explained the procedure. • Positioned patient in a sitting position, slightly reclined (or as directed) with a drape available (in case of bleeding).				
4	Handed provider equipment and supplies as needed.				
5	Discarded supplies according to OSHA standards; removed gloves and washed hands.				
6	Demonstrated professional behavior in manner, organization, and attire, including communicating clearly and comfortably with patient and provider.				
7	Correctly documented the procedure.				
Student's Total Points					
Points Possible					
Final Score (Student's Total Points/ Possible Points)					

Name ______________________________ **Date** ____________ **Score** ______

WORK DOCUMENTATION

Instructor's/Evaluator's Comments and Suggestions:

____

____

____

____

____

CHECK #1	
Evaluator's Signature:	Date:

CHECK #2	
Evaluator's Signature:	Date:

CHECK #3	
Evaluator's Signature:	Date:

ABHES Competency: VI.A.1.a.4.h Prepare patient for and assist physician with routine and specialty examinations and treatments and minor office surgeries

CAAHEP Curriculum: I.P.10 Assisting physician with patient care

Name ______________________________ Date ____________ Score ______

COMPETENCY ASSESSMENT

Procedure 18-14 Cautery Treatment of Epistaxis

Task: To assist the provider with treatment and control of nose bleeding.

Conditions: Nasal speculum, hands-free light source, gloves, kidney basin, bayonet forceps, silver nitrate applicators, cotton balls, nasal packing material, cotton-tipped applicators, 2 small syringes with large-gauge needles, epinephrine, 2 small medication cups, local anesthetic, antibiotic ointment, other medications as ordered by the provider, patient drape

Standards: Perform the Task within 20 minutes with a minimum score of _____ points.

Work Documentation: Patient chart entry

No.	Step	Points	Check #1	Check #2	Check #3
1	Organized supplies and room.				
2	Identified and greeted patient appropriately; washed hands and applied gloves.				
3	Prepared the patient for the procedure: • Explained the procedure. • Positioned patient in a sitting position slightly reclined (or as directed) with a drape and basin available.				
4	Prepared the anesthesia as directed by the provider by withdrawing it from the vial and putting it into a medication cup.				
5	Prepared the epinephrine as directed by the provider by withdrawing it from the vial and putting it into a medication cup.				
6	Handed provider equipment and supplies as needed.				
7	Discarded supplies according to OSHA standards; removed gloves and washed hands.				
8	Demonstrated professional behavior in manner, organization, and attire, including communicating clearly and comfortably with patient and provider.				
9	Correctly documented the procedure.				
Student's Total Points					
Points Possible					
Final Score (Student's Total Points/ Possible Points)					

Name ______________________________ **Date** __________ **Score** ______

WORK DOCUMENTATION

Instructor's/Evaluator's Comments and Suggestions:

____

____

____

____

____

CHECK #1
Evaluator's Signature: Date:

CHECK #2
Evaluator's Signature: Date:

CHECK #3
Evaluator's Signature: Date:

ABHES Competency: VI.A.1.a.4.h Prepare patient for and assist physician with routine and specialty examinations and treatments and minor office surgeries

CAAHEP Curriculum: I.P.10 Assisting physician with patient care

Name ______________________________ Date ____________ Score ______

COMPETENCY ASSESSMENT

Procedure 18-15 Performing Nasal Instillation

Task: To provide medication to the nasal tissues as ordered by the provider.

Conditions: Medication as ordered, sterile medicine dropper, tissues

Standards: Perform the Task within 15 minutes with a minimum score of _____ points.

Work Documentation: Patient chart entry

No.	Step	Points	Check #1	Check #2	Check #3
1	Organized supplies and room. Selected proper medication as ordered and carefully checked dose and expiration date.				
2	Identified and greeted patient appropriately; washed hands and applied gloves.				
3	Prepared the patient for the procedure: • Explained the procedure. • Positioned patient in supine position with head slightly lowered, or sitting with head tilted back. • Helped patient adjust for comfort.				
4	Checked the medication order carefully again including the dose and expiration date.				
5	Instilled the medication properly: • Drew medication into the dropper. • Applied the medication to the affected nostril or both nostrils as directed. • Did not touch the dropper to the nostril. • Handled medication using sterile technique. • Instructed patient to remain in position for 5 minutes. • Handed tissues to patient when head was tilted back or when patient sat up.				
6	Discarded supplies according to OSHA standards; removed gloves and washed hands.				
7	Demonstrated professional behavior in manner, organization, and attire, including communicating clearly and comfortably with patient and provider.				
8	Correctly documented the procedure.				
Student's Total Points					
Points Possible					
Final Score (Student's Total Points/ Possible Points)					

Name ______________________________ **Date** ____________ **Score** ______

WORK DOCUMENTATION

Instructor's/Evaluator's Comments and Suggestions:

____

____

____

____

____

CHECK #1

Evaluator's Signature: Date:

CHECK #2

Evaluator's Signature: Date:

CHECK #3

Evaluator's Signature: Date:

ABHES Competency: VI.A.1.a.4.h Prepare patient for and assist physician with routine and specialty examinations and treatments and minor office surgeries

CAAHEP Curriculum: I.P.10 Assisting physician with patient care

Name ______________________ Date __________ Score ______

COMPETENCY ASSESSMENT

Procedure 18-16 Administer Oxygen by Nasal Cannula for Minor Respiratory Distress

Task: To provide a low dose of concentrated oxygen to a patient during periods of respiratory distress.

Conditions: Portable oxygen tank with stand, disposable nasal cannula with connecting tube, flow meter, and pressure regulator

Standards: Perform the Task within 15 minutes with a minimum score of _____ points.

Work Documentation: Patient chart entry

No.	Step	Points	Check #1	Check #2	Check #3
1	Organized supplies and room.				
2	Identified and greeted patient appropriately; washed hands and applied gloves.				
3	Explained procedure to the patient.				
4	Prepared the oxygen equipment properly: • Opened the cylinder one full turn counterclockwise. • Checked the pressure gauge to be sure oxygen was available and flowing. • Attached the nasal cannula to the tubing and then to the flow meter. • Adjusted the flow rate according to the provider's orders. • Placed the tips in the patient's nostrils properly, adjusted around the patient's ears, and secured it under the chin.				
5	Cautioned the patient about safety around oxygen use, answered questions.				
6	Discarded supplies according to OSHA standards; removed gloves and washed hands.				
7	Demonstrated professional behavior in manner, organization, and attire, including communicating clearly and comfortably with patient and provider.				
8	Correctly documented the procedure.				
Student's Total Points					
Points Possible					
Final Score (Student's Total Points/ Possible Points)					

Name ______________________ **Date** __________ **Score** ______

WORK DOCUMENTATION

Instructor's/Evaluator's Comments and Suggestions:

____

____

____

____

____

CHECK #1	
Evaluator's Signature:	Date:

CHECK #2	
Evaluator's Signature:	Date:

CHECK #3	
Evaluator's Signature:	Date:

ABHES Competency: VI.A.1.a.4.h Prepare patient for and assist physician with routine and specialty examinations and treatments and minor office surgeries

CAAHEP Curriculum: I.P.10 Assisting physician with patient care

Name ______________________________ Date ____________ Score ______

COMPETENCY ASSESSMENT

Procedure 18-17 Instructing Patient in Use of Metered Dose Inhaler

Task: To instruct the patient in the correct use of a handheld metered dose inhaler.

Conditions: Handheld nebulizer containing medication ordered by the provider

Standards: Perform the Task within 20 minutes with a minimum score of _____ points.

Work Documentation: Patient chart entry

No.	Step	Points	Check #1	Check #2	Check #3
1	Organized supplies and room.				
2	Identified and greeted patient appropriately; washed hands.				
3	Checked medication order three times.				
4	Demonstrated the procedure to the patient, and asked the patient to repeat the demonstration.				
5	Administered the medication: • Instructed patient to sit upright and exhale fully. • Instructed patient to remove cap and shake MDI well. • Helped patient hold nebulizer to mouth, closing the lips and teeth around the mouthpiece. • Instructed patient to tilt head back and take a deep breath while pushing medication container against the mouthpiece. • Instructed patient to continue to inhale deeply until the lungs were full. • Had patient remove the mouthpiece and hold breath for 10 seconds. • Waited one minute and repeated the process (if the provider ordered more than one treatment). • Replaced cap. • If the MDI contained a steroid, instructed patient to rinse mouth well and gargle. • Checked patient for adverse reaction.				

No.	Step	Points	Check #1	Check #2	Check #3
6	Demonstrated professional behavior in manner, organization, and attire, including: • Communicated appropriately and comfortably with the patient				
7	Cleaned/disposed of supplies and equipment appropriately and washed hands.				
8	Documented correctly.				
Student's Total Points					
Points Possible					
Final Score (Student's Total Points/ Possible Points)					

Name ______________________________ Date ____________ Score ______

WORK DOCUMENTATION

Instructor's/Evaluator's Comments and Suggestions:

____

____

____

____

____

CHECK #1	
Evaluator's Signature:	Date:

CHECK #2	
Evaluator's Signature:	Date:

CHECK #3	
Evaluator's Signature:	Date:

ABHES Competency: VI.A.1.a.4.h Prepare patient for and assist physician with routine and specialty examinations and treatments and minor office surgeries

CAAHEP Curriculum: I.P.10 Assisting physician with patient care

Name ______________________________ Date ____________ Score ______

COMPETENCY ASSESSMENT

Procedure 18-18 Spirometry

Task: To test a patient's respiratory function.

Conditions: Spirometer, disposable mouthpiece

Standards: Perform the Task within 20 minutes with a minimum score of _____ points.

Work Documentation: Patient chart entry

No.	Step	Points	Check #1	Check #2	Check #3
1	Organized supplies and area for testing.				
2	Identified and greeted patient appropriately; washed hands.				
3	Prepared the patient and performed the test: • Explained the procedure. • Placed the patient in a comfortable position with instruction to loosen collar if appropriate. • Instructed the patient to not lean forward when blowing into the machine. • Reinforced the inhalation process. • Instructed the patient to continue blowing into the mouthpiece until instructed to stop or patient could not blow any longer. • Was supportive and encouraging throughout the test.				
4	Showed the results to the provider.				
5	Demonstrated professional behavior in manner, organization, and attire, including: • Communicated appropriately and comfortably with the patient.				
6	Cleaned/disposed of supplies and equipment appropriately and washed hands.				
7	Documented correctly.				
Student's Total Points					
Points Possible					
Final Score (Student's Total Points/ Possible Points)					

Name ______________________________ Date ____________ Score ______

WORK DOCUMENTATION

Instructor's/Evaluator's Comments and Suggestions:

____

____

____

____

____

CHECK #1
Evaluator's Signature: Date:

CHECK #2
Evaluator's Signature: Date:

CHECK #3
Evaluator's Signature: Date:

ABHES Competency: VI.A.1.a.4.ee Perform respiratory testing

CAAHEP Curriculum: I.P.10 Assisting physician with patient care

Name ______________________________ Date ____________ Score ______

COMPETENCY ASSESSMENT

Procedure 18-19 Pulse Oximetry

Task: To measure arterial oxyhemoglobin saturation within seconds by using an external sensor.

Conditions: Pulse oximeter, sensor, soap and water, alcohol wipes, nail polish remover (as needed)

Standards: Perform the Task within 20 minutes with a minimum score of _____ points.

Work Documentation: Patient chart entry

No.	Step	Points	Check #1	Check #2	Check #3
1	Organized supplies and area for testing.				
2	Identified and greeted patient appropriately; washed hands.				
3	Prepared the patient for the test: • Explained the procedure to the patient. • Selected a site for the sensor, cleaned the site with alcohol (removed nail polish if needed).				
4	Performed the test: • Applied sensor, connected sensor to oximeter. • Turned sensor on and adjusted volume. • Set alarm for abnormal readings. • Checked pulse manually and compared with oximeter, noting results for quality control. • Notified provider of any abnormal results.				
5	Demonstrated professional behavior in manner, organization, and attire, including: • Communicated appropriately and comfortably with the patient.				
6	Cleaned/disposed of supplies and equipment appropriately and washed hands.				
7	Documented correctly.				
Student's Total Points					
Points Possible					
Final Score (Student's Total Points/ Possible Points)					

Name ______________________ **Date** ____________ **Score** ______

WORK DOCUMENTATION

Instructor's/Evaluator's Comments and Suggestions:

____

____

____

____

____

CHECK #1

Evaluator's Signature: Date:

CHECK #2

Evaluator's Signature: Date:

CHECK #3

Evaluator's Signature: Date:

ABHES Competency: VI.A.1.a.4.h Prepare patient for and assist physician with routine and specialty examinations and treatments and minor office surgeries

CAAHEP Curriculum: I.P.10 Assisting physician with patient care; I.P.11 Perform quality control measures

Name ______________________________ Date ____________ Score ______

COMPETENCY ASSESSMENT

Procedure 18-20 Assisting with Plaster Cast Application

Task: To assist with cast application.

Conditions: Plaster bandage rolls or synthetic cast rolls (for small arm cast, use two to three 2- or 3-inch rolls. For short leg cast, use two to three 3- to 4-inch rolls. For long leg cast, use three to four 4- to 6-inch rolls), container of warm water that is lined with plastic or cloth to catch loose plaster, stockinette (3-inch width for arms, 4- to 6-inch width for legs, etc.), Webril padding rolls, bandage scissors, gloves, walking heel if needed, lotion if using synthetic casting

Standards: Perform the Task within 25 minutes with a minimum score of _____ points.

Work Documentation: Patient chart entry

No.	Step	Points	Check #1	Check #2	Check #3
1	Organized supplies and room.				
2	Identified and greeted patient appropriately; washed hands.				
3	Correctly prepared the patient: • Explained the procedure to the patient. • Properly positioned patient for cast being applied. • Carefully cleaned and dried area to be casted. • Noted open wounds and reported these to the provider.				
4	Correctly assisted the provider: • Prepared stockinette appropriate for the area being casted. • Prepared Webril appropriate for the area being casted. • Assisted provider and patient during the procedure.				
5	After cast application, cleaned patient's skin and provided oral and written instructions to the patient.				
6	Demonstrated professional behavior in manner, organization, and attire, including: • Communicated appropriately and comfortably with the patient and provider.				

No.	Step	Points	Check #1	Check #2	Check #3
7	Cleaned/disposed of supplies and equipment appropriately and washed hands.				
8	Documented correctly.				
Student's Total Points					
Points Possible					
Final Score (Student's Total Points/ Possible Points)					

Name ______________________________ Date ____________ Score ______

WORK DOCUMENTATION

Instructor's/Evaluator's Comments and Suggestions:

____

____

____

____

____

CHECK #1

Evaluator's Signature: Date:

CHECK #2

Evaluator's Signature: Date:

CHECK #3

Evaluator's Signature: Date:

ABHES Competency: VI.A.1.a.4.h Prepare patient for and assist physician with routine and specialty examinations and treatments and minor office surgeries

CAAHEP Curriculum: I.P.10 Assisting physician with patient care

Name ______________________________ Date ____________ Score ______

COMPETENCY ASSESSMENT

Procedure 18-21 Assisting with Cast Removal

Task: To assist with cast removal.

Conditions: Cast removal saw, cast spreader, cast scissors, patient drape

Standards: Perform the Task within 20 minutes with a minimum score of _____ points.

Work Documentation: Patient chart entry

No.	Step	Points	Check #1	Check #2	Check #3
1	Organized supplies and area.				
2	Identified and greeted patient appropriately; washed hands.				
3	Correctly prepared the patient: • Explained the procedure to the patient. • Reassured the patient. • Properly positioned patient for cast being removed.				
4	Removed the cast properly or assisted the provider as needed. Handed provider equipment as requested.				
5	After cast removal, helped clean patient's skin and provided oral and written instructions to the patient.				
6	Demonstrated professional behavior in manner, organization, and attire, including: • Communicated appropriately and comfortably with the patient and provider.				
7	Cleaned/disposed of supplies and equipment appropriately and washed hands.				
8	Documented correctly.				
Student's Total Points					
Points Possible					
Final Score (Student's Total Points/ Possible Points)					

Name ______________________________ **Date** ____________ **Score** ______

WORK DOCUMENTATION

Instructor's/Evaluator's Comments and Suggestions:

____

____

____

____

____

CHECK #1

Evaluator's Signature: Date:

CHECK #2

Evaluator's Signature: Date:

CHECK #3

Evaluator's Signature: Date:

ABHES Competency: VI.A.1.a.4.h Prepare patient for and assist physician with routine and specialty examinations and treatments and minor office surgeries

CAAHEP Curriculum: I.P.10 Assisting physician with patient care

Name ______________________ Date __________ Score ______

COMPETENCY ASSESSMENT

Procedure 18-22 Assisting the Physician during a Lumbar Puncture or Cerebrospinal Fluid Aspiration

Task: To position the patient and assist with removal of cerebrospinal fluid (CSF).

Conditions: Patient drape; Xylocaine 1–2%; syringe and needle for anesthetic; sterile gloves; disposable sterile lumbar puncture tray to include: skin antiseptic with applicator, adhesive bandage, spinal puncture needle, three to four test tubes with secure tops, laboratory requisition, specimen transport bag, patient gown and drape, manometer, laboratory requisition, examination light, gauze sponges

Standards: Perform the Task within 30 minutes with a minimum score of _____ points.

Work Documentation: Patient chart entry, laboratory requisition

No.	Step	Points	Check #1	Check #2	Check #3
1	Organized supplies and area for procedure.				
2	Identified and greeted patient appropriately; washed hands.				
3	Correctly prepared the patient: • Explained the procedure to the patient. • Instructed patient to empty bladder, bowel. • Verified that the patient signed a consent form. • Instructed patient to undress and gown; covered patient with additional drape. • Positioned patient on edge of table. • Applied gloves and cleansed puncture site. • Positioned patient in fetal position.				
4	Assisted the provider and patient during the procedure as needed: • Assisted the provider to aspirate anesthetic. • Helped the patient maintain position until needle was inserted into spinal canal. • Reminded patient to breathe evenly. • At the provider's direction, instructed patient to straighten the legs. • Assisted the physician in collecting CSF as needed. • When the puncture was completed, assisted the provider in applying dressing to the puncture site.				

No.	Step	Points	Check #1	Check #2	Check #3
5	Repositioned the patient into prone position for 2–3 hours, and had the patient drink fluids as directed.				
6	Applied gloves and labeled the specimens, put into transfer bag, and completed lab requisition.				
7	Demonstrated professional behavior in manner, organization, and attire, including: • Communicated appropriately and comfortably with the patient and provider.				
8	Cleaned/disposed of supplies and equipment appropriately and washed hands.				
9	Documented correctly.				
Student's Total Points					
Points Possible					
Final Score (Student's Total Points/ Possible Points)					

Name ______________________ Date __________ Score ______

WORK DOCUMENTATION

Instructor's/Evaluator's Comments and Suggestions:

____

____

____

____

____

CHECK #1	
Evaluator's Signature:	Date:

CHECK #2	
Evaluator's Signature:	Date:

CHECK #3	
Evaluator's Signature:	Date:

ABHES Competency: VI.A.1.a.4.h Prepare patient for and assist physician with routine and specialty examinations and treatments and minor office surgeries

CAAHEP Curriculum: I.P.10 Assisting physician with patient care

Name ______________________________ Date ____________ Score ______

COMPETENCY ASSESSMENT

Procedure 18-23 Assisting the Provider with a Neurologic Screening Examination

Task: To determine a patient's neurologic status.

Conditions: Percussion hammer, safety pin or sensory wheel, material for odor identification, cotton ball, tuning fork, flashlight, tongue blade, ophthalmoscope

Standards: Perform the Task within 20 minutes with a minimum score of _____ points.

Work Documentation: Patient chart entry

No.	Step	Points	Check #1	Check #2	Check #3
1	Organized supplies and area for procedure.				
2	Identified and greeted patient appropriately; washed hands.				
3	While taking patient's medical history, observed level of awareness, memory, cognition, and mood.				
4	Assisted the provider as needed during examination.				
5	Demonstrated professional behavior in manner, organization, and attire, including: • Communicated appropriately and comfortably with the patient and provider.				
6	Cleaned/disposed of supplies and equipment appropriately and washed hands.				
7	Documented correctly.				
Student's Total Points					
Points Possible					
Final Score (Student's Total Points/ Possible Points)					

Name ______________________________ **Date** ____________ **Score** ______

WORK DOCUMENTATION

Instructor's/Evaluator's Comments and Suggestions:

____

____

____

____

____

CHECK #1	
Evaluator's Signature:	Date:

CHECK #2	
Evaluator's Signature:	Date:

CHECK #3	
Evaluator's Signature:	Date:

ABHES Competency: VI.A.1.a.4.h Prepare patient for and assist physician with routine and specialty examinations and treatments and minor office surgeries

CAAHEP Curriculum: I.P.10 Assisting physician with patient care

Name ______________________________ Date ____________ Score ______

COMPETENCY ASSESSMENT

Procedure 19-1 Applying Sterile Gloves

Task: Applying sterile gloves.

Conditions: Packaged pair of sterile gloves of appropriate size and a flat, clean, dry surface

Standards: Perform the Task within 10 minutes with a minimum score of _____ points.

No.	Step	Points	Check #1	Check #2	Check #3
1	Removed ring(s) and watch and washed hands.				
2	Selected proper glove size and type, inspected package, and placed on a clean, dry, flat surface above waist level.				
3	Opened package properly: • Peeled open outer package. • Positioned inner package properly. • Opened inner package with care not to contaminate. • Determined that gloves were in position or adjusted.				
4	Applied both gloves properly without contamination.				
Student's Total Points					
Points Possible					
Final Score (Student's Total Points/ Possible Points)					

Name ______________________ **Date** ____________ **Score** ______

Instructor's/Evaluator's Comments and Suggestions:

____

____

____

____

____

CHECK #1	
Evaluator's Signature:	Date:

CHECK #2	
Evaluator's Signature:	Date:

CHECK #3	
Evaluator's Signature:	Date:

ABHES Competency: VI.A.1.a.4.c Apply principles of aseptic techniques and infection control

CAAHEP Curriculum: III.P.3 Select appropriate barrier/personal protective equipment (PPE) for potentially infectious situations

Name ______________________ Date ____________ Score ______

COMPETENCY ASSESSMENT

Procedure 19-2 Chemical "Cold" Sterilization of Endoscopes

Task: To sterilize heat-sensitive items such as fiber-optic endoscopes, using chemical solution.

Conditions: Chemical solution, timer, sterile water, airtight container, heavy-duty gloves, sterile towels, poly-lined sterile drapes

Standards: Perform the Task within 30 minutes with a minimum score of _____ points.

No.	Step	Points	Check #1	Check #2	Check #3
1	Sanitized and dried instrument/scope following manufacturer's instructions.				
2	Read manufacturer's instructions regarding use of sterilizing chemicals.				
3	Applied PPE.				
4	Prepared solution according to instructions. Recorded the solution and ratio. Poured solution into container with a tight-fitting lid.				
5	Placed scope into the solution, closed lid, timed properly.				
6	When time was up, prepared sterile field, applied PPE and sterile gloves, removed endoscope from solution, rinsed and applied to sterile tray without contaminating.				
Student's Total Points					
Points Possible					
Final Score (Student's Total Points/ Possible Points)					

Name ______________________ **Date** __________ **Score** ______

Instructor's/Evaluator's Comments and Suggestions:

____

____

____

____

____

CHECK #1

Evaluator's Signature: Date:

CHECK #2

Evaluator's Signature: Date:

CHECK #3

Evaluator's Signature: Date:

ABHES Competency: VI.A.1.a.4.p Perform sterilization techniques

CAAHEP Curriculum: III.P.3 Select appropriate barrier/personal protective equipment (PPE) for potentially infectious situations; III.P.6 Perform sterilization procedures

Name ______________________________ Date __________ Score ______

COMPETENCY ASSESSMENT

Procedure 19-3 Preparing Instruments for Sterilization in Autoclave

Task: To properly wrap sanitized instruments for sterilization in an autoclave.

Conditions: Sanitized instruments, wrapping materials (muslin, disposable wrapping paper), sterilization indicators, 2 × 2 gauze (if instrument has hinges), autoclave wrapping tape, tip protectors as indicated, marking pen for labeling

Standards: Perform the Task within 10 minutes with a minimum score of _____ points.

No.	Step	Points	Check #1	Check #2	Check #3
1	Washed hands. Prepared a clean, dry, flat surface of adequate size to lay the wrapping material on.				
2	Selected appropriate size and type of wrap.				
3	Wrapped first layer properly so it was snug and neat. Included sterilization indicator, tip protectors, and gauze as appropriate.				
4	Wrapped second layer properly so it was snug and neat.				
5	Taped package closed and labeled properly.				
Student's Total Points					
Points Possible					
Final Score (Student's Total Points/ Possible Points)					

Name ______________________________ **Date** ____________ **Score** ______

Instructor's/Evaluator's Comments and Suggestions:

____

____

____

____

____

CHECK #1	
Evaluator's Signature:	Date:

CHECK #2	
Evaluator's Signature:	Date:

CHECK #3	
Evaluator's Signature:	Date:

ABHES Competency: VI.A.1.a.4.o Wrap items for autoclaving

CAAHEP Curriculum: III.P.5 Prepare items for autoclaving

Name ______________________________ Date ____________ Score ______

COMPETENCY ASSESSMENT

Procedure 19-4 Sterilization of Instruments (Autoclave)

Task: To rid instruments of all forms of microbial (microorganism) life for use in invasive procedures.

Conditions: Steam sterilizer (autoclave), autoclave manufacturer procedure manual, wrapped sanitized instrument package(s) with sterilization indicators placed inside the package (or unwrapped item, if removed with sterile transfer forceps)

Standards: Perform the Task within 45 minutes with a minimum score of _____ points.

No.	Step	Points	Check #1	Check #2	Check #3
1	Washed hands. Checked water level in autoclave, and added distilled water, if necessary.				
2	Loaded packages into autoclave properly.				
3	Sealed door, turned on autoclave, and set proper time.				
4	When cycle completed, turned off autoclave and allowed instruments to cool before removing.				
5	When cooled, removed wrapped contents with dry, clean hands and stored in clean, dry, closed storage area.				
6	Removed unwrapped contents with sterile transfer forceps.				
Student's Total Points					
Points Possible					
Final Score (Student's Total Points/ Possible Points)					

Name ______________________ **Date** ____________ **Score** ______

Instructor's/Evaluator's Comments and Suggestions:

____

____

____

____

____

CHECK #1

Evaluator's Signature: Date:

CHECK #2

Evaluator's Signature: Date:

CHECK #3

Evaluator's Signature: Date:

ABHES Competency: VI.A.1.a.4.p Perform sterilization techniques

CAAHEP Curriculum: III.P.6 Perform sterilization procedures

Name ______________________________ Date ____________ Score ______

COMPETENCY ASSESSMENT

Procedure 19-5 Setting Up and Covering a Sterile Field

Task: To lay a sterile field onto a Mayo tray suitable for surgery or a sterile procedure, and to cover the sterile tray with another sterile drape.

Conditions: Disposable sterile poly-lined field drapes or sterile towels (two), Mayo instrument tray/stand positioned above the waist with stem to the right, at right angle to the counter

Standards: Perform the Task within 15 minutes with a minimum score of _____ points.

No.	Step	Points	Check #1	Check #2	Check #3
1	Washed hands.				
2	Sanitized and disinfected a Mayo instrument tray. Positioned tray above waist level with the stem to the right.				
3	Set up sterile field onto tray without contaminating it.				
4	Applied instruments and supplies properly without contamination, was able to problem-solve as needed.				
5	Covered tray using proper sterile technique.				
Student's Total Points					
Points Possible					
Final Score (Student's Total Points/ Possible Points)					

Name ______________________________ **Date** ____________ **Score** ______

Instructor's/Evaluator's Comments and Suggestions:

____

____

____

____

____

CHECK #1

Evaluator's Signature: Date:

CHECK #2

Evaluator's Signature: Date:

CHECK #3

Evaluator's Signature: Date:

ABHES Competency: VI.A.1.a.4.g Prepare and maintain examination and treatment area

Name ______________________________ Date ____________ Score ______

COMPETENCY ASSESSMENT

Procedure 19-6 Opening Sterile Packages of Instruments and Supplies and Applying Them to a Sterile Field

Task: To open sterile packages of surgical instruments and supplies and place them onto a sterile field using sterile technique.

Conditions: Mayo instrument tray draped with a sterile field, sterile gloves, wrapped-twice sterile surgical instruments, prepackaged sterile surgical supplies

Standards: Perform the Task within 20 minutes with a minimum score of _____ points.

No.	Step	Points	Check #1	Check #2	Check #3
1	Washed hands and assembled supplies.				
2	Set up sterile tray correctly.				
3	Properly opened packages without contaminating contents.				
4	Transferred sterile instruments and supplies to sterile tray using sterile technique.				
5	Applied sterile gloves and arranged instruments and supplies on the tray in an organized and logical manner according to the provider's preference.				
6	Applied the sterile cover (as described in Procedure 19-5).				
Student's Total Points					
Points Possible					
Final Score (Student's Total Points/ Possible Points)					

Name ______________________________ **Date** __________ **Score** ______

Instructor's/Evaluator's Comments and Suggestions:

____

____

____

____

____

CHECK #1	
Evaluator's Signature:	Date:

CHECK #2	
Evaluator's Signature:	Date:

CHECK #3	
Evaluator's Signature:	Date:

ABHES Competency: VI.A.1.a.4.g Prepare and maintain examination and treatment area

Name ______________________________ Date ____________ Score ________

COMPETENCY ASSESSMENT

Procedure 19-7 Pouring a Sterile Solution into a Cup on a Sterile Field

Task: To pour a sterile solution into a cup on a sterile tray in a sterile manner.

Conditions: Covered sterile surgical tray with a sterile cup in upper right corner, container of sterile scrub solution (as ordered)

Standards: Perform the Task within 5 minutes with a minimum score of _____ points.

No.	Step	Points	Check #1	Check #2	Check #3
1	Washed hands.				
2	Selected the appropriate solution, read the label of the solution container two times, and checked expiration date.				
3	Transported the covered surgical tray to the surgical area before pouring solution.				
4	Read the label again just before pouring to ensure accuracy. Palmed the label and handled the cap properly.				
5	Exposed the cup and poured the solution without splashing or contaminating the sterile field.				
Student's Total Points					
Points Possible					
Final Score (Student's Total Points/ Possible Points)					

Name ______________________ **Date** ____________ **Score** ______

Instructor's/Evaluator's Comments and Suggestions:

____

____

____

____

____

CHECK #1	
Evaluator's Signature:	Date:

CHECK #2	
Evaluator's Signature:	Date:

CHECK #3	
Evaluator's Signature:	Date:

ABHES Competency: VI.A.1.a.4.g Prepare and maintain examination and treatment area

Name ______________________________ Date ____________ Score ______

COMPETENCY ASSESSMENT

Procedure 19-8 Assisting with Office/Ambulatory Surgery

Task: To maintain sterility while assisting with office surgery.

Conditions: *On Mayo stand:* sterile field and cover drapes (two), gauze sponges, scalpel (handle and blade), operating scissors, thumb forceps, hemostats (curved and straight), dressing forceps, suture pack, needle holder, skin retractor, transfer forceps. *May be on sterile field or on the side (provider preference):* fenestrated drape, needles and syringe for anesthesia, prep bowl/cup, Betadine® solution. *On counter or side table:* sterile gloves in package, labeled biopsy containers with formalin, laboratory requisition, anesthesia vial, alcohol wipes, dressings, tape, bandages, biohazard container, extra gauze in sterile package

Standards: Perform the Task within 30 minutes with a minimum score of _____ points.

Work Documentation: Laboratory requisition (if appropriate)

No.	Step	Points	Check #1	Check #2	Check #3
1	Checked room for equipment, readiness, cleanliness, and washed hands.				
2	Set up side table or counter for nonsterile items.				
3	Performed surgical asepsis hand washing and applied appropriate PPE.				
4	Set up sterile surgical tray.				
5	Prepared the patient: • Greeted and identified patient, introduced self, and explained the procedure. • Checked for signed informed consent form. • Identified health concerns, allergies, tetanus status, possible complications, and current medications. • Positioned and prepped the patient.				
6	Assisted the physician and patient as needed.				
7	Prepared lab specimens and requisitions as needed.				
8	Demonstrated professional behavior in manner, organization, and attire, including: • Communicatied appropriately and comfortably with the patient and provider.				

No.	Step	Points	Check #1	Check #2	Check #3
9	Cleaned/disposed of supplies and equipment appropriately and washed hands.				
Student's Total Points					
Points Possible					
Final Score (Student's Total Points/ Possible Points)					

Name ______________________ **Date** __________ **Score** ______

WORK DOCUMENTATION

*Also attach lab requisition.

Instructor's/Evaluator's Comments and Suggestions:

____

____

____

____

____

CHECK #1	
Evaluator's Signature:	Date:

CHECK #2	
Evaluator's Signature:	Date:

CHECK #3	
Evaluator's Signature:	Date:

ABHES Competency: VI.A.1.a.4.g Prepare and maintain examination and treatment area; VI.A.1.a.4.h Prepare patient for and assist physician with routine and specialty examinations and treatments and minor office surgeries

CAAHEP Curriculum: I.P.10 Assist physician with patient care; III.P.4 Select appropriate barrier/personal protective equipment (PPE) for potentially infectious situations

Name ______________________________ Date ____________ Score ______

COMPETENCY ASSESSMENT

Procedure 19-9 Dressing Change

Task: To remove a wound dressing, clean the wound, and apply a dry, sterile dressing.

Conditions: *On the sterile field:* several sterile gauze sponges and other dressing material as needed, sterile bowl/cup with Betadine® solution or prepared sterile Betadine swab sticks, sterile dressing forceps, sterile sponge forceps. *On counter side area:* nonsterile gloves, sterile gloves in package, container of sterile water, sterile cotton-tipped applicators in package, sterile adhesive strips, antibacterial ointment/cream as ordered, tape, sponge forceps, bandage scissors, waterproof waste bag, biohazard waste container

Standards: Perform the Task within 20 minutes with a minimum score of _____ points.

Work Documentation: Patient chart entry

No.	Step	Points	Check #1	Check #2	Check #3
1	Checked provider's orders and washed hands.				
2	Prepared the supplies and room: • Prepared sterile field, added supplies using sterile technique. • Positioned a waterproof bag and biohazard container away from the sterile area. • Prepared Betadine® solution into sterile bowl or used swab sticks.				
3	Greeted and identified the patient, introduced self, and explained the procedure.				
4	Correctly removed old bandage and cleaned the wound: • Applied gloves. • Removed dressing and/or bandage, placing into biohazard container. • Assessed wound and noted any drainage or signs of infection. • Cleaned the wound with antiseptic solution as ordered. • Applied topical medication as ordered.				
5	Correctly applied sterile dressing: • Removed gloves, washed hands, applied sterile gloves. • Applied sterile dressing and bandaging as appropriate. • Disposed of contaminated supplies properly, washed hands.				

No.	Step	Points	Check #1	Check #2	Check #3
6	Demonstrated professional behavior in manner, organization, and attire, including: • Communicated appropriately and comfortably with the patient.				
7	Cleaned/disposed of supplies and equipment appropriately and washed hands.				
8	Correctly documented the procedure.				
Student's Total Points					
Points Possible					
Final Score (Student's Total Points/ Possible Points)					

Name ______________________ Date __________ Score ______

WORK DOCUMENTATION

Instructor's/Evaluator's Comments and Suggestions:

____

____

____

____

____

CHECK #1
Evaluator's Signature: Date:

CHECK #2
Evaluator's Signature: Date:

CHECK #3
Evaluator's Signature: Date:

ABHES Competency: VI.A.1.a.4.h Prepare patient for and assist physician with routine and specialty examinations and treatments and minor office surgeries

CAAHEP Curriculum: I.P.10 Assist physician with patient care; III.P.4 Select appropriate barrier/personal protective equipment (PPE) for potentially infectious situations

Name ____________________ Date __________ Score ______

COMPETENCY ASSESSMENT

Procedure 19-10 Wound Irrigation

Task: To irrigate a wound to remove the accumulation of excessive exudates, which impair and delay healing.

Conditions: Sterile gloves, sterile irrigation kit, sterile dressing material, waterproof pad, sterile solution (according to doctor's orders), nonsterile gloves, waterproof waste bag

Standards: Perform the Task within 20 minutes with a minimum score of _____ points.

Work Documentation: Patient chart entry

No.	Step	Points	Check #1	Check #2	Check #3
1	Checked provider's order. Selected the appropriate solution, verifying expiration date.				
2	Greeted and identified the patient, introduced self. Explained the procedure.				
3	Washed hands.				
4	Removed old dressing properly: • Applied nonsterile gloves, removed the dressing, and disposed of it into waterproof waste bag. • Noted the wound's appearance, color, amount of discharge, and odor of discharge. • Removed and discarded gloves into biohazard container and washed hands, applied sterile gloves.				
5	Irrigated the wound properly: • Checked the irrigation solution order again, verifying amount and expiration date. • Maintained sterile technique. • Prepared the irrigation supplies. • Irrigated the wound. • Dried with sterile gauze. • Applied sterile dressing and bandage as appropriate.				
6	Demonstrated professional behavior in manner, organization, and attire, including: • Communicated appropriately and comfortably with the patient.				
7	Cleaned/disposed of supplies and equipment appropriately and washed hands.				
8	Correctly documented the procedure.				
Student's Total Points					
Points Possible					
Final Score (Student's Total Points/ Possible Points)					

Name ______________________________ **Date** ____________ **Score** ______

WORK DOCUMENTATION

Instructor's/Evaluator's Comments and Suggestions:

____

____

____

____

____

CHECK #1	
Evaluator's Signature:	Date:

CHECK #2	
Evaluator's Signature:	Date:

CHECK #3	
Evaluator's Signature:	Date:

ABHES Competency: VI.A.1.a.4.h Prepare patient for and assist physician with routine and specialty examinations and treatments and minor office surgeries

CAAHEP Curriculum: I.P.10 Assist physician with patient care; III.P.4 Select appropriate barrier/personal protective equipment (PPE) for potentially infectious situations

Name ______________________________ Date __________ Score ______

COMPETENCY ASSESSMENT

Procedure 19-11 Preparation of Patient's Skin before Surgery

Task: To remove as many microorganisms as possible from the patient's skin before surgery.

Conditions: Absorbent pad, sterile drapes (two), one fenestrated drape if doctor prefers, disposable skin prep kit (includes antiseptic soap, several sponges, razor, and a container for water), sterile water, antiseptic solution (as ordered), sterile bowl, sterile gloves (two pair)

Standards: Perform the Task within 20 minutes with a minimum score of _____ points.

No.	Step	Points	Check #1	Check #2	Check #3
1	Assembled supplies and washed hands.				
2	Greeted and identified the patient, introduced self, explained the procedure, and checked for signed informed consent.				
3	Positioned patient for comfort and access to site. Laid protective absorbent pad under site. Provided good lighting.				
4	Washed hands and applied sterile gloves.				
5	Applied antiseptic soap with gauze sponges, beginning in center of operative site and moving in concentric circles outward. Shaved hair as indicated, washed skin again, rinsed and dried area using sterile technique.				
6	Removed and discarded absorbent pad, gauze sponges, disposable prep kit, and gloves. Washed hands again.				
7	Using sterile technique, placed sterile towel/drape under operative site. Covered site with another sterile drape. Instructed the patient not to touch the area. Explained rationale.				
8	Poured antiseptic solution into bowl for provider to apply with sterile gauze. Used fenestrated drape according to provider's preference.				
9	Demonstrated professional behavior in manner, organization, and attire, including: • Communicated appropriately and comfortably with the patient.				
Student's Total Points					
Points Possible					
Final Score (Student's Total Points/ Possible Points)					

Name ______________________________ **Date** ____________ **Score** ______

Instructor's/Evaluator's Comments and Suggestions:

____

____

____

____

____

CHECK #1

Evaluator's Signature: Date:

CHECK #2

Evaluator's Signature: Date:

CHECK #3

Evaluator's Signature: Date:

ABHES Competency: VI.A.1.a.4.h Prepare patient for and assist physician with routine and specialty examinations and treatments and minor office surgeries

CAAHEP Curriculum: I.P.10 Assist physician with patient care

Name ______________________ **Date** ____________ **Score** _______

COMPETENCY ASSESSMENT

Procedure 19-12 Suturing of Laceration or Incision Repair

Task: To set up and assist with the procedure of suturing a wound.

Conditions: *On the sterile tray:* syringe and needle for anesthetic, hemostats (curved), Adson with teeth or thumb tissue forceps, needle holder with cutting edge or plain needle holder and curved iris scissors, suture pack (suture material and needle, sized and typed according to provider's preference), gauze sponges. *On the counter:* anesthetic as ordered by the physician, dressings, bandages, tape, splint/brace/sling (optional), sterile gloves in package

Standards: Perform the Task within 30 minutes with a minimum score of _____ points.

Work Documentation: Patient chart entry

No.	Step	Points	Check #1	Check #2	Check #3
1	Assembled the supplies and washed hands.				
2	Greeted and identified the patient, introduced self, explained the procedure, checked for signed informed consent form.				
3	Prepared the patient for the procedure: • Identified known allergies, tetanus status, health concerns. • Positioned patient for comfort and safety and accessed the site. • Reassured the patient as needed. • Assessed the cause of wound and severity. • Soaked or irrigated wound in antiseptic solution as ordered. • Cleaned and dried wound.				
4	Assisted the provider and patient as needed.				
5	Provided post-op care: • Applied sterile gloves. • Cleaned area around the wound and dried the wound. • Dressed/bandaged/splinted the area, following provider's orders. • Removed gloves and washed hands. • Checked patient's color and blood pressure. • Gave wound care instructions, both orally and written, symptoms of infection, after-hours phone numbers. • Assisted the patient with concerns and questions. • Arranged for follow-up care, medications, and scheduled return appointment.				

No.	Step	Points	Check #1	Check #2	Check #3
6	Demonstrated professional behavior in manner, organization, and attire, including: • Communicated appropriately and comfortably with the patient.				
7	Cleaned/disposed of supplies and equipment appropriately and washed hands.				
8	Correctly documented the procedure.				
Student's Total Points					
Points Possible					
Final Score (Student's Total Points/ Possible Points)					

Name ______________________ **Date** __________ **Score** ______

WORK DOCUMENTATION

Instructor's/Evaluator's Comments and Suggestions:

____

____

____

____

____

CHECK #1

Evaluator's Signature: Date:

CHECK #2

Evaluator's Signature: Date:

CHECK #3

Evaluator's Signature: Date:

ABHES Competency: VI.A.1.a.4.h Prepare patient for and assist physician with routine and specialty examinations and treatments and minor office surgeries

CAAHEP Curriculum: I.P.10 Assist physician with patient care

Name ______________________________ **Date** ____________ **Score** ______

COMPETENCY ASSESSMENT

Procedure 19-13 Sebaceous Cyst Excision

Task: To remove an inflamed or infected sebaceous cyst or to remove a sebaceous cyst that is not inflamed or infected but is located on an area of the body where the cyst is unsightly or where it may become irritated from rubbing.

Conditions: *On the sterile field:* syringe and needle for anesthesia, iris scissors (curved), mosquito hemostat (curved), scalpel blade and handle, tissue forceps (two), suture material with needle, needle holder, Mayo scissors (curved). *On the counter:* skin prep supplies, extra sterile gauze (in package), fenestrated drape in package, antiseptic solution as ordered, gloves (sterile in package and nonsterile), personal protective equipment, anesthesia as directed, sterile dressing in package, bandages, tape, biohazard waste container, alcohol pledgets, sterile culture tube, requisition and transport bag (optional), wicking material (optional)

Standards: Perform the Task within 30 minutes with a minimum score of _____ points.

Work Documentation: Patient chart entry, lab requisition

No.	Step	Points	Check #1	Check #2	Check #3
1	Washed hands, assembled the supplies, and set up the sterile tray.				
2	Greeted and identified the patient, introduced self, explained the procedure, and checked for signed informed consent form.				
3	Prepared the patient for the procedure: • Identified known allergies, tetanus status, health concerns. • Positioned patient for comfort and safety and accessed the site. • Applied PPE and prepared the patient's skin as directed.				
4	Assisted the provider during the procedure: • Assisted with drawing up anesthesia as needed. • Blotted surgical site as needed. • Handed and received supplies and equipment as directed. • Supported the patient during surgery. • Prepared lab specimen and requisition as directed.				

No.	Step	Points	Check #1	Check #2	Check #3
5	Provided post-op care: • Applied sterile gloves. • Cleaned area around the wound and dried the wound. • Dressed and bandaged the wound. • Removed gloves and washed hands. • Checked patient's color and blood pressure. • Gave wound care instructions, both orally and written, symptoms of infection, after-hours phone numbers. • Assisted the patient with concerns and questions. • Arranged for follow-up care, medications, and scheduled return appointment.				
6	Demonstrated professional behavior in manner, organization, and attire, including: • Communicated appropriately and comfortably with the patient.				
7	Cleaned/disposed of supplies and equipment appropriately and washed hands.				
8	Correctly documented the procedure.				
Student's Total Points					
Points Possible					
Final Score (Student's Total Points/ Possible Points)					

Name ______________________________ **Date** ____________ **Score** ______

WORK DOCUMENTATION

*Also attach lab requisition.

Instructor's/Evaluator's Comments and Suggestions:

____

____

____

____

____

CHECK #1	
Evaluator's Signature:	Date:

CHECK #2	
Evaluator's Signature:	Date:

CHECK #3	
Evaluator's Signature:	Date:

ABHES Competency: VI.A.1.a.4.h Prepare patient for and assist physician with routine and specialty examinations and treatments and minor office surgeries

CAAHEP Curriculum: I.P.10 Assist physician with patient care

Name ______________________________ Date ____________ Score ______

COMPETENCY ASSESSMENT

Procedure 19-14 Incision and Drainage of Localized Infection

Task: To assist with the incision and drainage of an abscess (localized infection).

Conditions: *On sterile tray:* syringe/needle for anesthesia; instruments as determined by physician: scalpel blade and handle, tissue forceps (two), thumb dressing forceps, Mayo scissors (curved), iris scissors (curved), mosquito hemostat (curved), gauze sponges (many), fenestrated drape, antiseptic solution in sterile cup. *On side area:* skin prep supplies, gloves (sterile unopened and nonsterile), personal protective equipment (PPE), anesthesia as directed, sterile dressing unopened, bandages, tape, culture container, requisition
and transport bag (optional), biohazard waste container, extra gauze sponges unopened, iodoform gauze wicking, alcohol pledgets, antiseptic solution

Standards: Perform the Task within 30 minutes with a minimum score of _____ points.

Work Documentation: Patient chart entry, lab requisition

No.	Step	Points	Check #1	Check #2	Check #3
1	Washed hands, assembled the supplies, and set up the sterile tray.				
2	Greeted and identified the patient, introduced self, explained the procedure, and checked for signed informed consent form.				
3	Prepared the patient for the procedure: • Identified known allergies, tetanus status, health concerns. • Positioned patient for comfort and safety and accessed the site. • Applied PPE and prepared the patient's skin as directed.				
4	Assisted the provider during the procedure: • Assisted with drawing up anesthesia as needed. • Blotted surgical site as needed. • Handed and received supplies and equipment as directed. • Supported the patient during surgery. • Prepared lab specimen and requisition as directed.				

No.	Step	Points	Check #1	Check #2	Check #3
5	Provided post-op care: • Applied sterile gloves. • Cleaned area around the wound and dried the wound. • Dressed and bandaged the wound. • Removed gloves and washed hands. • Checked patient's color and blood pressure. • Gave wound care instructions, both orally and written, symptoms of infection, after-hours phone numbers. • Assisted the patient with concerns and questions. • Arranged for follow-up care, medications, and scheduled return appointment.				
6	Demonstrated professional behavior in manner, organization, and attire, including: • Communicated appropriately and comfortably with the patient.				
7	Cleaned/disposed of supplies and equipment appropriately and washed hands.				
8	Correctly documented the procedure.				
Student's Total Points					
Points Possible					
Final Score (Student's Total Points/ Possible Points)					

Name ______________________________ **Date** ____________ **Score** ______

WORK DOCUMENTATION

*Also attach lab requisition.

Instructor's/Evaluator's Comments and Suggestions:

CHECK #1

Evaluator's Signature: Date:

CHECK #2

Evaluator's Signature: Date:

CHECK #3

Evaluator's Signature: Date:

ABHES Competency: VI.A.1.a.4.h Prepare patient for and assist physician with routine and specialty examinations and treatments and minor office surgeries

CAAHEP Curriculum: I.P.10 Assist physician with patient care

Name ______________________________ Date ____________ Score ______

COMPETENCY ASSESSMENT

Procedure 19-15 Aspiration of Joint Fluid

Task: To remove excess synovial fluid from a joint after injury.

Conditions: *On surgical field:* syringe/needle for anesthesia (size and gauge as directed), syringe/needle for drainage (size and gauge as directed), sturdy hemostat or needle driver (to remove needle from syringe), gauze sponges (many, sterile), sterile basin for aspirated fluid, fenestrated drape (optional). *On side counter:* skin prep supplies, gloves (sterile, in package and nonsterile), personal protective equipment (PPE), anesthesia as directed, cortisone medication as directed, culture tube, specimen container, pathology requisition, biohazard specimen transfer bag, alcohol swabs, dressings, bandages, tape, biohazard waste container

Standards: Perform the Task within 30 minutes with a minimum score of _____ points.

Work Documentation: Patient chart entry, lab requisition

No.	Step	Points	Check #1	Check #2	Check #3
1	Washed hands, assembled the supplies, and set up the sterile tray.				
2	Greeted and identified the patient, introduced self, explained the procedure, and checked for signed informed consent form.				
3	Prepared the patient for the procedure: • Identified known allergies, tetanus status, health concerns. • Positioned patient for comfort and safety and accessed the site. • Applied PPE and prepared the patient's skin as directed.				
4	Assisted the provider during the procedure: • Assisted with drawing up anesthesia as needed. • Blotted surgical site as needed. • Handed and received supplies and equipment as directed. • Supported the patient during surgery. • Prepared lab specimen and requisition as directed.				

No.	Step	Points	Check #1	Check #2	Check #3
5	Provided post-op care: • Applied sterile gloves. • Cleaned area around the wound and dried the wound. • Dressed and bandaged the wound. • Removed gloves and washed hands. • Checked patient's color and blood pressure. • Gave wound care instructions, both orally and written, symptoms of infection, after-hours phone numbers. • Assisted the patient with concerns and questions. • Arranged for follow-up care, medications, and scheduled return appointment.				
6	Demonstrated professional behavior in manner, organization, and attire, including: • Communicated appropriately and comfortably with the patient.				
7	Cleaned/disposed of supplies and equipment appropriately and washed hands.				
8	Correctly documented the procedure.				
Student's Total Points					
Points Possible					
Final Score (Student's Total Points/ Possible Points)					

Name ______________________________ **Date** ____________ **Score** ______

WORK DOCUMENTATION

*Also attach lab requisition.

Instructor's/Evaluator's Comments and Suggestions:

____

____

____

____

____

CHECK #1

Evaluator's Signature: Date:

CHECK #2

Evaluator's Signature: Date:

CHECK #3

Evaluator's Signature: Date:

ABHES Competency: VI.A.1.a.4.h Prepare patient for and assist physician with routine and specialty examinations and treatments and minor office surgeries

CAAHEP Curriculum: I.P.10 Assist physician with patient care

Name ______________________________ Date ____________ Score ______

COMPETENCY ASSESSMENT

Procedure 19-16 Hemorrhoid Thrombectomy

Task: To incise inflamed hemorrhoids and remove thrombus. To remove hemorrhoids with laser, electrosurgery, cryosurgery, or banding.

Conditions: *On surgical field:* syringe/needle for anesthesia, mosquito hemostat (curved), sterile basin, gauze sponges, rubber bands (optional), fenestrated drape. *On side counter:* skin prep supplies, gloves (sterile in package and nonsterile), personal protective equipment (PPE), anesthesia as directed, biohazard waste container, extra gauze sponges, soft absorbent pad (similar to sanitary napkin), T-bandage (to hold pad in place)

Standards: Perform the Task within 30 minutes with a minimum score of _____ points.

Work Documentation: Patient chart entry

No.	Step	Points	Check #1	Check #2	Check #3
1	Washed hands, assembled the supplies, and set up the sterile tray.				
2	Greeted and identified the patient, introduced self, explained the procedure, and checked for signed informed consent form.				
3	Prepared the patient for the procedure: • Identified known allergies, tetanus status, health concerns. • Positioned the patient for comfort, safety, and access to the site. • Applied PPE and prepared the surgical site as directed.				
4	Assisted the provider during the procedure: • Assisted with drawing up anesthesia as needed. • Blotted surgical site as needed. • Handed and received supplies and equipment as directed. • Supported the patient during surgery. • Prepared lab specimen and requisition as directed.				

No.	Step	Points	Check #1	Check #2	Check #3
5	Provided post-op care: • Applied sterile gloves. • Cleaned area around the wound and dried the wound. • Applied absorbent pad as necessary. • Removed gloves and washed hands. • Checked patient's color and blood pressure. • Gave wound care instructions, both orally and written, symptoms of infection, after-hours phone numbers. • Assisted the patient with concerns and questions. • Arranged for follow-up care, medications, and scheduled return appointment.				
6	Demonstrated professional behavior in manner, organization, and attire, including: • Communicated appropriately and comfortably with the patient.				
7	Cleaned/disposed of supplies and equipment appropriately and washed hands.				
8	Correctly documented the procedure.				
Student's Total Points					
Points Possible					
Final Score (Student's Total Points/ Possible Points)					

Name ______________________ **Date** ____________ **Score** ______

WORK DOCUMENTATION

Instructor's/Evaluator's Comments and Suggestions:

____

____

____

____

____

CHECK #1	
Evaluator's Signature:	Date:

CHECK #2	
Evaluator's Signature:	Date:

CHECK #3	
Evaluator's Signature:	Date:

ABHES Competency: VI.A.1.a.4.h Prepare patient for and assist physician with routine and specialty examinations and treatments and minor office surgeries

CAAHEP Curriculum: I.P.10 Assist physician with patient care

Name ______________________________ Date ____________ Score ______

COMPETENCY ASSESSMENT

Procedure 19-17 Suture/Staple Removal

Task: To remove sutures or staples from a healed surgical wound.

Conditions: *To remove bandage:* bandage scissors, gloves. *To remove sutures/staples:* sterile gloves, suture/staple removal kit (suture scissors and thumb dressing forceps, or staple remover, and 4 × 4 pads) *To redress:* antibiotic cream if ordered, cotton-tipped applicators, gauze sponges, and tape or adhesive strip. *Clean up:* sharps container for staples, biohazard waste container

Standards: Perform the Task within 15 minutes with a minimum score of _____ points.

Work Documentation: Patient chart entry

No.	Step	Points	Check #1	Check #2	Check #3
1	Checked provider's orders, washed hands, assembled the supplies, set up the sterile field.				
2	Greeted and identified the patient, introduced self, explained the procedure, and positioned patient properly for comfort and safety.				
3	Performed the removal of all sutures and staples using proper technique.				
4	Cleaned and bandaged the wound, explained follow-up care as directed.				
5	Demonstrated professional behavior in manner, organization, and attire, including: • Communicated appropriately and comfortably with the patient.				
6	Cleaned/disposed of supplies and equipment appropriately and washed hands.				
7	Correctly documented the procedure.				
Student's Total Points					
Points Possible					
Final Score (Student's Total Points/ Possible Points)					

Name ______________________________ Date ____________ Score ______

WORK DOCUMENTATION

Instructor's/Evaluator's Comments and Suggestions:

____

____

____

____

____

CHECK #1	
Evaluator's Signature:	Date:

CHECK #2	
Evaluator's Signature:	Date:

CHECK #3	
Evaluator's Signature:	Date:

ABHES Competency: VI.A.1.a.4.h Prepare patient for and assist physician with routine and specialty examinations and treatments and minor office surgeries

CAAHEP Curriculum: I.P.10 Assist physician with patient care

Name ______________________________ **Date** ____________ **Score** _______

COMPETENCY ASSESSMENT

Procedure 19-18 Application of Sterile Adhesive Skin Closure Strips

Task: To approximate the edges of a wound after the removal of sutures. Sometimes used in lieu of sutures or to give additional support together with sutures.

Conditions: *On sterile field:* suture removal instruments and supplies (as indicated), sterile adhesive skin closure strips, iris scissors (straight), Adson dressing forceps, tincture of benzoin (optional), sterile cotton-tipped applicators (for tincture of benzoin). *On side area:* sterile gloves in package, dressings, bandages, tape

Standards: Perform the Task within 15 minutes with a minimum score of _____ points.

Work Documentation: Patient chart entry

No.	Step	Points	Check #1	Check #2	Check #3
1	Checked provider's orders, washed hands, assembled the supplies, set up the sterile field.				
2	Greeted and identified the patient, introduced self, explained the procedure, and positioned patient properly for comfort and safety.				
3	Applied sterile adhesive skin closure strips using proper technique.				
4	Cleaned and bandaged the wound, explained follow-up care as directed.				
5	Demonstrated professional behavior in manner, organization, and attire, including: • Communicated appropriately and comfortably with the patient.				
6	Cleaned/disposed of supplies and equipment appropriately and washed hands.				
7	Correctly documented the procedure.				
Student's Total Points					
Points Possible					
Final Score (Student's Total Points/ Possible Points)					

Name ________________________________ **Date** ____________ **Score** ______

WORK DOCUMENTATION

Instructor's/Evaluator's Comments and Suggestions:

____

____

____

____

____

CHECK #1	
Evaluator's Signature:	Date:

CHECK #2	
Evaluator's Signature:	Date:

CHECK #3	
Evaluator's Signature:	Date:

ABHES Competency: VI.A.1.a.4.h Prepare patient for and assist physician with routine and specialty examinations and treatments and minor office surgeries

CAAHEP Curriculum: I.P.10 Assist physician with patient care

Name ______________________________ Date ____________ Score ______

COMPETENCY ASSESSMENT

Procedure 21-1 Transferring Patient from Wheelchair to Examination Table

Task: To safely transfer a patient from a wheelchair to an examination table using a one-person transfer technique, and then using a two-person transfer technique.

Conditions: Wheelchair, examination table, gait belt, step stool with rubber tips and a handle for gripping

Standards: Perform the Task within 15 minutes with a minimum score of _____ points.

No.	Step	Points	Check #1	Check #2	Check #3
1	Checked provider's orders, checked room for cleanliness, equipment, and readiness, and washed hands.				
2	Greeted and identified the patient, introduced self, and explained the procedure.				
3	Transferred the patient correctly and safely by self.				
4	Transferred the patient correctly and safely with the assistance of another person.				
5	Demonstrated professional behavior in manner, organization, and attire, including: • Communicated appropriately and comfortably with the patient.				
Student's Total Points					
Points Possible					
Final Score (Student's Total Points/ Possible Points)					

Name ______________________ **Date** __________ **Score** ______

Instructor's/Evaluator's Comments and Suggestions:

____

____

____

____

____

CHECK #1

Evaluator's Signature: Date:

CHECK #2

Evaluator's Signature: Date:

CHECK #3

Evaluator's Signature: Date:

ABHES Competency: VI.A.1.a.4.h Prepare patient for and assist physician with routine and specialty examinations and treatments and minor office surgeries

CAAHEP Curriculum: XI.P.11 Use proper body mechanics

Name ______________________ Date __________ Score ______

COMPETENCY ASSESSMENT

Procedure 21-2 Transferring Patient from Examination Table to Wheelchair

Task: To safely transfer a patient from the examination table to a wheelchair.

Conditions: Wheelchair, examination table, gait belt, step stool with rubber tips and a handle for gripping

Standards: Perform the Task within 15 minutes with a minimum score of _____ points.

No.	Step	Points	Check #1	Check #2	Check #3
1	Checked provider's orders, checked room for cleanliness, equipment, and readiness, and washed hands.				
2	Greeted and identified the patient, introduced self, and explained the procedure.				
3	Transferred the patient correctly and safely by self.				
4	Transferred the patient correctly and safely with the assistance of another person.				
5	Demonstrated professional behavior in manner, organization, and attire, including: • Communicated appropriately and comfortably with the patient.				
Student's Total Points					
Points Possible					
Final Score (Student's Total Points/ Possible Points)					

Name ____________________ **Date** __________ **Score** ______

Instructor's/Evaluator's Comments and Suggestions:

CHECK #1

Evaluator's Signature: Date:

CHECK #2

Evaluator's Signature: Date:

CHECK #3

Evaluator's Signature: Date:

ABHES Competency: VI.A.1.a.4.h Prepare patient for and assist physician with routine and specialty examinations and treatments and minor office surgeries

CAAHEP Curriculum: XI.P.11 Use proper body mechanics

Name ______________________________ Date ____________ Score ______

COMPETENCY ASSESSMENT

Procedure 21-3 Assisting the Patient to Stand and Walk

Task: To help a patient ambulate safely.

Conditions: Gait belt, chair, or wheelchair

Standards: Perform the Task within 20 minutes with a minimum score of _____ points.

Work Documentation: Patient chart entry

No.	Step	Points	Check #1	Check #2	Check #3
1	Checked provider's orders, checked room for cleanliness, equipment, and readiness, and washed hands.				
2	Greeted and identified the patient, introduced self, and explained the procedure.				
3	Assisted the patient to stand and walk correctly and safely.				
4	Demonstrated professional behavior in manner, organization, and attire, including: • Communicated appropriately and comfortably with the patient.				
5	Documented the procedure correctly.				
Student's Total Points					
Points Possible					
Final Score (Student's Total Points/ Possible Points)					

Name ______________________________ **Date** ____________ **Score** ______

WORK DOCUMENTATION

Instructor's/Evaluator's Comments and Suggestions:

____

____

____

____

____

CHECK #1	
Evaluator's Signature:	Date:

CHECK #2	
Evaluator's Signature:	Date:

CHECK #3	
Evaluator's Signature:	Date:

ABHES Competency: VI.A.1.a.4.h Prepare patient for and assist physician with routine and specialty examinations and treatments and minor office surgeries

CAAHEP Curriculum: XI.P.11 Use proper body mechanics

Name ______________________________ Date ____________ Score ______

COMPETENCY ASSESSMENT

Procedure 21-4 Care of the Falling Patient

Task: To help a patient fall safely to avoid injury.

Conditions: Gait belt may already be on the patient.

Standards: Perform the Task within 5 minutes with a minimum score of _____ points.

Work Documentation: Patient chart entry, incident report

No.	Step	Points	Check #1	Check #2	Check #3
1	Assisted the patient to fall gently, safely, and without harm to either the patient or self.				
2	Alerted the provider for patient examination before further moving the fallen patient.				
3	Demonstrated professional behavior in manner, organization, and attire, including: • Communicated appropriately and comfortably with the patient.				
4	Documented correctly and completed an accident report per clinic policy.				
	Student's Total Points				
	Points Possible				
	Final Score (Student's Total Points/ Possible Points)				

Name ______________________________ Date ____________ Score ______

WORK DOCUMENTATION

*Also attach incident report.

Instructor's/Evaluator's Comments and Suggestions:

____

____

____

____

____

CHECK #1	
Evaluator's Signature:	Date:

CHECK #2	
Evaluator's Signature:	Date:

CHECK #3	
Evaluator's Signature:	Date:

ABHES Competency: VI.A.1.a.4.e Recognize emergencies; VI.A.1.a.5.a Determine needs for documentation and reporting; VI.A.1.a.5.h Perform risk management procedures

CAAHEP Curriculum: IX.P.6 Complete an incident report; XI.P.11 Use proper body mechanics

Name ______________________ Date ____________ Score ______

COMPETENCY ASSESSMENT

Procedure 21-5 Assisting a Patient to Ambulate with a Walker

Task: To help a patient to ambulate safely and independently with a walker.

Conditions: Gait belt, walker

Standards: Perform the Task within 20 minutes with a minimum score of _____ points.

Work Documentation: Patient chart entry

No.	Step	Points	Check #1	Check #2	Check #3
1	Checked provider's orders, checked area for cleanliness, equipment, and readiness, and washed hands.				
2	Greeted and identified the patient, introduced self, and explained the procedure.				
3	Assisted the patient to stand and walk correctly and safely using a walker. Demonstrated proper technique, then assisted the patient to follow the instructions. Provided the patient with written instructions.				
4	Demonstrated professional behavior in manner, organization, and attire, including: • Communicated appropriately and comfortably with the patient.				
5	Documented the procedure correctly.				
Student's Total Points					
Points Possible					
Final Score (Student's Total Points/ Possible Points)					

Name ______________________________ Date ____________ Score ______

WORK DOCUMENTATION

Instructor's/Evaluator's Comments and Suggestions:

____

____

____

____

____

CHECK #1	
Evaluator's Signature:	Date:

CHECK #2	
Evaluator's Signature:	Date:

CHECK #3	
Evaluator's Signature:	Date:

ABHES Competency: VI.A.1.a.7.b Instruct patients with special needs

CAAHEP Curriculum: IV.P.5 Instruct patients according to their needs to promote health maintenance and disease prevention

Name ______________________ Date ____________ Score ______

COMPETENCY ASSESSMENT

Procedure 21-6 Teaching the Patient to Ambulate with Crutches

Task: To help a patient to ambulate safely using crutches.

Conditions: Gait belt, crutches

Standards: Perform the Task within 20 minutes with a minimum score of _____ points.

Work Documentation: Patient chart entry

No.	Step	Points	Check #1	Check #2	Check #3
1	Checked provider's orders, checked area for cleanliness, equipment, and readiness, and washed hands.				
2	Greeted and identified the patient, introduced self, and explained the procedure.				
3	Assisted the patient to stand and walk correctly and safely using crutches. Demonstrated proper technique, then assisted the patient to follow the instructions. Provided the patient with written instructions.				
4	Demonstrated professional behavior in manner, organization, and attire, including: • Communicated appropriately and comfortably with the patient.				
5	Documented the procedure correctly.				
Student's Total Points					
Points Possible					
Final Score (Student's Total Points/ Possible Points)					

Name ______________________ **Date** ____________ **Score** ______

WORK DOCUMENTATION

Instructor's/Evaluator's Comments and Suggestions:

CHECK #1	
Evaluator's Signature:	Date:

CHECK #2	
Evaluator's Signature:	Date:

CHECK #3	
Evaluator's Signature:	Date:

ABHES Competency: VI.A.1.a.7.b Instruct patients with special needs

CAAHEP Curriculum: IV.P.5 Instruct patients according to their needs to promote health maintenance and disease prevention

Name ______________________ Date ____________ Score ______

COMPETENCY ASSESSMENT

Procedure 21-7 Assisting a Patient to Ambulate with a Cane

Task: To help a patient to ambulate safely with a cane.

Conditions: Gait belt, appropriate cane for patient

Standards: Perform the Task within 20 minutes with a minimum score of _____ points.

Work Documentation: Patient chart entry

No.	Step	Points	Check #1	Check #2	Check #3
1	Checked provider's orders, checked area for cleanliness, equipment, and readiness, and washed hands.				
2	Greeted and identified the patient, introduced self, and explained the procedure.				
3	Assisted the patient to stand and walk correctly and safely using crutches. Demonstrated proper technique, then assisted the patient to follow the instructions. Provided the patient with written instructions.				
4	Demonstrated professional behavior in manner, organization, and attire, including: • Communicated appropriately and comfortably with the patient.				
5	Documented the procedure correctly.				
Student's Total Points					
Points Possible					
Final Score (Student's Total Points/ Possible Points)					

Name ______________________________ **Date** ______________ **Score** ________

WORK DOCUMENTATION

Instructor's/Evaluator's Comments and Suggestions:

CHECK #1	
Evaluator's Signature:	Date:

CHECK #2	
Evaluator's Signature:	Date:

CHECK #3	
Evaluator's Signature:	Date:

ABHES Competency: VI.A.1.a.7.b Instruct patients with special needs

CAAHEP Curriculum: IV.P.5 Instruct patients according to their needs to promote health maintenance and disease prevention

Name ______________________________ Date ____________ Score ______

COMPETENCY ASSESSMENT

Procedure 22-1 Provide Instruction for Health Maintenance and Disease Prevention

Task: To instruct patients about how to exercise more responsibly and control their health in order to extend their lives and enjoy healthy years.

Conditions: Discussion, DVDs, videos, print material, authentic Web-based interactive information, community resources directories

Standards: Perform the Task within 20 minutes with a minimum score of _____ points.

Work Documentation: Patient chart entry

No.	Step	Points	Check #1	Check #2	Check #3
1	Checked provider's orders, gathered materials and supplies for education, and arranged for a quiet area.				
2	Greeted and identified the patient and introduced self.				
3	Discussed the patient education topic per the provider's orders.				
4	Reinforced discussion by giving patient written materials and resources.				
5	Demonstrated professional behavior in manner, organization, and attire, including: • Communicated appropriately and comfortably with the patient.				
6	Documented patient education session on the patient's chart.				
Student's Total Points					
Points Possible					
Final Score (Student's Total Points/ Possible Points)					

Name ______________________ **Date** ____________ **Score** ________

WORK DOCUMENTATION

Instructor's/Evaluator's Comments and Suggestions:

____

____

____

____

____

CHECK #1	
Evaluator's Signature:	Date:

CHECK #2	
Evaluator's Signature:	Date:

CHECK #3	
Evaluator's Signature:	Date:

ABHES Competency: VI.A.1.a.7.c Teach patients methods of health promotion and disease prevention

CAAHEP Curriculum: IV.P.5 Instruct patients according to their needs to promote health maintenance and disease prevention

Name ______________________________ **Date** ____________ **Score** ______

COMPETENCY ASSESSMENT

Procedure 23-1 Proper Disposal of Drugs

Task: To properly dispose of drugs that have reached their expiration dates.

Conditions: Drugs (oral and parenteral) that have reached their expiration dates

Standards: Perform the Task within 10 minutes with a minimum score of _____ points.

Work Documentation: Medication disposal log

No.	Step	Points	Check #1	Check #2	Check #3
1	Gathered all expired drugs.				
2	Properly disposed of the drugs per agency policy and state law.				
3	Documented instructions in the office log that the drugs with expired use-by dates were disposed of either by returning them to the pharmacy or by having the contracted agency incinerate them. Saved all receipts associated with disposal.				
Student's Total Points					
Points Possible					
Final Score (Student's Total Points/ Possible Points)					

Name ______________________ **Date** ____________ **Score** ______

WORK DOCUMENTATION

*Attach medication disposal log.

Instructor's/Evaluator's Comments and Suggestions:

____

____

____

____

____

CHECK #1	
Evaluator's Signature:	Date:

CHECK #2	
Evaluator's Signature:	Date:

CHECK #3	
Evaluator's Signature:	Date:

ABHES Competency: VI.A.1.a.5.e Dispose of controlled substances in compliance with government regulations

CAAHEP Curriculum: IX.P.8 Apply local, state and federal health care legislation and regulation appropriate to the medical assisting practice setting

Name ______________________________ Date ____________ Score ______

COMPETENCY ASSESSMENT

Procedure 24-1 Administration of Oral Medications

Task: To correctly administer an oral medication after receiving a physician's order.

Conditions: Patient chart, medication order from provider, medication, medicine tray, medicine cup, water

Standards: Perform the Task within 10 minutes with a minimum score of _____ points.

Work Documentation: Patient chart entry

No.	Step	Points	Check #1	Check #2	Check #3
1	Checked provider's orders; organized equipment and supplies; checked room for cleanliness, equipment, and readiness; washed hands.				
2	Correctly prepared the medication: • Selected the proper medication, checked the expiration date. • Calculated the proper dosage according to the provider's order. • Prepared the medication tray for transport to the exam room.				
3	Correctly prepared the patient: • Greeted and identified patient and introduced self. • Identified health concerns, allergies, tetanus status, possible complications, and current medications. • Positioned the patient appropriately and comfortably.				
4	Administered the medication correctly and safely: • Followed the six rights of medication administration. • Checked the medication order, dosage calculation, and expiration date again. • Gave the patient adequate water to swallow the medication.				
5	Demonstrated professional behavior in manner, organization, and attire, including: • Communicated appropriately and comfortably with the patient.				
6	Documented correctly and returned medication bottle to storage.				
Student's Total Points					
Points Possible					
Final Score (Student's Total Points/ Possible Points)					

Name ______________________ **Date** ____________ **Score** ______

WORK DOCUMENTATION

Instructor's/Evaluator's Comments and Suggestions:

____

____

____

____

____

CHECK #1

Evaluator's Signature: Date:

CHECK #2

Evaluator's Signature: Date:

CHECK #3

Evaluator's Signature: Date:

ABHES Competency: VI.A.1.a.4.m Prepare and administer oral and parenteral medications as directed by physician

CAAHEP Curriculum: I.P.8 Administer oral medications; II.P.1 Prepare proper dosages of medication for administration

Name ______________________________ Date __________ Score ______

COMPETENCY ASSESSMENT

Procedure 24-2 Withdrawing Medication from a Vial

Task: To correctly withdraw medication from a vial with 100% accuracy.

Conditions: Medication order by provider, vial of medication, medication note, appropriately sized safety syringe and needle, alcohol wipes, gloves, sharps container

Standards: Perform the Task within 5 minutes with a minimum score of _____ points.

No.	Step	Points	Check #1	Check #2	Check #3
1	Checked provider's orders; organized equipment and supplies; washed hands.				
2	Correctly prepared and withdrew the medication: • Selected the proper medication and checked the expiration date. • Calculated the proper dosage according to the provider's order. • Prepared the syringe and needle using sterile technique. • Prepped the vial properly. • Withdrew the appropriate amount of medication, releasing any bubbles, and recapped safely. • Changed needles according to office protocol.				
3	Performed the six rights of medication administration as appropriate.				
4	Demonstrated professional behavior in manner, organization, and attire.				
5	Documented correctly.				
Student's Total Points					
Points Possible					
Final Score (Student's Total Points/ Possible Points)					

Name ________________________ **Date** ____________ **Score** ______

Instructor's/Evaluator's Comments and Suggestions:

CHECK #1	
Evaluator's Signature:	Date:

CHECK #2	
Evaluator's Signature:	Date:

CHECK #3	
Evaluator's Signature:	Date:

ABHES Competency: VI.A.1.a.4.m Prepare and administer oral and parenteral medications as directed by physician

CAAHEP Curriculum: II.P.1 Prepare proper dosages of medication for administration

Name ______________________________ **Date** ____________ **Score** _______

COMPETENCY ASSESSMENT

Procedure 24-3 Withdrawing Medication from an Ampule

Task: To properly withdraw medication from an ampule with 100% accuracy.

Conditions: Medicine tray, medication order by physician, ampule of medication, medication note, appropriately sized safety syringe and filter needle and regular needle, antiseptic wipes (alcohol), sharps container

Standards: Perform the Task within 5 minutes with a minimum score of _____ points.

No.	Step	Points	Check #1	Check #2	Check #3
1	Checked provider's orders; organized equipment and supplies; washed hands.				
2	Correctly prepared and withdrew the medication: • Selected the proper medication and checked the expiration date. • Calculated the proper dosage according to the provider's order. • Prepared the syringe and needle using sterile technique. • Prepped the ampule properly. • Withdrew the appropriate amount of medication, releasing any bubbles and recapped safely. • Changed filter needle to a regular needle.				
3	Performed the six rights of medication administration as appropriate.				
4	Demonstrated professional behavior in manner, organization, and attire.				
5	Documented correctly.				
Student's Total Points					
Points Possible					
Final Score (Student's Total Points/ Possible Points)					

Name ______________________ **Date** ____________ **Score** ______

Instructor's/Evaluator's Comments and Suggestions:

____

____

____

____

____

CHECK #1	
Evaluator's Signature:	Date:

CHECK #2	
Evaluator's Signature:	Date:

CHECK #3	
Evaluator's Signature:	Date:

ABHES Competency: VI.A.1.a.4.m Prepare and administer oral and parenteral medications as directed by physician

CAAHEP Curriculum: II.P.1 Prepare proper dosages of medication for administration

Name ____________________ Date __________ Score ______

COMPETENCY ASSESSMENT

Procedure 24-4 Administration of Subcutaneous, Intramuscular, and Intradermal Injections

Task: To correctly administer subcutaneous, intramuscular, and intradermal injections with 100% accuracy.

Conditions: Medication order by provider, medication vial or ampule, medication note, appropriately sized safety needle-syringe unit, antiseptic (alcohol) wipes, gloves, cotton balls, adhesive strip, sharps container

Standards: Perform the Task within 10 minutes with a minimum score of _____ points.

Work Documentation: Patient chart entry

No.	Step	Points	Check #1	Check #2	Check #3
1	Checked provider's orders; organized equipment and supplies; checked room for cleanliness, equipment, and readiness; washed hands.				
2	Properly and accurately selected and withdrew the medication using all safety precautions.				
3	Correctly prepared the patient: • Greeted and identified patient and introduced self; explained procedure and checked for signed informed consent form. • Identified health concerns, allergies, tetanus status, possible complications, and current medications. • Positioned patient appropriately and comfortably. • Exposed, calculated, and prepped the appropriate site. • Reassured the patient as needed.				
4	Administered medication properly and safely: • Followed the six rights of medication administration. • Correctly administered medication. • Activated safety mechanism immediately and disposed of syringe/needle unit properly.				

No.	Step	Points	Check #1	Check #2	Check #3
5	Checked patient for adverse reactions, applied adhesive strip as needed, and instructed the patient about precautions to watch for as appropriate.				
6	Demonstrated professional behavior in manner, organization, and attire, including: • Communicated appropriately and comfortably with the patient.				
7	Documented correctly.				
Student's Total Points					
Points Possible					
Final Score (Student's Total Points/ Possible Points)					

Name ______________________________ Date ____________ Score ______

WORK DOCUMENTATION

Instructor's/Evaluator's Comments and Suggestions:

____

____

____

____

____

CHECK #1	
Evaluator's Signature:	Date:

CHECK #2	
Evaluator's Signature:	Date:

CHECK #3	
Evaluator's Signature:	Date:

ABHES Competency: VI.A.1.a.4.m Prepare and administer oral and parenteral medications as directed by physician

CAAHEP Curriculum: I.P.9 Administer parenteral (excluding IV) medications; II.P.1 Prepare proper dosages of medication for administration

Name ____________________ Date __________ Score ______

COMPETENCY ASSESSMENT

Procedure 24-5 Administering a Subcutaneous Injection

Task: To correctly administer a subcutaneous injection with 100% accuracy.

Conditions: Medication order by provider, medication vial or ampule, medication note, appropriately sized safety needle-syringe unit, antiseptic (alcohol) wipes, gloves, cotton balls, adhesive strip, sharps container

Standards: Perform the Task within 10 minutes with a minimum score of _____ points.

Work Documentation: Patient chart entry

No.	Step	Points	Check #1	Check #2	Check #3
1	Checked provider's orders; organized equipment and supplies; checked room for cleanliness, equipment, and readiness; washed hands.				
2	Properly and accurately selected and withdrew the medication using all safety precautions.				
3	Correctly prepared the patient: • Greeted and identified patient and introduced self; explained procedure and checked for signed informed consent form. • Identified health concerns, allergies, tetanus status, possible complications, and current medications. • Positioned patient appropriately and comfortably. • Exposed, calculated, and prepped the appropriate site. • Reassured the patient as needed.				
4	Administered medication properly and safely: • Followed the six rights of medication administration. • Correctly administered medication. • Activated safety mechanism immediately and disposed of syringe/needle unit properly.				
5	Checked patient for adverse reactions, applied adhesive strip as needed, and instructed the patient about precautions to watch for as appropriate.				

No.	Step	Points	Check #1	Check #2	Check #3
6	Demonstrated professional behavior in manner, organization, and attire, including: • Communicated appropriately and comfortably with the patient.				
7	Documented correctly.				
Student's Total Points					
Points Possible					
Final Score (Student's Total Points/ Possible Points)					

Name ______________________ **Date** ____________ **Score** ______

WORK DOCUMENTATION

Instructor's/Evaluator's Comments and Suggestions:

____

____

____

____

____

CHECK #1	
Evaluator's Signature:	Date:

CHECK #2	
Evaluator's Signature:	Date:

CHECK #3	
Evaluator's Signature:	Date:

ABHES Competency: VI.A.1.a.4.m Prepare and administer oral and parenteral medications as directed by physician

CAAHEP Curriculum: I.P.9 Administer parenteral (excluding IV) medications; II.P.1 Prepare proper dosages of medication for administration

Name ______________________ **Date** __________ **Score** ______

COMPETENCY ASSESSMENT

Procedure 24-6 Administering an Intramuscular Injection

Task: To correctly administer an intramuscular injection with 100% accuracy.

Conditions: Medication order by provider, medication vial or ampule, medication note, appropriately sized safety needle-syringe unit, antiseptic (alcohol) wipes, gloves, cotton balls, adhesive strip, sharps container

Standards: Perform the Task within 10 minutes with a minimum score of _____ points.

Work Documentation: Patient chart entry

No.	Step	Points	Check #1	Check #2	Check #3
1	Checked provider's orders; organized equipment and supplies; checked room for cleanliness, equipment, and readiness; washed hands.				
2	Properly and accurately selected and withdrew the medication using all safety precautions.				
3	Correctly prepared the patient: • Greeted and identified patient and introduced self; explained procedure and checked for signed informed consent form. • Identified health concerns, allergies, tetanus status, possible complications, and current medications. • Positioned patient appropriately and comfortably. • Exposed, calculated, and prepped the appropriate site. • Reassured the patient as needed.				
4	Administered medication properly and safely: • Followed the six rights of medication administration. • Correctly administered medication. • Activated safety mechanism immediately and disposed of syringe/needle unit properly.				
5	Checked patient for adverse reactions, applied adhesive strip as needed, and instructed the patient about precautions to watch for as appropriate.				

No.	Step	Points	Check #1	Check #2	Check #3
6	Demonstrated professional behavior in manner, organization, and attire, including: • Communicated appropriately and comfortably with the patient.				
7	Documented correctly.				
Student's Total Points					
Points Possible					
Final Score (Student's Total Points/ Possible Points)					

Name ______________________________ Date ____________ Score ______

WORK DOCUMENTATION

Instructor's/Evaluator's Comments and Suggestions:

____

____

____

____

____

CHECK #1	
Evaluator's Signature:	Date:

CHECK #2	
Evaluator's Signature:	Date:

CHECK #3	
Evaluator's Signature:	Date:

ABHES Competency: VI.A.1.a.4.m Prepare and administer oral and parenteral medications as directed by physician

CAAHEP Curriculum: I.P.9 Administer parenteral (excluding IV) medications; II.P.1 Prepare proper dosages of medication for administration

Name ______________________ Date __________ Score ______

COMPETENCY ASSESSMENT

Procedure 24-7 Administering an Intradermal Injection of Purified Protein Derivative (PPD)

Task: To correctly administer an intradermal injection of PPD with 100% accuracy.

Conditions: Medication order by provider, medication vial, medication note, appropriately sized safety needle-syringe unit, antiseptic (alcohol) wipes, gloves, cotton balls, adhesive strip, sharps container, disclosure form

Standards: Perform the Task within 15 minutes with a minimum score of _____ points.

Work Documentation: Patient chart entry

No.	Step	Points	Check #1	Check #2	Check #3
1	Checked provider's orders; organized equipment and supplies; checked room for cleanliness, equipment, and readiness; washed hands.				
2	Properly and accurately selected and withdrew the medication using all safety precautions.				
3	Correctly prepared the patient: • Greeted and identified patient and introduced self, explained procedure. • Determined if patient could return for the TB reading in 48 hours; checked for signed disclosure form. • Identified health concerns, allergies, tetanus status, possible complications, and current medications. • Positioned patient appropriately and comfortably. • Exposed, calculated, and prepped the appropriate site. • Reassured the patient as needed.				
4	Administered medication properly and safely: • Followed the six rights of medication administration. • Correctly administered medication. • Activated safety mechanism immediately and disposed of syringe/needle unit properly.				

No.	Step	Points	Check #1	Check #2	Check #3
5	Checked patient for adverse reactions, applied adhesive strip as needed, and instructed the patient about precautions to watch for as appropriate.				
6	Scheduled follow-up appointment for reading the TB test.				
7	Demonstrated professional behavior in manner, organization, and attire, including: • Communicated appropriately and comfortably with the patient.				
8	Documented correctly.				
Student's Total Points					
Points Possible					
Final Score (Student's Total Points/ Possible Points)					

Name ______________________________ **Date** ____________ **Score** ______

WORK DOCUMENTATION

Instructor's/Evaluator's Comments and Suggestions:

____

____

____

____

____

CHECK #1	
Evaluator's Signature:	Date:

CHECK #2	
Evaluator's Signature:	Date:

CHECK #3	
Evaluator's Signature:	Date:

ABHES Competency: VI.A.1.a.4.m Prepare and administer oral and parenteral medications as directed by physician

CAAHEP Curriculum: I.P.9 Administer parenteral (excluding IV) medications; II.P.1 Prepare proper dosages of medication for administration

Name ______________________________ Date ____________ Score ______

COMPETENCY ASSESSMENT

Procedure 24-8 Reconstituting a Powder Medication for Administration

Task: To correctly reconstitute a powder medication and calculate correct dosage with 100% accuracy.

Conditions: Medication order by provider, vial of medication, vial of diluent, medication note, two appropriately sized safety syringes and needles, alcohol wipes, gloves, sharps container

Standards: Perform the Task within 10 minutes with a minimum score of _____ points.

No.	Step	Points	Check #1	Check #2	Check #3
1	Checked provider's orders; organized equipment and supplies; washed hands.				
2	Correctly prepared the medication: • Selected proper medication and diluent, checked the expiration dates. • Calculated proper strength and dosage according to the provider's order. • Prepared syringe and needle using sterile technique. • Prepped the vials properly. • Withdrew appropriate amount of diluent and injected it properly into the powdered medication. • Mixed well. • Drew up correct dosage of mixed medication, releasing any bubbles, and recapped safely. • Changed needles according to office protocol.				
3	Performed the six rights of medication administration as appropriate.				
4	Demonstrated professional behavior in manner, organization, and attire.				
5	Documented correctly.				
Student's Total Points					
Points Possible					
Final Score (Student's Total Points/ Possible Points)					

Name ______________________ **Date** ____________ **Score** ______

Instructor's/Evaluator's Comments and Suggestions:

____

____

____

____

____

CHECK #1	
Evaluator's Signature:	Date:

CHECK #2	
Evaluator's Signature:	Date:

CHECK #3	
Evaluator's Signature:	Date:

ABHES Competency: VI.A.1.a.4.m Prepare and administer oral and parenteral medications as directed by physician

CAAHEP Curriculum: II.P.1 Prepare proper dosages of medication for administration

Name ______________________________ Date ____________ Score ______

COMPETENCY ASSESSMENT

Procedure 24-9 Z-Track Intramuscular Injection Technique

Task: To correctly administer a Z-track intramuscular injection with 100% accuracy.

Conditions: Medication order by provider, medication note, medication vial, appropriately sized safety needle-syringe unit, antiseptic (alcohol) wipes, gloves, cotton balls, adhesive strip, sharps container

Standards: Perform the Task within 10 minutes with a minimum score of _____ points.

Work Documentation: Patient chart entry

No.	Step	Points	Check #1	Check #2	Check #3
1	Checked provider's orders; organized equipment and supplies; checked room for cleanliness, equipment, and readiness; washed hands.				
2	Properly and accurately selected and withdrew the medication using all safety precautions.				
3	Correctly prepared the patient: • Greeted and identified patient and introduced self; explained procedure and checked for signed informed consent form. • Identified health concerns, allergies, tetanus status, possible complications, and current medications. • Positioned patient appropriately and comfortably. • Exposed, calculated, and prepped the appropriate site. • Reassured the patient as needed.				
4	Administered medication properly and safely: • Followed the six rights of medication administration. • Correctly administered medication. • Activated safety mechanism immediately and disposed of syringe/needle unit properly.				

No.	Step	Points	Check #1	Check #2	Check #3
5	Checked patient for adverse reactions, applied adhesive strip as needed, and instructed the patient about precautions to watch for as appropriate.				
6	Demonstrated professional behavior in manner, organization, and attire, including: • Communicated appropriately and comfortably with the patient.				
7	Documented correctly.				
Student's Total Points					
Points Possible					
Final Score (Student's Total Points/ Possible Points)					

Name ______________________ **Date** __________ **Score** ______

WORK DOCUMENTATION

Instructor's/Evaluator's Comments and Suggestions:

____

____

____

____

____

CHECK #1	
Evaluator's Signature:	Date:

CHECK #2	
Evaluator's Signature:	Date:

CHECK #3	
Evaluator's Signature:	Date:

ABHES Competency: VI.A.1.a.4.m Prepare and administer oral and parenteral medications as directed by physician

CAAHEP Curriculum: I.P.9 Administer parenteral (excluding IV) medications; II.P.1 Prepare proper dosages of medication for administration

Name ______________________________ Date ____________ Score ______

COMPETENCY ASSESSMENT

Procedure 25-1 Perform Single-Channel or Multichannel Electrocardiogram

Task: To perform a standard 12-lead electrocardiogram (ECG).

Conditions: Electrocardiograph machine, lead wires with end clips, tabbed adhesive electrodes, tracing paper, patient gown, small pillow, blanket/sheet, alcohol, razor (optional), mounting card/paper

Standards: Perform the Task within 20 minutes with a minimum score of _____ points.

Work Documentation: Patient chart entry, output from ECG machine

No.	Step	Points	Check #1	Check #2	Check #3
1	Checked provider's orders; organized equipment and supplies, ensuring ECG machine is ready; checked room for cleanliness, equipment, and readiness; washed hands.				
2	Correctly prepared the patient: • Greeted and identified patient and introduced self; explained procedure and checked for signed informed consent form. • Identified health concerns, allergies, tetanus status, possible complications, and current medications; obtained blood pressure. • Positioned patient appropriately and comfortably. • Exposed chest, arms, and legs, shaving hair if needed. • Reassured the patient as needed.				
3	Performed the ECG properly, mounting it if needed.				
4	Alerted provider immediately if any abnormalities were shown; otherwise, showed ECG to provider before removing the electrodes, following clinic protocol.				
5	Demonstrated professional behavior in manner, organization, and attire, including: • Communicated appropriately and comfortably with the patient.				
6	Documented correctly.				
Student's Total Points					
Points Possible					
Final Score (Student's Total Points/ Possible Points)					

Name ______________________________ Date ____________ Score ______

WORK DOCUMENTATION

*Also attach ECG output.

Instructor's/Evaluator's Comments and Suggestions:

____

____

____

____

____

CHECK #1	
Evaluator's Signature:	Date:

CHECK #2	
Evaluator's Signature:	Date:

CHECK #3	
Evaluator's Signature:	Date:

ABHES Competency: VI.A.1.a.4.l Screen and follow up patient test results; VI.A.1.a.4.dd Perform electrocardiograms

CAAHEP Curriculum: I.P.5 Perform electrocardiography; I.P.16 Screen test results

Name ______________________ Date __________ Score _______

COMPETENCY ASSESSMENT

Procedure 25-2 Holter Monitor Application (Cassette and Digital)

Task: To apply a Holter or cardiac event monitor and teach the patient how to wear the monitor, record the incidents, keep the activity log/diary, and when to return.

Conditions: Holter or cardiac event monitor, patient activity diary/log, blank magnetic tape cassette, disposable electrodes, alcohol, razor, gauze, carrying case, belt or shoulder strap

Standards: Perform the Task within 20 minutes with a minimum score of _____ points.

Work Documentation: Patient chart entry

No.	Step	Points	Check #1	Check #2	Check #3
1	Checked provider's orders; organized equipment and supplies, ensuring monitor is in working order; checked room for cleanliness, equipment, and readiness; washed hands.				
2	Correctly prepared the patient: • Greeted and identified patient and introduced self; explained procedure and checked for signed informed consent form. • Identified health concerns, allergies, tetanus status, possible complications, and current medications; obtained blood pressure. • Positioned patient appropriately and comfortably. • Exposed chest, shaving hair if needed. • Reassured the patient as needed.				
3	Performed the procedure properly: • Applied monitor properly. • Instructed patient clearly in the proper use of the monitor and provided written instruction. • Instructed patient clearly in the use of activity log. • Answered patient questions as needed, discussed solutions to any problems that could arise. • Provided patient with 24-hour numbers to call if needed. • Arranged for follow-up appointment.				
4	Demonstrated professional behavior in manner, organization, and attire, including: • Communicated appropriately and comfortably with the patient.				
5	Documented correctly.				
Student's Total Points					
Points Possible					
Final Score (Student's Total Points/ Possible Points)					

Name ____________________ **Date** __________ **Score** ______

WORK DOCUMENTATION

Instructor's/Evaluator's Comments and Suggestions:

CHECK #1
Evaluator's Signature: Date:

CHECK #2
Evaluator's Signature: Date:

CHECK #3
Evaluator's Signature: Date:

ABHES Competency: VI.A.1.a.4.dd Perform electrocardiograms

CAAHEP Curriculum: I.P.5 Perform electrocardiography

Name ______________________________ Date ____________ Score _______

COMPETENCY ASSESSMENT

Procedure 27-1 Using the Microscope

Task: To properly use a microscope to view organisms using the coarse and fine adjustments, as well as the low- and high-power and oil-immersion objectives.

Conditions: Microscope, lens paper, lens cleaner, prepared slides, immersion oil, disinfectant

Standards: Perform the Task within 15 minutes with a minimum score of _____ points.

No.	Step	Points	Check #1	Check #2	Check #3
1	Washed hands.				
2	Set up the microscope, cleaned lens, turned on light, adjusted as needed.				
3	Placed slide properly, adjusted vision.				
4	Handled objectives properly, moved away from the field while using coarse adjustments.				
5	Examined the slide, turned off the light, notified the provider that the slide was ready.				
6	When provider completed the PPMP, cleaned microscope properly and disposed of slide(s) and other samples according to OSHA standards.				
7	Demonstrated professional behavior in manner, organization, and attire, including: • Communicated appropriately and comfortably with the physician.				
Student's Total Points					
Points Possible					
Final Score (Student's Total Points/ Possible Points)					

Name ______________________________ **Date** ____________ **Score** ______

Instructor's/Evaluator's Comments and Suggestions:

____

____

____

____

____

CHECK #1	
Evaluator's Signature:	Date:

CHECK #2	
Evaluator's Signature:	Date:

CHECK #3	
Evaluator's Signature:	Date:

ABHES Competency: VI.A.1.a.4.g Prepare and maintain examination and treatment area

Name ______________________________ Date ____________ Score ______

COMPETENCY ASSESSMENT

Procedure 28-1 Palpating a Vein and Preparing a Patient for Venipuncture

Task: To palpate for an appropriate vein for venipuncture using a tourniquet.

Conditions: Gloves, alcohol swab, tourniquet

Standards: Perform the Task within 5 minutes with a minimum score of _____ points.

No.	Step	Points	Check #1	Check #2	Check #3
1	Organized equipment and supplies; checked room for cleanliness, equipment, and readiness; washed hands.				
2	Greeted and identified patient and introduced self.				
3	Performed the procedure correctly and safely: • Positioned patient correctly for proper body mechanics. • Exposed arm appropriately. • Applied tourniquet correctly. • Palpated veins to determine depth, direction, characteristics. • Ruled out a pulse that would indicate an artery rather than a vein. • Released tourniquet. • Repeated procedure on other arm if needed.				
4	Demonstrated professional behavior in manner, organization, and attire, including: • Communicated appropriately and comfortably with the patient.				
5	Washed hands.				
Student's Total Points					
Points Possible					
Final Score (Student's Total Points/ Possible Points)					

Name ______________________________ **Date** ____________ **Score** ______

Instructor's/Evaluator's Comments and Suggestions:

____

____

____

____

____

CHECK #1	
Evaluator's Signature:	Date:

CHECK #2	
Evaluator's Signature:	Date:

CHECK #3	
Evaluator's Signature:	Date:

ABHES Competency: VI.A.1.a.4.b Prepare patients for procedures

Name ______________________________ Date __________ Score ______

COMPETENCY ASSESSMENT

Procedure 28-2 Venipuncture by Syringe

Task: Using a syringe to obtain venous blood acceptable for laboratory testing as requisitioned by a physician.

Conditions: Gloves, goggles, and mask, 10-mL syringe, 21-gauge safety needle, vacuum tube(s) or special collection tube(s), vacuum tube safety holder, tourniquet, 70% isopropyl alcohol swab, cotton balls, gauze, adhesive bandage or tape, sharps container, test tube rack

Standards: Perform the Task within 15 minutes with a minimum score of _____ points.

Work Documentation: Patient chart entry, lab requisition

No.	Step	Points	Check #1	Check #2	Check #3
1	Checked provider's orders; organized equipment and supplies; checked room for cleanliness, equipment, and readiness; washed hands.				
2	Correctly prepared the patient: • Greeted and identified patient and introduced self, explained procedure, washed hands. • Identified health concerns, allergies, tetanus status, possible complications, and current medications. • Positioned patient appropriately and comfortably. • Reassured the patient as needed.				
3	Applied appropriate PPE.				
4	Performed the procedure correctly and safely: • Applied tourniquet correctly. • Palpated veins correctly, ruled out artery, planned approach. • Prepped skin. • Performed puncture correctly and safely with minimum of discomfort to patient, did not unduly move the needle during the procedure. • Released tourniquet. • Removed needle safely and comfortably while applying pressure on site. • Selected correct tubes in order and filled them correctly using a rack. • Implemented safety mechanism on syringe/needle unit and disposed of properly. • Applied appropriate dressing.				

No.	Step	Points	Check #1	Check #2	Check #3
5	Disposed of contaminated supplies following OSHA regulations and washed hands.				
6	Demonstrated professional behavior in manner, organization, and attire, including: • Communicated appropriately and comfortably with the patient.				
7	Labeled tubes properly, completed requisition correctly and completely, packaged specimens for transport correctly.				
8	Documented correctly.				
Student's Total Points					
Points Possible					
Final Score (Student's Total Points/ Possible Points)					

Name ______________________ Date ____________ Score ________

WORK DOCUMENTATION

*Also attach lab requisition.

Instructor's/Evaluator's Comments and Suggestions:

CHECK #1

Evaluator's Signature: Date:

CHECK #2

Evaluator's Signature: Date:

CHECK #3

Evaluator's Signature: Date:

ABHES Competency: VI.A.1.a.4.s Perform venipuncture

CAAHEP Curriculum: I.P.2 Perform venipuncture; III.P.3 Select appropriate barrier/personal protective equipment (PPE) for potentially infectious situations

Name ______________________ Date __________ Score ______

COMPETENCY ASSESSMENT

Procedure 28-3 Venipuncture by Vacuum Tube System

Task: Using a vacuum tube system to obtain venous blood acceptable for laboratory testing as requisitioned by a physician.

Conditions: Gloves, goggles, and mask, vacuum tube adapter/holder, 21-gauge multidraw needle, vacuum tube(s) or special collection tube(s), tourniquet, 70% isopropyl alcohol swab, cotton balls, adhesive bandage or tape, sharps container

Standards: Perform the Task within 15 minutes with a minimum score of _____ points.

Work Documentation: Patient chart entry, lab requisition

No.	Step	Points	Check #1	Check #2	Check #3
1	Checked provider's orders; organized equipment and supplies; checked room for cleanliness, equipment, and readiness; washed hands.				
2	Correctly prepared the patient: • Greeted and identified patient and introduced self, explained procedure, washed hands. • Identified health concerns, allergies, tetanus status, possible complications, and current medications. • Positioned patient appropriately and comfortably. • Reassured the patient as needed.				
3	Applied appropriate PPE.				
4	Performed the procedure correctly and safely: • Applied tourniquet correctly. • Palpated veins correctly, ruled out artery, planned approach. • Prepped skin. • Performed puncture correctly and safely with minimum of discomfort to the patient, did not move needle during tube changes. • Selected correct tubes in order and filled them correctly. • Released tourniquet. • Removed needle safely and comfortably while applying pressure on site. • Implemented safety mechanism and disposed of properly. • Applied appropriate dressing.				

No.	Step	Points	Check #1	Check #2	Check #3
5	Disposed of contaminated supplies following OSHA regulations; washed hands.				
6	Demonstrated professional behavior in manner, organization, and attire, including: • Communicated appropriately and comfortably with the patient.				
7	Labeled tubes properly, completed requisition correctly and completely, packaged specimens for transport correctly.				
8	Documented correctly.				
Student's Total Points					
Points Possible					
Final Score (Student's Total Points/ Possible Points)					

Name ________________________________ Date ____________ Score ______

WORK DOCUMENTATION

*Also attach lab requisition.

Instructor's/Evaluator's Comments and Suggestions:

____

____

____

____

____

CHECK #1

Evaluator's Signature: Date:

CHECK #2

Evaluator's Signature: Date:

CHECK #3

Evaluator's Signature: Date:

ABHES Competency: VI.A.1.a.4.s Perform venipuncture

CAAHEP Curriculum: I.P.2 Perform venipuncture; III.P.3 Select appropriate barrier/personal protective equipment (PPE) for potentially infectious situations

Name ______________________________ Date __________ Score ______

COMPETENCY ASSESSMENT

Procedure 28-4 Venipuncture by Butterfly Needle System

Task: Using a butterfly needle system to obtain venous blood acceptable for laboratory testing as requisitioned by a provider.

Conditions: Gloves, goggles, and mask, vacuum tube adapter/holder (if using a vacuum tube connection), a 10- to 15-mL syringe (if using a syringe connection), butterfly needle system with 21-gauge needle (use a multi-sample needle system with a luer adapter for attaching to the vacuum tube and a hypodermic needle for syringe attachment), vacuum tube rack (syringe collection), vacuum tubes, tourniquet, 70% isopropyl alcohol swab, gauze or cotton balls, adhesive bandage or tape, sharps container

Standards: Perform the Task within 15 minutes with a minimum score of _____ points.

Work Documentation: Patient chart entry, lab requisition

No.	Step	Points	Check #1	Check #2	Check #3
1	Checked provider's orders; organized equipment and supplies; checked room for cleanliness, equipment, and readiness; washed hands.				
2	Correctly prepared the patient: • Greeted and identified patient and introduced self, explained procedure, washed hands. • Identified health concerns, allergies, tetanus status, possible complications, and current medications. • Positioned patient appropriately and comfortably. • Reassured the patient as needed.				
3	Applied appropriate PPE.				
4	Performed the procedure correctly and safely: • Applied tourniquet correctly. • Palpated veins correctly, ruled out artery, planned approach. • Prepped skin. • Performed puncture correctly and safely with minimum of discomfort to the patient, did not move needle during procedure. • If using vacuum system: Selected correct tubes in order and filled them correctly. • Released tourniquet.				

No.	Step	Points	Check #1	Check #2	Check #3
	• Removed needle safely and comfortably while applying pressure on site. • If transferring blood to tubes from syringe: Selected correct tubes in order and filled them correctly using a rack. • Implemented safety mechanism on butterfly unit and disposed of properly. • Applied appropriate dressing.				
5	Disposed of contaminated supplies following OSHA regulations; washed hands.				
6	Demonstrated professional behavior in manner, organization, and attire, including: • Communicated appropriately and comfortably with the patient.				
7	Labeled tubes properly, completed requisition correctly and completely, packaged specimens for transport correctly.				
8	Documented correctly.				
Student's Total Points					
Points Possible					
Final Score (Student's Total Points/ Possible Points)					

Name ______________________________ **Date** __________ **Score** ______

WORK DOCUMENTATION

*Also attach lab requisition.

Instructor's/Evaluator's Comments and Suggestions:

____

____

____

____

____

CHECK #1	
Evaluator's Signature:	Date:

CHECK #2	
Evaluator's Signature:	Date:

CHECK #3	
Evaluator's Signature:	Date:

ABHES Competency: VI.A.1.a.4.s Perform venipuncture

CAAHEP Curriculum: I.P.2 Perform venipuncture; III.P.3 Select appropriate barrier/personal protective equipment (PPE) for potentially infectious situations

Name ______________________________ Date ____________ Score _______

COMPETENCY ASSESSMENT

Procedure 28-5 Capillary Puncture

Task: To obtain capillary blood acceptable for laboratory testing as required by a provider.

Conditions: Gloves, goggles, and mask (optional), alcohol swab, microcollection tubes, capillary tubes or specific test kit, safety lancet, gauze, cotton balls, adhesive bandage or tape, sharps container

Standards: Perform the Task within 20 minutes with a minimum score of _____ points.

Work Documentation: Patient chart entry, lab requisition

No.	Step	Points	Check #1	Check #2	Check #3
1	Checked provider's orders; organized equipment and supplies; checked room for cleanliness, equipment, and readiness; washed hands.				
2	Correctly prepared the patient: • Greeted and identified patient and introduced self, explained procedure, washed hands. • Identified health concerns, allergies, tetanus status, possible complications, and current medications. • Positioned patient appropriately and comfortably.				
3	Applied appropriate PPE.				
4	Performed the procedure correctly and safely: • Encouraged good blood flow: Had patient wash hands in warm water. If needed, applied warming pack to fingers. • Encouraged patient to relax and provided a comfortable, relaxing atmosphere. • Selected an appropriate puncture site. • Cleansed the site with alcohol. • Held the finger securely and comfortably. • Performed the puncture correctly and safely with minimum of discomfort to the patient. • Disposed of puncture lancet safely and properly. • Disposed of first drop. • Acquired specimen as needed for test(s). • Applied appropriate dressing to puncture site and held pressure as needed.				

No.	Step	Points	Check #1	Check #2	Check #3
5	Demonstrated professional behavior in manner, organization, and attire, including: • Communicated appropriately and comfortably with the patient.				
6	Disposed of contaminated supplies following OSHA regulations; washed hands.				
7	Processed specimens as requisitioned or labeled containers properly, completed requisition correctly and completely, packaged specimens for transport correctly.				
8	Documented correctly.				
Student's Total Points					
Points Possible					
Final Score (Student's Total Points/ Possible Points)					

Name ____________________ **Date** ____________ **Score** ______

WORK DOCUMENTATION

*Also attach lab requisition.

Instructor's/Evaluator's Comments and Suggestions:

____

____

____

____

____

CHECK #1	
Evaluator's Signature:	Date:

CHECK #2	
Evaluator's Signature:	Date:

CHECK #3	
Evaluator's Signature:	Date:

ABHES Competency: VI.A.1.a.4.t Perform capillary puncture

CAAHEP Curriculum: I.P.3 Perform capillary puncture; III.P.3 Select appropriate barrier/personal protective equipment (PPE) for potentially infectious situations

Name ______________________ Date __________ Score ______

COMPETENCY ASSESSMENT

Procedure 28-6 Obtaining a Capillary Specimen for Transport Using a Microtainer Transport Unit

Task: To obtain a specimen of capillary blood for transport to a laboratory for testing, using a Microtainer transport unit.

Standards: Capillary puncture supplies (gloves, alcohol pad, safety lancet, cotton ball, adhesive bandage), Microtainer transport unit, laboratory requisition, small sturdy container with a tightly fitting lid (such as a urine specimen cup), pen, biohazard specimen transport bag

Standards: Perform the Task within 20 minutes with a minimum score of _____ points.

Work Documentation: Patient chart entry

No.	Step	Points	Check #1	Check #2	Check #3
1	Checked provider's orders; organized equipment and supplies; checked room for cleanliness, equipment, and readiness; washed hands.				
2	Correctly prepared the patient: • Greeted and identified patient and introduced self, explained procedure, washed hands. • Identified health concerns, allergies, tetanus status, possible complications, and current medications. • Positioned patient appropriately and comfortably.				
3	Applied appropriate PPE.				
4	Performed the procedure correctly and safely: • Encouraged good blood flow: Had patient wash hands in warm water. If needed, applied warming pack to the fingers. • Encouraged the patient to relax and provided a comfortable, relaxing atmosphere. • Selected an appropriate puncture site. • Cleansed the site with alcohol. • Held the finger securely and comfortably. • Performed puncture correctly and safely with minimum of discomfort to patient.				

No.	Step	Points	Check #1	Check #2	Check #3
	• Disposed of puncture lancet safely and properly. • Disposed of first drop. • Scooped the blood drops into Microtainer tube properly, agitating tube after each drop to mix well. Filled Microtainer tube as needed for tests. • Removed scoop and capped tube. • Applied appropriate dressing to puncture site and held pressure as needed.				
5	Disposed of contaminated supplies following OSHA regulations.				
6	Placed tube into capped transport container and washed hands.				
7	Demonstrated professional behavior in manner, organization, and attire, including: • Communicated appropriately and comfortably with the patient.				
8	Labeled containers properly, completed requisition correctly and completely, packaged specimens for transport correctly.				
9	Documented correctly.				
Student's Total Points					
Points Possible					
Final Score (Student's Total Points/ Possible Points)					

Name ______________________ **Date** __________ **Score** ______

WORK DOCUMENTATION

Instructor's/Evaluator's Comments and Suggestions:

CHECK #1	
Evaluator's Signature:	Date:

CHECK #2	
Evaluator's Signature:	Date:

CHECK #3	
Evaluator's Signature:	Date:

ABHES Competency: VI.A.1.a.4.t Perform capillary puncture

CAAHEP Curriculum: I.P.3 Perform capillary puncture; III.P.3 Select appropriate barrier/personal protective equipment (PPE) for potentially infectious situations

Name ______________________ Date __________ Score ______

COMPETENCY ASSESSMENT

Procedure 28-7 Obtaining Blood for Blood Culture

Task: While performing venipuncture from two separate sites, prepare two culture bottles of blood from each site for culture (four total).

Conditions: Nonsterile gloves for use with povidone-iodine solution; sterile gloves; laboratory requisition; blood cultures, anaerobic and aerobic (usually four: two bottles each for two sets of cultures); 70% isopropyl alcohol; povidone-iodine solution swabs or towelettes; venipuncture supplies (according to method used) for two separate sites; biohazard red bag; biohazard sharps container; labeling pen

Standards: Perform the Task within 20 minutes with a minimum score of _____ points.

Work Documentation: Patient chart entry, lab requisition, bottle labels

No.	Step	Points	Check #1	Check #2	Check #3
1	Checked provider's orders; organized equipment and supplies; checked room for cleanliness, equipment, and readiness; washed hands.				
2	Correctly prepared the patient: • Greeted and identified patient and introduced self, explained procedure, washed hands. • Identified health concerns, allergies, tetanus status, possible complications, and current medications. • Determined that the patient has not already started antibiotic therapy. • Positioned patient appropriately and comfortably.				
3	Applied appropriate PPE.				
4	Performed the procedures correctly and safely: • Prepped the skin with iodine surgical prep, allowing the prep to air dry for 1 full minute. • Did not touch the prepped area. • Cleansed the culture bottle tops with surgical prep solution. • Applied sterile gloves. • Performed venipuncture properly and safely. • Mixed the specimens into the culture media by inverting 8–10 times. • Repeated procedure at a second site within 30 minutes.				

No.	Step	Points	Check #1	Check #2	Check #3
5	Disposed of contaminated supplies following OSHA regulations, disinfected surfaces, and washed hands.				
6	Demonstrated professional behavior in manner, organization, and attire, including: • Communicated appropriately and comfortably with the patient.				
7	Labeled bottles correctly and completed the requisitions correctly according to the laboratory manual instructions. Provided all the information required and held pressure as needed.				
8	Documented correctly.				
Student's Total Points					
Points Possible					
Final Score (Student's Total Points/ Possible Points)					

Name ______________________ Date __________ Score ______

WORK DOCUMENTATION

*Also attach lab requisition.

Instructor's/Evaluator's Comments and Suggestions:

CHECK #1	
Evaluator's Signature:	Date:

CHECK #2	
Evaluator's Signature:	Date:

CHECK #3	
Evaluator's Signature:	Date:

ABHES Competency: VI.A.1.a.4.s Perform venipuncture

CAAHEP Curriculum: I.P.2 Perform venipuncture; III.P.3 Select appropriate barrier/personal protective equipment (PPE) for potentially infectious situations

Name ______________________________ Date __________ Score ______

COMPETENCY ASSESSMENT

Procedure 29-1 Hemoglobin Determination Using a CLIA Waived Hemoglobin Analyzer

Task: To properly and safely perform an automated hemoglobin determination to evaluate the oxygen capacity of the blood.

Conditions: Gloves, disinfectant, capillary puncture equipment or blood samples collected in EDTA, HemoCue® system or other hemoglobin analyzer with supplies appropriate for the analyzer, biohazard red bag, biohazard sharps container

Standards: Perform the Task within 20 minutes with a minimum score of _____ points.

Work Documentation: Patient chart entry, lab report

No.	Step	Points	Check #1	Check #2	Check #3
1	Checked provider's orders; organized equipment and supplies, turned on instrument; checked room for cleanliness, equipment, and readiness.				
2	Correctly prepared the patient: • Greeted and identified patient and introduced self, explained procedure, washed hands. • Identified health concerns, allergies, tetanus status, possible complications, and current medications. • Positioned patient appropriately and comfortably.				
3	Applied appropriate PPE.				
4	Performed the procedure correctly and safely: • Performed capillary puncture correctly and safely. • Obtained specimen properly. • Inserted specimen into machine following manufacturer's instructions. • Performed test according to instructions. • Recorded the results.				
5	Disposed of contaminated supplies following OSHA regulations; cleaned and stored machine, disinfected surfaces, washed hands.				

No.	Step	Points	Check #1	Check #2	Check #3
6	Demonstrated professional behavior in manner, organization, and attire, including: • Communicated appropriately and comfortably with the patient.				
7	Documented correctly.				
Student's Total Points					
Points Possible					
Final Score (Student's Total Points/ Possible Points)					

Name ______________________ **Date** ____________ **Score** ______

WORK DOCUMENTATION

*Also attach lab report.

Instructor's/Evaluator's Comments and Suggestions:

____

____

____

____

____

CHECK #1	
Evaluator's Signature:	Date:

CHECK #2	
Evaluator's Signature:	Date:

CHECK #3	
Evaluator's Signature:	Date:

ABHES Competency: VI.A.1.a.4.j Collect and process specimens; VI.A.1.a.4.t Perform capillary puncture; VI.A.1.a.4.z Perform hematology

CAAHEP Curriculum: I.P.3 Perform capillary puncture; I.P.12 Perform hematology testing

Name ______________________________ Date ____________ Score ______

COMPETENCY ASSESSMENT

Procedure 29-2 Microhematocrit Determination

Task: To properly and safely perform the microhematocrit procedure using a few microliters of blood in a capillary tube to separate the cellular elements of the blood from the plasma by centrifugation.

Conditions: Gloves, capillary tubes (heparinized), sealing clay, microhematocrit centrifuge and reader, alcohol swabs, gauze and cotton balls, safety lancets, adhesive strip, disinfectant, biohazard red bag, sharps container. OPTIONAL: If obtaining blood from a vacuum tube: vacuum tube of anticoagulated blood, safety shield for cap removal, face shield

Standards: Perform the Task within 15 minutes with a minimum score of _____ points.

Work Documentation: Patient chart entry, lab report

No.	Step	Points	Check #1	Check #2	Check #3
1	Checked provider's orders; organized equipment and supplies, turned on instrument; checked room for cleanliness, equipment, and readiness.				
2	Correctly prepared the patient: • Greeted and identified patient and introduced self, explained procedure, washed hands. • Identified health concerns, allergies, tetanus status, possible complications, and current medications. • Positioned patient appropriately and comfortably.				
3	Applied appropriate PPE.				
4	Performed the procedure correctly and safely: • Performed capillary puncture correctly and safely. • Filled two tubes using proper technique. • Loaded tubes into machine correctly. • Centrifuged correctly. • Read and recorded the averaged results.				
5	Disposed of contaminated supplies following OSHA regulations; cleaned and stored machine, disinfected surfaces, washed hands.				
6	Demonstrated professional behavior in manner, organization, and attire, including: • Communicated appropriately and comfortably with the patient.				
7	Documented correctly.				
Student's Total Points					
Points Possible					
Final Score (Student's Total Points/ Possible Points)					

Name ______________________________ **Date** ____________ **Score** ______

WORK DOCUMENTATION

*Also attach lab report.

Instructor's/Evaluator's Comments and Suggestions:

____

____

____

____

____

CHECK #1

Evaluator's Signature: Date:

CHECK #2

Evaluator's Signature: Date:

CHECK #3

Evaluator's Signature: Date:

ABHES Competency: VI.A.1.a.4.j Collect and process specimens; VI.A.1.a.4.t Perform capillary puncture; VI.A.1.a.4.z Perform hematology

CAAHEP Curriculum: I.P.3 Perform capillary puncture; I.P.12 Perform hematology testing

Name ______________________ Date __________ Score _______

COMPETENCY ASSESSMENT

Procedure 29-3 Erythrocyte Sedimentation Rate

Task: To properly and safely perform an erythrocyte sedimentation rate (ESR).

Conditions: Gloves, sample of venous blood collected in EDTA, Sediplast® or other ESR kit (sedivial and sedirack, Sediplast® autozeroing pipette, pipette capable of delivering up to 1.0 mL), Wintrobe method (Wintrobe sedimentation tube, Wintrobe sedimentation rack, long-stem Pasteur-type pipette with rubber bulb), timer, 10% chlorine bleach solution/disinfectant, face shield or goggles and mask, biohazard red bag for waste, sharps container

Standards: Perform the Task within 75 minutes with a minimum score of _____ points.

Work Documentation: Patient chart entry, lab report

No.	Step	Points	Check #1	Check #2	Check #3
1	Checked provider's orders; organized equipment and supplies, turned on instrument; checked room for cleanliness, equipment, and readiness.				
2	Correctly prepared the patient: • Greeted and identified patient and introduced self, explained procedure, washed hands. • Identified health concerns, allergies, tetanus status, possible complications, and current medications. • Positioned patient appropriately and comfortably.				
3	Applied appropriate PPE.				
4	Performed the procedure correctly and safely: • Performed venipuncture correctly and safely. • Performed either the Sediplast ESR or Wintrobe method correctly, following manufacturer's and lab manual instructions. • After 1 hour of undisturbed sedimentation, observed and recorded the ESR results.				
5	Disposed of contaminated supplies following OSHA regulations; cleaned and stored equipment, disinfected surfaces, washed hands.				
6	Demonstrated professional behavior in manner, organization, and attire, including: • Communicated appropriately and comfortably with the patient.				
7	Documented correctly.				
Student's Total Points					
Points Possible					
Final Score (Student's Total Points/ Possible Points)					

Name ______________________________ **Date** ____________ **Score** ______

WORK DOCUMENTATION

*Also attach lab report.

Instructor's/Evaluator's Comments and Suggestions:

____

____

____

____

____

CHECK #1	
Evaluator's Signature:	Date:

CHECK #2	
Evaluator's Signature:	Date:

CHECK #3	
Evaluator's Signature:	Date:

ABHES Competency: VI.A.1.a.4.j Collect and process specimens; VI.A.1.a.4.s Perform venipuncture; VI.A.1.a.4.z Perform hematology

CAAHEP Curriculum: I.P.2 Perform venipuncture; I.P.12 Perform hematology testing

Name ______________________ Date ____________ Score ______

COMPETENCY ASSESSMENT

Procedure 29-4 Prothrombin Time (Using CLIA Waived ProTime Analyzer)

Task: Properly and safely perform an automated prothrombin time determination to evaluate the clotting time of a drop of blood.

Condition: Gloves, biohazard container, sharps container, capillary puncture equipment, alcohol wipes, safety lancet, cotton ball, gauze 2 × 2, adhesive bandage, CLIA Waived ProTime Analyzer with accessories

Standards: Perform the Task within 15 minutes with a minimum score of _____ points.

Work Documentation: Patient chart entry, lab report

No.	Step	Points	Check #1	Check #2	Check #3
1	Checked provider's orders; checked room for cleanliness, equipment, and readiness; organized equipment and supplies, turned on and prepared instrument.				
2	Correctly prepared the patient: • Greeted and identified patient and introduced self, explained procedure, washed hands. • Identified health concerns, allergies, tetanus status, possible complications, and current medications. • Positioned patient appropriately and comfortably.				
3	Applied appropriate PPE.				
4	Performed the procedure correctly and safely: • Performed capillary puncture correctly and safely. • Filled Tenderlett lancet cup to fill line and placed onto the cuvette; pressed start. • Applied cotton ball to patient's arm and held pressure for 3–5 minutes. • When prompted by machine, removed device and discarded into sharps container. • Read and recorded clotting time and INR.				
	Alerted provider immediately if results fell into critical range.				

No.	Step	Points	Check #1	Check #2	Check #3
5	Disposed of contaminated supplies following OSHA regulations; cleaned and stored equipment, disinfected surfaces, washed hands.				
6	Demonstrated professional behavior in manner, organization, and attire, including: • Communicated appropriately and comfortably with the patient.				
7	Documented correctly.				
Student's Total Points					
Points Possible					
Final Score (Student's Total Points/ Possible Points)					

Name ______________________ **Date** ____________ **Score** ______

WORK DOCUMENTATION

*Also attach lab report.

Instructor's/Evaluator's Comments and Suggestions:

CHECK #1
Evaluator's Signature: Date:

CHECK #2
Evaluator's Signature: Date:

CHECK #3
Evaluator's Signature: Date:

ABHES Competency: VI.A.1.a.4.j Collect and process specimens; VI.A.1.a.4.t Perform capillary puncture; VI.A.1.a.4.z Perform hematology

CAAHEP Curriculum: I.P.3 Perform capillary puncture; I.P.12 Perform hematology testing

Name ______________________________ Date ____________ Score ______

COMPETENCY ASSESSMENT

Procedure 30-1 Assessing Urine Volume, Color, and Clarity

Task: Determine and document the volume, color, and clarity of a urine sample.

Conditions: Gloves, urine specimen in labeled, clear urine cup with secure lid, biohazard container, disinfectant cleaner, laboratory report form

Standards: Perform the Task within 5 minutes with a minimum score of _____ points.

Work Documentation: Patient chart entry, lab report

No.	Step	Points	Check #1	Check #2	Check #3
1	Washed hands, organized supplies and equipment, and applied appropriate PPE.				
2	Examined specimen for proper labeling. With lid tightly sealed, mixed urine well.				
3	Noted the amount of urine in the cup (in milliliters).				
4	Assessed and noted the urine color against a white background with good lighting.				
5	Assessed the clarity of the urine using the white background. Recorded any cloudiness as appropriate.				
6	Disposed of contaminated supplies following OSHA regulations; disinfected surfaces; washed hands.				
7	Demonstrated professional behavior in manner, organization, and attire.				
8	Documented correctly.				
Student's Total Points					
Points Possible					
Final Score (Student's Total Points/ Possible Points)					

Name ____________________ **Date** __________ **Score** ______

WORK DOCUMENTATION

*Also attach lab report.

Instructor's/Evaluator's Comments and Suggestions:

____

____

____

____

____

CHECK #1

Evaluator's Signature: Date:

CHECK #2

Evaluator's Signature: Date:

CHECK #3

Evaluator's Signature: Date:

ABHES Competency: VI.A.1.a.4.j Collect and process specimens; VI.A.1.a.4.y Perform urinalysis

CAAHEP Curriculum: I.P.14 Perform urinalysis

Name ______________________________ Date ____________ Score ______

COMPETENCY ASSESSMENT

Procedure 30-2 Using the Refractometer to Measure Specific Gravity

Task: Measure and record the specific gravity of a urine specimen.

Conditions: Refractometer, gloves, urine sample, pipettes, distilled water, lint-free (lens) tissues, biohazard container, disinfectant, laboratory report form

Standards: Perform the Task within 5 minutes with a minimum score of _____ points.

Work Documentation: Patient chart entry

No.	Step	Points	Check #1	Check #2	Check #3
1	Washed hands, organized supplies and equipment, and applied appropriate PPE.				
2	Performed quality control on the refractometer by checking it using distilled water. Calibrated as needed.				
3	Examined specimen for proper labeling. With lid tightly sealed, mixed urine well.				
4	Applied urine to the refractometer according to manufacturer's instructions. Read and noted the specific gravity.				
5	Disposed of contaminated supplies following OSHA regulations; cleaned and stored equipment; disinfected surfaces; washed hands.				
6	Demonstrated professional behavior in manner, organization, and attire.				
7	Documented correctly.				
Student's Total Points					
Points Possible					
Final Score (Student's Total Points/ Possible Points)					

Name ______________________________ **Date** ____________ **Score** ______

WORK DOCUMENTATION

Instructor's/Evaluator's Comments and Suggestions:

____

____

____

____

____

CHECK #1	
Evaluator's Signature:	Date:

CHECK #2	
Evaluator's Signature:	Date:

CHECK #3	
Evaluator's Signature:	Date:

ABHES Competency: VI.A.1.a.4.i Use quality control; VI.A.1.a.4.j Collect and process specimens; VI.A.1.a.4.y Perform urinalysis

CAAHEP Curriculum: I.P.11 Perform quality control measures; I.P.14 Perform urinalysis

Name ______________________________ Date ____________ Score ______

COMPETENCY ASSESSMENT

Procedure 30-3 Performing a Urinalysis Chemical Examination

Task: Detect any abnormal chemical constituents of a urine specimen.

Conditions: Gloves, urine test strips, urine specimen, paper towel, biohazard container, disinfectant cleaner, laboratory report form

Standards: Perform the Task within 15 minutes with a minimum score of _____ points.

Work Documentation: Patient chart entry, lab report

No.	Step	Points	Check #1	Check #2	Check #3
1	Washed hands, organized supplies and equipment, checked expiration date on bottle of test strips, applied appropriate PPE.				
2	Examined specimen for proper labeling. With lid tightly sealed, mixed urine well.				
3	Performed the procedure correctly and safely: • Opened container of test strips, set lid down properly. Selected one test strip properly without contaminating other strips. Secured lid back onto container. • Dipped the strip into the urine completely, tapped edge onto paper towel. • Held strip close to color chart but did not touch it. Timed each test properly while comparing strip with chart, noting results.				
4	Disposed of contaminated supplies following OSHA regulations; disinfected surfaces; washed hands.				
5	Demonstrated professional behavior in manner, organization, and attire.				
6	Documented correctly.				
Student's Total Points					
Points Possible					
Final Score (Student's Total Points/ Possible Points)					

Name ______________________________ **Date** ____________ **Score** ______

WORK DOCUMENTATION

*Also attach lab report.

Instructor's/Evaluator's Comments and Suggestions:

____

____

____

____

____

CHECK #1	
Evaluator's Signature:	Date:

CHECK #2	
Evaluator's Signature:	Date:

CHECK #3	
Evaluator's Signature:	Date:

ABHES Competency: VI.A.1.a.4.j Collect and process specimens; VI.A.1.a.4.y Perform urinalysis

CAAHEP Curriculum: I.P.14 Perform urinalysis

Name ______________________________ Date ____________ Score ______

COMPETENCY ASSESSMENT

Procedure 30-4 Preparing Slide for Microscopic Examination of Urine Sediment

Task: Prepare a slide for a microscopic examination of urine sediment.

Conditions: Gloves, microscope, centrifuge, microscope slides, cover slips, disposable pipette, centrifuge tubes and holder, urine specimen, urine atlas guide, disinfectant cleaner, biohazard container, sharps container, Sedi-Stain® (optional)

Standards: Perform the Task within 15 minutes with a minimum score of _____ points.

Work Documentation: Patient chart entry, lab report

No.	Step	Points	Check #1	Check #2	Check #3
1	Washed hands, organized supplies and equipment, set up microscope, applied appropriate PPE.				
2	Examined specimen for proper labeling. With lid tightly sealed, mixed urine well.				
3	Correctly processed specimen in centrifuge: • Labeled centrifuge tube. • Poured 12–15 mL of urine into tube. • Placed tube into centrifuge, balancing as needed. • Secured lid on centrifuge. • Centrifuged specimen at 1500 rpm for 5 minutes.				
4	Poured off supernatant.				
5	Correctly prepared slide: • Mixed sediment to dislodge and evenly disperse. Applied 2 drops of Sedi-Stain® to sediment if desired. Mixed well. • Used pipette to apply one drop of sediment to center of microscope slide. Applied cover slip smoothly, without air bubbles. • Placed slide onto microscope stage, adjusting for provider viewing. Turned light off until provider was ready. If medical assistant viewed slide for educational purposes, prepared fresh slide for provider.				

No.	Step	Points	Check #1	Check #2	Check #3
6	Removed PPE, washed hands, and prepared lab report for provider to complete.				
7	Disposed of contaminated supplies following OSHA regulations; disinfected surfaces; washed hands.				
8	Demonstrated professional behavior in manner, organization, and attire.				
9	Documented correctly.				
Student's Total Points					
Points Possible					
Final Score (Student's Total Points/ Possible Points)					

Name ______________________ **Date** ____________ **Score** ______

WORK DOCUMENTATION

*Also attach lab report.

Instructor's/Evaluator's Comments and Suggestions:

____

____

____

____

____

CHECK #1

Evaluator's Signature: Date:

CHECK #2

Evaluator's Signature: Date:

CHECK #3

Evaluator's Signature: Date:

ABHES Competency: VI.A.1.a.4.j Collect and process specimens; VI.A.1.a.4.y Perform urinalysis

CAAHEP Curriculum: I.P.14 Perform urinalysis

Name ______________________ Date __________ Score ______

COMPETENCY ASSESSMENT

Procedure 30-5 Performing a Complete Urinalysis

Task: Perform a complete urinalysis, including the physical and chemical examinations, and prepare for the microscopic examination test within 30 minutes of obtaining the specimen.

Conditions: Gloves, patient preparation supplies and information, urine specimen, pipettes, centrifuge tube, centrifuge, microscope, microscope slides, cover slip, permanent marker, urine test strips, urine atlas, refractometer, distilled water, lint-free tissues, biohazard container, sharps container, disinfectant cleaner, laboratory report form, Sedi-Stain® (optional)

Standards: Perform the Task within 15 minutes with a minimum score of _____ points.

Work Documentation: Patient chart entry, lab report

No.	Step	Points	Check #1	Check #2	Check #3
1	Washed hands, organized supplies and equipment, set up microscope, applied appropriate PPE.				
2	Examined specimen for proper labeling. With lid tightly sealed, mixed urine well.				
3	Properly performed centrifugation of 12–15 mL of urine.				
4	While specimen was spinning, properly performed physical and chemical examination of urine, documenting results correctly and completely.				
5	After specimen was spun, prepared microscope slide for provider. Turned light off to preserve specimen. If desired, prepared another slide for self to view for educational purposes.				
6	Disposed of contaminated supplies following OSHA regulations; disinfected surfaces; removed PPE; washed hands.				
7	Demonstrated professional behavior in manner, organization, and attire.				
8	Documented correctly.				
Student's Total Points					
Points Possible					
Final Score (Student's Total Points/ Possible Points)					

Name ______________________________ **Date** ____________ **Score** ______

WORK DOCUMENTATION

*Also attach lab report.

Instructor's/Evaluator's Comments and Suggestions:

____

____

____

____

____

CHECK #1	
Evaluator's Signature:	Date:

CHECK #2	
Evaluator's Signature:	Date:

CHECK #3	
Evaluator's Signature:	Date:

ABHES Competency: VI.A.1.a.4.i Use quality control; VI.A.1.a.4.j Collect and process specimens; VI.A.1.a.4.y Perform urinalysis

CAAHEP Curriculum: I.P.11 Perform quality control measures; I.P.14 Perform urinalysis

Name ______________________________ **Date** ____________ **Score** ______

COMPETENCY ASSESSMENT

Procedure 30-6 Utilizing a Urine Transport System for C&S

Task: Perform a complete urinalysis, including the physical and chemical examinations, and prepare for the microscopic examination test within 30 minutes of obtaining the specimen.

Conditions: Gloves, patient preparation supplies and information, urine specimen, pipettes, centrifuge tube, centrifuge, microscope, microscope slides, cover slip, permanent marker, urine test strips, urine atlas, refractometer, distilled water, lint-free tissues, biohazard container, sharps container, disinfectant cleaner, laboratory report form, Sedi-Stain® (optional)

Standards: Perform the Task within 15 minutes with a minimum score of _____ points.

Work Documentation: Patient chart entry, lab requisition, practice label

No.	Step	Points	Check #1	Check #2	Check #3
1	Washed hands, organized supplies and equipment, set up microscope, applied appropriate PPE.				
2	Examined specimen for proper labeling. With lid tightly sealed, mixed urine well.				
3	Correctly performed the procedure: • Checked the urine culture and sensitivity transport kit expiration date. • Followed the manufacturer's instructions exactly, which will vary, depending on the system being used. • Secured and labeled the transport container and placed it into biohazard transport bag.				
4	Completed requisition correctly and placed it into biohazard transport bag.				
5	Disposed of contaminated supplies following OSHA regulations; disinfected surfaces; removed PPE; washed hands.				
6	Demonstrated professional behavior in manner, organization, and attire.				
7	Documented correctly.				
Student's Total Points					
Points Possible					
Final Score (Student's Total Points/ Possible Points)					

Name ________________________ **Date** ____________ **Score** ______

WORK DOCUMENTATION

*Also attach lab requisition.

Instructor's/Evaluator's Comments and Suggestions:

CHECK #1

Evaluator's Signature: Date:

CHECK #2

Evaluator's Signature: Date:

CHECK #3

Evaluator's Signature: Date:

ABHES Competency: VI.A.1.a.4.j Collect and process specimens; VI.A.1.a.4.y Perform urinalysis

CAAHEP Curriculum: I.P.14 Perform urinalysis

Name ______________________ Date __________ Score ______

COMPETENCY ASSESSMENT

Procedure 30-7 Instructing a Patient in the Collection of a Clean-Catch, Midstream Urine Specimen

Task: To instruct a patient in the proper technique of collecting a urine specimen suitable for urinalysis testing.

Conditions: Gloves, urine cup with a secure lid, cleansing towelettes, marking pen, written instructions posted appropriately in the bathroom

Standards: Perform the Task within 15 minutes with a minimum score of _____ points.

No.	Step	Points	Check #1	Check #2	Check #3
1	Checked room for cleanliness, equipment, and readiness; organized supplies and equipment; washed hands.				
2	Greeted and identified the patient and introduced self. Explained the procedure. Provided patient with written instructions so she could read along as medical assistant instructs.				
3	Provided patient with cleansing wipes, gloves, and labeled urine container with lid.				
4	Escorted patient to restroom and pointed out the written instructions on the wall beside the toilet. Instructed her where to place specimen when finished and how to get back to the examination room if not available to escort her. If possible, escorted patient back to examination room.				
5	Demonstrated professional behavior in manner, organization, and attire, including: • Communicated appropriately and comfortably with the patient.				
Student's Total Points					
Points Possible					
Final Score (Student's Total Points/ Possible Points)					

Name ______________________________ **Date** ____________ **Score** ______

Instructor's/Evaluator's Comments and Suggestions:

____

____

____

____

____

CHECK #1	
Evaluator's Signature:	Date:

CHECK #2	
Evaluator's Signature:	Date:

CHECK #3	
Evaluator's Signature:	Date:

ABHES Competency: VI.A.1.a.4.w Instruct patients in the collection of a clean-catch mid-stream urine specimen

CAAHEP Curriculum: IV.P.2 Report relevant information to others succinctly and accurately; IV.P.6 Prepare a patient for procedures and/or treatments

Name ______________________ Date __________ Score ______

COMPETENCY ASSESSMENT

Procedure 31-1 Procedure for Obtaining a Throat Specimen for Culture

Task: To obtain secretions from the nasopharnyx and tonsillar area as a means of identifying pathogenic microorganisms.

Conditions: Tongue depressor, culture tube with applicator stick or commercially prepared culture collection system (culturette), label and requisition form, gloves and face shield, good light source, emesis basin and tissues

Standards: Perform the Task within 15 minutes with a minimum score of _____ points.

Work Documentation: Patient chart entry, lab report

No.	Step	Points	Check #1	Check #2	Check #3
1	Washed hands; checked room for cleanliness, equipment, and readiness; organized supplies and equipment.				
2	Greeted and identified the patient and introduced self. Explained the procedure and washed hands.				
3	Provided the patient with emesis basin and tissues and positioned the patient appropriately. Applied appropriate PPE.				
4	Obtained the specimen properly.				
5	Handled and labeled the specimen properly.				
6	Disposed of contaminated supplies following OSHA regulations; disinfected surfaces; washed hands.				
7	Demonstrated professional behavior in manner, organization, and attire, including: • Communicated appropriately and comfortably with the patient.				
8	Documented correctly.				
Student's Total Points					
Points Possible					
Final Score (Student's Total Points/ Possible Points)					

Name ______________________________ **Date** ____________ **Score** ______

WORK DOCUMENTATION

*Also attach lab report.

Instructor's/Evaluator's Comments and Suggestions:

____

____

____

____

____

CHECK #1	
Evaluator's Signature:	Date:

CHECK #2	
Evaluator's Signature:	Date:

CHECK #3	
Evaluator's Signature:	Date:

ABHES Competency: VI.A.1.a.4.u Obtain throat specimen for microbiological testing

CAAHEP Curriculum: III.P.7 Obtain specimens for microbiological testing

Name ______________________________ Date ____________ Score _______

COMPETENCY ASSESSMENT

Procedure 31-2 Wet Mount and Hanging Drop Slide Preparations

Task: To prepare a slide for viewing live microorganisms for motility and identifying characteristics.

Conditions: Gloves, glass slide and cover slip, special slide with a well, petroleum jelly, dropper

Standards: Perform the Task within 15 minutes with a minimum score of _____ points.

No.	Step	Points	Check #1	Check #2	Check #3
1	Washed hands; organized supplies and equipment; applied appropriate PPE.				
2	Prepared the wet mount appropriately.				
3	Prepared the hanging drop slide appropriately.				
4	Obtained the specimen properly.				
5	Disposed of contaminated supplies following OSHA regulations; disinfected surfaces; washed hands.				
6	Demonstrated professional behavior in manner, organization, and attire.				
Student's Total Points					
Points Possible					
Final Score (Student's Total Points/ Possible Points)					

Name ______________________________ **Date** ____________ **Score** ______

Instructor's/Evaluator's Comments and Suggestions:

____

____

____

____

____

CHECK #1	
Evaluator's Signature:	Date:

CHECK #2	
Evaluator's Signature:	Date:

CHECK #3	
Evaluator's Signature:	Date:

ABHES Competency: VI.A.1.a.4.j Collect and process specimens

Name ______________________ Date __________ Score ______

COMPETENCY ASSESSMENT

Procedure 31-3 Performing Strep Throat Testing

Task: To test for streptococcus infection of the throat for diagnostic purposes. The following steps are intentionally general, so a variety of kits can be used.

Conditions: Gloves, commercial strep throat testing kit including controls and standards, disinfectant, tongue blade, adjustable light source, biohazard container

Standards: Perform the Task within 15 minutes with a minimum score of _____ points.

Work Documentation: Patient chart entry, lab report

No.	Step	Points	Check #1	Check #2	Check #3
1	Washed hands; checked room for cleanliness, equipment, and readiness; organized supplies and equipment.				
2	Greeted and identified the patient and introduced self. Explained the procedure and washed hands.				
3	Provided the patient with emesis basin and tissues and positioned the patient appropriately. Applied appropriate PPE.				
4	Obtained the specimen properly.				
5	Handled and labeled the specimen properly.				
6	Tested the specimen according to the test kit's manufacturer's instructions, following instructions exactly.				
7	Disposed of contaminated supplies following OSHA regulations; disinfected surfaces; washed hands.				
8	Demonstrated professional behavior in manner, organization, and attire, including: • Communicated appropriately and comfortably with the patient.				
9	Documented correctly.				
Student's Total Points					
Points Possible					
Final Score (Student's Total Points/ Possible Points)					

Name ______________________ **Date** __________ **Score** ______

WORK DOCUMENTATION

*Also attach lab report.

Instructor's/Evaluator's Comments and Suggestions:

____

____

____

____

____

CHECK #1	
Evaluator's Signature:	Date:

CHECK #2	
Evaluator's Signature:	Date:

CHECK #3	
Evaluator's Signature:	Date:

ABHES Competency: VI.A.1.a.4.u Obtain throat specimen for microbiological testing; VI.A.1.a.4.cc Perform microbiology testing

CAAHEP Curriculum: III.P.7 Obtain specimens for microbiological testing; III.P.8 Perform CLIA waived microbiology testing

Name ______________________ Date __________ Score ______

COMPETENCY ASSESSMENT

Procedure 31-4 Instructing a Patient on Obtaining a Fecal Specimen

Task: To instruct a patient in the correct collection of a fecal sample.

Condition: Gloves, biohazard container, sturdy and opaque waterproof specimen container with a securely fitting lid, special laboratory manual instructions if needed

Standards: Perform the Task within 15 minutes with a minimum score of _____ points.

Work Documentation: Patient chart entry

No.	Step	Points	Check #1	Check #2	Check #3
1	Checked room for cleanliness, equipment, and readiness; organized supplies and equipment; washed hands.				
2	Greeted and identified the patient and introduced self. Explained the procedure and provided patient with written instructions as well.				
3	Handed patient the labeled specimen container and instructed patient to deposit a sample of stool into the cup, then securely set the lid. Cautioned patient not to contaminate specimen with urine.				
4	Gave the patient a biohazard transport bag and instructions on which pocket to put the specimen into and how to secure the bag.				
5	Instructed patient to transport the specimen as soon as possible to the lab, keeping the specimen at or just below body temperature.				
6	Demonstrated professional behavior in manner, organization, and attire, including: • Communicated appropriately and comfortably with the patient.				
7	Documented correctly.				
Student's Total Points					
Points Possible					
Final Score (Student's Total Points/ Possible Points)					

Name ______________________ **Date** __________ **Score** ______

WORK DOCUMENTATION

Instructor's/Evaluator's Comments and Suggestions:

____

____

____

____

____

CHECK #1	
Evaluator's Signature:	Date:

CHECK #2	
Evaluator's Signature:	Date:

CHECK #3	
Evaluator's Signature:	Date:

ABHES Competency: VI.A.1.a.4.x Instruct patient in the collection of fecal specimen

CAAHEP Curriculum: IV.P.2 Report relevant information to others succinctly and accurately

Name ______________________________ **Date** ____________ **Score** ______

COMPETENCY ASSESSMENT

Procedure 32-1 Pregnancy Test

Task: To perform the enzyme immunoassay or agglutination inhibition test to detect human chorionic gonadotropin (hCG) in urine to determine positive or negative pregnancy results.

Conditions: Gloves, urine specimen, timer, surface disinfectant, biohazard container, hCG negative and positive urine control, pregnancy test kit

Standards: Perform the Task within 15 minutes with a minimum score of _____ points.

Work Documentation: Patient chart entry, lab report

No.	Step	Points	Check #1	Check #2	Check #3
1	Washed hands; organized supplies and equipment; applied appropriate PPE.				
2	Performed urine pregnancy test properly.				
3	Disposed of contaminated supplies following OSHA regulations; disinfected surfaces; washed hands.				
4	Demonstrated professional behavior in manner, organization, and attire.				
5	Documented correctly.				
Student's Total Points					
Points Possible					
Final Score (Student's Total Points/ Possible Points)					

Name ______________________________ **Date** ____________ **Score** ______

WORK DOCUMENTATION

*Also attach lab report.

Instructor's/Evaluator's Comments and Suggestions:

____

____

____

____

____

CHECK #1

Evaluator's Signature: Date:

CHECK #2

Evaluator's Signature: Date:

CHECK #3

Evaluator's Signature: Date:

ABHES Competency: VI.A.1.a.4.k Perform selected CLIA-waived tests (i.e. kit tests such as pregnancy, quick strep, dip sticks) that assist with diagnosis and treatment

Name ______________________________ **Date** ____________ **Score** ______

COMPETENCY ASSESSMENT

Procedure 32-2 Performing Infectious Mononucleosis Test

Task: To perform an accurate test of serum or plasma to detect the presence or absence of antibodies of mononucleosis.

Conditions: Gloves, goggles (optional), safety lancet, alcohol swabs, cotton balls, gauze, adhesive strip, glucose analyzer, control solutions for glucose analyzer, test strips for glucose analyzer, laboratory tissue

Standards: Perform the Task within 15 minutes with a minimum score of _____ points.

Work Documentation: Patient chart entry, lab report

No.	Step	Points	Check #1	Check #2	Check #3
1	Washed hands; organized supplies and equipment; applied appropriate PPE.				
2	Performed infectious mononucleosis test properly.				
3	Disposed of contaminated supplies following OSHA regulations; disinfected surfaces; washed hands.				
4	Demonstrated professional behavior in manner, organization, and attire.				
5	Documented correctly.				
Student's Total Points					
Points Possible					
Final Score (Student's Total Points/ Possible Points)					

Name ______________________________ **Date** ____________ **Score** ______

WORK DOCUMENTATION

*Also attach lab report.

Instructor's/Evaluator's Comments and Suggestions:

____

____

____

____

____

CHECK #1	
Evaluator's Signature:	Date:

CHECK #2	
Evaluator's Signature:	Date:

CHECK #3	
Evaluator's Signature:	Date:

ABHES Competency: VI.A.1.a.4.bb Perform immunology testing

CAAHEP Curriculum: I.P.15 Perform immunology testing

Name ______________________________ Date ____________ Score ______

COMPETENCY ASSESSMENT

Procedure 32-3 Obtaining Blood Specimen for Phenylketonuria (PKU) Test

Task: To obtain a blood specimen using a PKU test card or "filter paper" to determine phenylalanine levels in newborns who are at least 3 days old.

Conditions: Gloves, PKU filter paper test card and mailing envelope, alcohol swabs, cotton balls or gauze pad, sterile pediatric-sized lancet, biohazard waste container

Standards: Perform the Task within 20 minutes with a minimum score of _____ points.

Work Documentation: Patient chart entry, PKU card

No.	Step	Points	Check #1	Check #2	Check #3
1	Washed hands; checked room for cleanliness, equipment, and readiness; organized supplies and equipment.				
2	Greeted and identified the patient and parents, and introduced self.				
3	Explained the procedure, gave parents information documents, obtained written informed consent, obtained patient information as required for PKU forms.				
4	Washed hands; positioned the patient properly for comfort and safety; applied PPE.				
5	Obtained the blood specimens properly and safely, filling the appropriate areas on the card as required for proper testing. Comforted the patient and assisted the parents as needed.				
6	Completed the forms properly, packaged the specimen for mailing, following manufacturer's instructions exactly.				
7	Disposed of contaminated supplies following OSHA regulations; disinfected surfaces; washed hands.				
8	Demonstrated professional behavior in manner, organization, and attire, including: • Communicated appropriately and comfortably with the patient.				
9	Documented correctly.				
Student's Total Points					
Points Possible					
Final Score (Student's Total Points/ Possible Points)					

Name ____________________ **Date** __________ **Score** ______

WORK DOCUMENTATION

*Also attach PKU card.

Instructor's/Evaluator's Comments and Suggestions:

CHECK #1

Evaluator's Signature: Date:

CHECK #2

Evaluator's Signature: Date:

CHECK #3

Evaluator's Signature: Date:

ABHES Competency: VI.A.1.a.4.aa Perform chemistry testing

CAAHEP Curriculum: I.P.13 Perform chemistry testing

Name ______________________________ Date ____________ Score ______

COMPETENCY ASSESSMENT

Procedure 32-4 Screening Test for PKU

Task: Test a urine specimen using the diaper test or the Phenistik test to determine phenylalanine levels in infants who are at least 6 weeks old. This is a quick screening test only and *does not* take the place of the blood test.

Conditions: Gloves, 10% ferric chloride for the diaper test or Phenistik Method Test, biohazard waste container

Standards: Perform the Task within 5 minutes with a minimum score of _____ points.

Work Documentation: Patient chart entry

No.	Step	Points	Check #1	Check #2	Check #3
1	Washed hands; checked room for cleanliness, equipment, and readiness; organized supplies and equipment.				
2	Greeted and identified the patient and parents, and introduced self.				
3	Explained the procedure and that this does not take the place of the PKU blood test. Determined that the patient was at least 6 weeks of age. Applied PPE.				
4	Removed diaper from the infant, replaced with clean diaper. Performed the test on urine in the diaper safely and away from patient and parent(s).				
5	If the test was positive, alerted the physician and followed up with the PKU test.				
6	Disposed of contaminated supplies following OSHA regulations; disinfected surfaces; washed hands.				
7	Demonstrated professional behavior in manner, organization, and attire, including: • Communicated appropriately and comfortably with the patient.				
8	Documented correctly.				
Student's Total Points					
Points Possible					
Final Score (Student's Total Points/ Possible Points)					

Name ______________________ **Date** __________ **Score** ______

WORK DOCUMENTATION

___

Instructor's/Evaluator's Comments and Suggestions:

___
___
___
___
___

CHECK #1
Evaluator's Signature: Date:

CHECK #2
Evaluator's Signature: Date:

CHECK #3
Evaluator's Signature: Date:

ABHES Competency: VI.A.1.a.4.l Screen and follow up patient test results; VI.A.1.a.4.aa Perform chemistry testing

CAAHEP Curriculum: I.P.13 Perform chemistry testing; I.P.16 Screen test results

Name ______________________ Date __________ Score ______

COMPETENCY ASSESSMENT

Procedure 32-5 Measurement of Blood Glucose Using an Automated Analyzer

Task: To measure blood glucose.

Conditions: Gloves, goggles (optional), safety lancet, alcohol swabs, cotton balls, gauze, adhesive strip, glucose analyzer, control solutions for glucose analyzer, test strips for glucose analyzer, laboratory tissue

Standards: Perform the Task within 15 minutes with a minimum score of _____ points.

Work Documentation: Patient chart entry, lab report

No.	Step	Points	Check #1	Check #2	Check #3
1	Washed hands; organized supplies and equipment; applied appropriate PPE.				
2	Performed instrument calibrations and quality controls.				
3	Obtained blood specimen using proper technique.				
4	Tested specimen following the manufacturer's instructions exactly. Repeated test if indicated.				
5	Disposed of contaminated supplies following OSHA regulations; disinfected surfaces; washed hands.				
6	Demonstrated professional behavior in manner, organization, and attire.				
7	Documented correctly.				
Student's Total Points					
Points Possible					
Final Score (Student's Total Points/ Possible Points)					

Name ______________________ Date ____________ Score ______

WORK DOCUMENTATION

*Also attach lab report.

Instructor's/Evaluator's Comments and Suggestions:

____

____

____

____

____

CHECK #1
Evaluator's Signature: Date:

CHECK #2
Evaluator's Signature: Date:

CHECK #3
Evaluator's Signature: Date:

ABHES Competency: VI.A.1.a.4.k Perform selected CLIA-waived tests (i.e. kit tests such as pregnancy, quick strep, dip sticks) that assist with diagnosis and treatment; VI.A.1.a.4.i Use quality control; VI.A.1.a.4.aa Perform chemistry testing

CAAHEP Curriculum: I.P.11 Perform quality control measures; I.P.13 Perform chemistry testing

Name ________________________________ Date ____________ Score ______

COMPETENCY ASSESSMENT

Procedure 32-6 Cholesterol Testing

Task: To test for cholesterol, high-density lipoprotein, or triglyceride level for monitoring purposes. The following steps are intentionally general, so a variety of kits can be used.

Conditions: Gloves, blood collection equipment, pipettes with disposable tips, chlorine bleach, commercial kit for manual determination of cholesterol, controls and standards, marking pen, biohazard container

Standards: Perform the Task within 15 minutes with a minimum score of _____ points.

Work Documentation: Patient chart entry, lab report

No.	Step	Points	Check #1	Check #2	Check #3
1	Washed hands; organized supplies and equipment; applied appropriate PPE.				
2	Performed instrument calibrations and quality controls.				
3	Obtained blood specimen using proper technique.				
4	Tested specimen following the manufacturer's instructions exactly.				
5	Disposed of contaminated supplies following OSHA regulations; disinfected surfaces; washed hands.				
6	Demonstrated professional behavior in manner, organization, and attire.				
7	Documented correctly.				
Student's Total Points					
Points Possible					
Final Score (Student's Total Points/ Possible Points)					

Name ______________________ Date __________ Score ______

WORK DOCUMENTATION

*Also attach lab report.

Instructor's/Evaluator's Comments and Suggestions:

____

____

____

____

____

CHECK #1

Evaluator's Signature: Date:

CHECK #2

Evaluator's Signature: Date:

CHECK #3

Evaluator's Signature: Date:

ABHES Competency: VI.A.1.a.4.k Perform selected CLIA-waived tests (i.e. kit tests such as pregnancy, quick strep, dip sticks) that assist with diagnosis and treatment; VI.A.1.a.4.i Use quality control; VI.A.1.a.4.aa Perform chemistry testing

CAAHEP Curriculum: I.P.11 Perform quality control measures; I.P.13 Perform chemistry testing

Name ______________________________ Date ____________ Score ______

COMPETENCY ASSESSMENT

Procedure 33-1 Completing a Medical Incident Report

Task: To complete a medical incident report and submit it in a timely manner.

Condition: Appropriate medical incident report form or computer with Incident Report Software

Standards: Perform the Task within 15 minutes with a minimum score of _____ points.

Work Documentation: Completed incident report form

No.	Step	Points	Check #1	Check #2	Check #3
1	Accurately completed the incident report form, filling in each section of the report, including: • Used quotes when referring to un-witnessed statements. • Wrote the names of all witnesses to the incident in the report.				
2	Submitted the completed incident report to the appropriate person.				
Student's Total Points					
Points Possible					
Final Score (Student's Total Points/ Possible Points)					

Name ______________________________ **Date** ______________ **Score** ________

WORK DOCUMENTATION

*Attach completed incident report form.

Instructor's/Evaluator's Comments and Suggestions:

____

____

____

____

____

CHECK #1	
Evaluator's Signature:	Date:

CHECK #2	
Evaluator's Signature:	Date:

CHECK #3	
Evaluator's Signature:	Date:

ABHES Competency: VI.A.1.a.5.h Perform risk management procedures

CAAHEP Curriculum: IX.P.6 Complete an incident report

Name ______________________________ **Date** ____________ **Score** ______

COMPETENCY ASSESSMENT

Procedure 33-2 Preparing a Meeting Agenda

Task: To prepare a meeting agenda with an established list of specific items to be discussed or acted on, or both.

Condition: List of participants, the order of business, names of individuals giving reports, names of any guest speakers, a computer, paper on which to print agendas

Standards: Perform the Task within 20 minutes with a minimum score of _____ points.

Work Documentation: Printed agenda

No.	Step	Points	Check #1	Check #2	Check #3
1	Confirmed the proposed dates and place of meeting.				
2	Prepared and typed agenda: • Collected information from previous meetings' minutes for old agenda items. • Checked with others for report items and determined any new business.				
3	When completed, had agenda approved by the meeting chair.				
4	Sent agenda to participants.				
5	Reserved meeting room and arranged for food items, equipment, and supplies that may be needed.				
Student's Total Points					
Points Possible					
Final Score (Student's Total Points/ Possible Points)					

Name ______________________ Date ____________ Score ______

WORK DOCUMENTATION

*Attach printed agenda.

Instructor's/Evaluator's Comments and Suggestions:

____

____

____

____

____

CHECK #1

Evaluator's Signature: Date:

CHECK #2

Evaluator's Signature: Date:

CHECK #3

Evaluator's Signature: Date:

ABHES Competency: VI.A.1.a.2.j Use correct grammar, spelling and formatting techniques in written works; VI.A.1.a.2.o Fundamental writing skills; VI.A.1.a.3.a Perform basic secretarial skills

CAAHEP Curriculum: IV.P.2 Report relevant information to others succinctly and accurately

Name ______________________________ Date ____________ Score ______

COMPETENCY ASSESSMENT

Procedure 33-3 Supervising a Student Practicum

Task: To prepare a training path for a student extern being assigned to the office, make the involved personnel aware of their responsibilities, preplan the jobs the student will perform and in what sequence they will be assigned, and try to make the externship successful by providing as much supervision and assistance as necessary.

Condition: A schedule log, calendar, office procedures manual, any criteria presented by the program director

Standards: Perform the Task within 30 minutes with a minimum score of _____ points.

No.	Step	Points	Check #1	Check #2	Check #3
1	Reviewed the clinical practicum contract between your agency and the educational institution.				
2	Identified student's supervisor, planned tasks that the student will perform, and created a schedule for the student and staff.				
3	Oriented the student to the facility and staff upon arrival.				
4	Maintained an accurate record of hours the student worked, including missed days and late arrivals.				
5	Consulted with providers, staff, and the student for feedback.				
6	Reported student progress to the medical assistants program director and prepared student's evaluation report using input from all who worked with student.				
Student's Total Points					
Points Possible					
Final Score (Student's Total Points/ Possible Points)					

Name ______________________ **Date** ____________ **Score** ______

Instructor's/Evaluator's Comments and Suggestions:

CHECK #1
Evaluator's Signature: Date:

CHECK #2
Evaluator's Signature: Date:

CHECK #3
Evaluator's Signature: Date:

ABHES Competency: VI.A.1.a.2.m Adaptation for individualized needs; VI.A.1.a.7.d orient and train personnel

CAAHEP Curriculum: IV.P.4 Explain general office policies

Name ______________________________ Date ____________ Score ______

COMPETENCY ASSESSMENT

Procedure 33-4 Developing and Maintaining a Procedure Manual

Task: To develop and maintain a comprehensive, up-to-date procedures manual covering each medical, technical, and administrative procedure in the office with step-by-step directions and rationale for performing each task.

Condition: A computer, three-ring binder, paper, procedures, and criteria

Standards: Perform the Task within 20 minutes with a minimum score of _____ points.

Work Documentation: Binder with procedure entries

No.	Step	Points	Check #1	Check #2	Check #3
1	Wrote detailed, step-by-step procedures and rationale for each medical, technical, and administrative function. Each procedure was written by experienced employees close to the function and reviewed by a supervisor or the office manager.				
2	Included regular maintenance (cleaning, servicing, and calibrating) instructions and flow sheets for all office equipment, both in the clinical area and in the office/business areas.				
3	Included step-by-step procedures on how to accomplish each task, both in the clinical area and in the office/business areas.				
4	Included local and out of the area resources for clinical staff, office/business staff, physicians/providers, and patients. Provided a listing in each area with contact information and services available.				
5	Included basic rules and regulations, state and federal, which are related to processes performed in both clinical and office/business areas.				
6	Included the clinic procedures and flow sheets for taking inventory in each of the areas, and instructions on ordering procedures.				
7	Collected the procedures into the office procedures manual.				
Student's Total Points					
Points Possible					
Final Score (Student's Total Points/ Possible Points)					

Name ______________________ **Date** __________ **Score** ______

WORK DOCUMENTATION

*Attach completed procedure manual entries.

Instructor's/Evaluator's Comments and Suggestions:

____

____

____

____

____

CHECK #1	
Evaluator's Signature:	Date:

CHECK #2	
Evaluator's Signature:	Date:

CHECK #3	
Evaluator's Signature:	Date:

ABHES Competency: VI.A.1.a.6.a Maintain physical plant; VI.A.1.a.7.d Orient and train personnel

CAAHEP Curriculum: IX.P.5 Incorporate the Patient's Bill of Rights into personal practice and medical office policies and procedures; IX.P.8 Apply local, state and federal health care legislation and regulation appropriate to the medical assisting practice setting

Name ______________________________ Date ____________ Score ______

COMPETENCY ASSESSMENT

Procedure 33-5 Making Travel Arrangements with a Travel Agent

Task: To make travel arrangements for the provider.

Condition: A travel plan/preferences, telephone, directory, computer, and the provider's or office credit card to secure reservations

Standards: Perform the Task within 20 minutes with a minimum score of _____ points.

Work Documentation: Completed itinerary

No.	Step	Points	Check #1	Check #2	Check #3
1	Confirmed the details of the trip: dates, times, places of departures and arrivals, preferred transportation method, number of travelers, preferred lodging type, and price range.				
2	Telephoned travel agent.				
3	Picked up tickets or arranged for delivery or secured confirmation of electronic tickets. Checked that flight, rental car, room arrangements were accurate and confirmed.				
4	Made copies of itinerary, forwarded one to the provider and maintained one copy in the office.				
Student's Total Points					
Points Possible					
Final Score (Student's Total Points/ Possible Points)					

Name ______________________________ **Date** ____________ **Score** ______

WORK DOCUMENTATION

*Attach completed itinerary.

Instructor's/Evaluator's Comments and Suggestions:

____

____

____

____

____

CHECK #1	
Evaluator's Signature:	Date:

CHECK #2	
Evaluator's Signature:	Date:

CHECK #3	
Evaluator's Signature:	Date:

ABHES Competency: VI.A.1.a.3.f Manage physician's professional schedule and travel

Name ______________________________ Date ____________ Score ______

COMPETENCY ASSESSMENT

Procedure 33-6 Making Travel Arrangements via the Internet

Task: To make travel arrangements for the provider using the Internet.

Condition: A travel plan/preferences, computer, and the provider's or office credit card to secure reservations

Standards: Perform the Task within 20 minutes with a minimum score of _____ points.

Work Documentation: Completed itinerary

No.	Step	Points	Check #1	Check #2	Check #3
1	Confirmed the details of the trip: dates, times, places of departures and arrivals, preferred transportation method, number of travelers, preferred lodging type, and price range.				
2	Made arrangements using the Internet.				
3	Picked up tickets or arranged for delivery or secured confirmation of electronic tickets. Checked that flight, rental car, room arrangements were accurate and confirmed.				
4	Made copies of itinerary, forwarded one to the provider and maintained one copy in the office.				
Student's Total Points					
Points Possible					
Final Score (Student's Total Points/ Possible Points)					

Name ______________________ **Date** ____________ **Score** ______

WORK DOCUMENTATION

*Attach completed itinerary.

Instructor's/Evaluator's Comments and Suggestions:

____

____

____

____

____

CHECK #1	
Evaluator's Signature:	Date:

CHECK #2	
Evaluator's Signature:	Date:

CHECK #3	
Evaluator's Signature:	Date:

ABHES Competency: VI.A.1.a.3.f Manage physician's professional schedule and travel

CAAHEP Curriculum: V.P.7 Use internet to access information related to the medical office

Name ______________________________ Date ____________ Score ______

COMPETENCY ASSESSMENT

Procedure 33-7 Processing Employee Payroll

Task: To process payroll compensating employees, calculating all deductions accurately.

Condition: Computer and payroll software or checkbook; tax withholding tables; Federal Employers Tax Guide

Standards: Perform the Task within 45 minutes with a minimum score of _____ points.

No.	Step	Points	Check #1	Check #2	Check #3
1	Reviewed time cards and determined each employee's time away from the office.				
2	Calculated the salary or hourly wages owed to each employee; calculated the deductions that must be withheld form the paycheck for each employee.				
3	Used computer and payroll software or handwrote the payroll checks for each employee, with explanation of deductions.				
4	Mailed each payroll check to the appropriate employee.				
Student's Total Points					
Points Possible					
Final Score (Student's Total Points/ Possible Points)					

Name ______________________ **Date** ____________ **Score** ______

Instructor's/Evaluator's Comments and Suggestions:

____

____

____

____

____

CHECK #1	
Evaluator's Signature:	Date:

CHECK #2	
Evaluator's Signature:	Date:

CHECK #3	
Evaluator's Signature:	Date:

ABHES Competency: VI.A.1.a.8.f Process employee payroll

Name ______________________________ Date ____________ Score ______

COMPETENCY ASSESSMENT

Procedure 33-8 Perform an Inventory of Equipment and Supplies

Task: To develop an inventory of expendable administrative and clinical supplies in a medical office.

Condition: Printout of most recent inventory spreadsheet, clipboard, pad of reorder forms, pen or pencil

Standards: Perform the Task within 15 minutes with a minimum score of _____ points.

Work Documentation: Completed inventory list

No.	Step	Points	Check #1	Check #2	Check #3
1	Assembled equipment and supplies to be inventoried.				
2	Accurately counted and recorded the quantity of each item and completed an inventory form.				
3	If a supply or equipment was below the minimum amount, indicated that reordering was necessary.				
4	Signed form and gave to person responsible for ordering supplies. Or filled out an order form for the additional supplies.				
Student's Total Points					
Points Possible					
Final Score (Student's Total Points/ Possible Points)					

Name ______________________________ **Date** ____________ **Score** ______

WORK DOCUMENTATION

*Attach completed inventory list.

Instructor's/Evaluator's Comments and Suggestions:

____

____

____

____

____

CHECK #1

Evaluator's Signature: Date:

CHECK #2

Evaluator's Signature: Date:

CHECK #3

Evaluator's Signature: Date:

ABHES Competency: VI.A.1.a.6.c Inventory equipment and supplies; VI.A.1.a.6.d Evaluate and recommend equipment and supplies for practice

CAAHEP Curriculum: V.P.10 Perform an office inventory

Name ______________________________ Date __________ Score ______

COMPETENCY ASSESSMENT

Procedure 33-9 Perform Routine Maintenance or Calibration of Administrative and Clinical Equipment

Task: To ensure the operability and calibration of administrative and clinical equipment.

Condition: Equipment list with maintenance or calibration requirements; clipboard, pen, maintenance record sheets, and deficiency tags; access to operation and service manuals of equipment to be serviced; access to any necessary maintenance tools and supplies

Standards: Perform the Task within 30 minutes with a minimum score of _____ points.

Work Documentation: Maintenance record form

No.	Step	Points	Check #1	Check #2	Check #3
1	Inspected appropriate administrative and clinical equipment. Inspected for cleanliness, safety, and operability. Noted and recorded equipment that required repairs.				
2	Properly completed maintenance checklist: • Included date. • Documented whether maintenance or repairs were needed. • Signed the form.				
Student's Total Points					
Points Possible					
Final Score (Student's Total Points/ Possible Points)					

Name ______________________________ **Date** ____________ **Score** ______

WORK DOCUMENTATION

*Attach maintenance record form.

Instructor's/Evaluator's Comments and Suggestions:

____

____

____

____

____

CHECK #1	
Evaluator's Signature:	Date:

CHECK #2	
Evaluator's Signature:	Date:

CHECK #3	
Evaluator's Signature:	Date:

ABHES Competency: VI.A.1.a.6.b Operate and maintain facilities and perform routine maintenance of administrative and clinical equipment safely

CAAHEP Curriculum: V.P.9 Perform routine maintenance of office equipment with documentation

Name ______________________________ Date ____________ Score ______

COMPETENCY ASSESSMENT

Procedure 34-1 Develop and Maintain a Policy Manual

Task: To develop and maintain a comprehensive, up-to-date policy manual of all office policies relating to employee practices, benefits, office conduct, and so forth.

Condition: Computer, three-ring binder, paper, standard policy format

Standards: Perform the Task within 20 minutes with a minimum score of _____ points.

Work Documentation: Printed policy manual entries

No.	Step	Points	Check #1	Check #2	Check #3
1	Following office format, developed precise, written office policies detailing all necessary information pertaining to the staff and their positions. Included benefits, vacation, sick leave, hours, dress codes, evaluations, rules of conduct, and grounds for dismissal.				
2	Identified procedures for reimbursing overtime, preventing discrimination and harassment, creating a safe workplace, and allowing for jury duty.				
3	Included a policy statement related to smoking and other substances.				
4	Identified steps to follow should an employee become disabled during employment.				
5	Determined what employee opportunities for continuing education would be reimbursed and included requirements for certification and licensures.				
6	Provided a copy of the policy manual for each employee.				
7	Reviewed and updated the policy manual regularly. Added or deleted items as necessary, dating each revision.				
Student's Total Points					
Points Possible					
Final Score (Student's Total Points/ Possible Points)					

Name ______________________ **Date** ____________ **Score** ______

WORK DOCUMENTATION

*Attach printed policy manual entries.

Instructor's/Evaluator's Comments and Suggestions:

____

____

____

____

____

CHECK #1

Evaluator's Signature: Date:

CHECK #2

Evaluator's Signature: Date:

CHECK #3

Evaluator's Signature: Date:

ABHES Competency: VI.A.1.a.7.d Orient and train personnel

CAAHEP Curriculum: IV.P.4 Explain general office policies

Name ______________________________ Date ____________ Score ______

COMPETENCY ASSESSMENT

Procedure 34-2 Prepare a Job Description

Task: To develop a precise definition of the tasks assigned to a job, to determine the expectations and level of competency required, and to specify the experience, training, and education needed to perform the job for purposes of recruiting and performance evaluation.

Condition: Computer, three-ring binder, paper, standard job description format

Standards: Perform the Task within 20 minutes with a minimum score of _____ points.

Work Documentation: Printout of job description, or job description written in documentation area

No.	Step	Points	Check #1	Check #2	Check #3
1	Detailed each task that creates the job.				
2	Listed special medical, technical, or clerical skills needed.				
3	Determined the level of education, training, and experience required for the position.				
4	Determined where the job fits into the overall structure of the office.				
5	Specified any unusual working conditions (hours, locations, etc.) that may apply.				
6	Described career path opportunities.				
7	Reviewed and updated the policy manual regularly. Added or deleted items as necessary, dating each revision.				
Student's Total Points					
Points Possible					
Final Score (Student's Total Points/ Possible Points)					

Name ______________________ **Date** __________ **Score** ______

WORK DOCUMENTATION

Instructor's/Evaluator's Comments and Suggestions:

____

____

____

____

____

CHECK #1	
Evaluator's Signature:	Date:

CHECK #2	
Evaluator's Signature:	Date:

CHECK #3	
Evaluator's Signature:	Date:

ABHES Competency: VI.A.1.a.6.a Maintain physical plant

CAAHEP Curriculum: IV.P.4 Explain general office policies

Name ______________________ **Date** __________ **Score** ______

COMPETENCY ASSESSMENT

Procedure 34-3 Conduct Interviews

Task: To screen applicants for training, experience, and characteristics to select the best candidate to fill the position vacancy.

Condition: Interview questions; policy manual (for referencing); applicant's résumé, application, and cover letter

Standards: Perform the Task within 40 minutes with a minimum score of _____ points.

No.	Step	Points	Check #1	Check #2	Check #3
1	Reviewed résumés and applications received and selected candidates who had the skills being sought. Created an interview worksheet for each candidate, listing the points to cover, and identified who on staff would be part of the interview team.				
2	Screened the applicant over the phone.				
3	Conducted the in-office interview of the applicant: • Provided an overview about the practice and staff, describing the job and answering preliminary questions. • Asked questions about the applicant's work experience and educational background. • Informed the applicants when a decision would be made, and thanked each applicant for participating in the interview.				
4	Checked references of all prospective employees.				
5	Established a second interview for the qualified candidate if necessary.				
6	Confirmed accepted job offers in writing, specifying the details of the offer and acceptance, and notified all unsuccessful applicants by letter when the position was filled.				
Student's Total Points					
Points Possible					
Final Score (Student's Total Points/ Possible Points)					

Name ______________________ **Date** ____________ **Score** ________

Instructor's/Evaluator's Comments and Suggestions:

____

____

____

____

____

CHECK #1
Evaluator's Signature: Date:

CHECK #2
Evaluator's Signature: Date:

CHECK #3
Evaluator's Signature: Date:

ABHES Competency: VI.A.1.a.2.f Interview effectively; VI.A.1.a.2.i Recognize and respond to verbal and non-verbal communication; VI.A.1.a.2.k Principles of verbal and nonverbal communication; VI.A.1.a.2.l Recognition and response to verbal and non-verbal communication

CAAHEP Curriculum: IV.P.2 Report relevant information to others succinctly and accurately; IV.P.4 Explain general office policies

Name ______________________________ Date ____________ Score ______

COMPETENCY ASSESSMENT

Procedure 34-4 Orient Personnel

Task: To acquaint new employees with office policies, staff, what the job encompasses, procedures to be performed, and job performance expectations.

Condition: Policy manual

Standards: Perform the Task within 30 minutes with a minimum score of _____ points.

No.	Step	Points	Check #1	Check #2	Check #3
1	Toured the facilities and introduced the office staff. Assigned a mentor from the staff to help with the orientation.				
2	Completed employee-related documents and explained their purpose. Explained the benefits program.				
3	Presented the office policy manual and discussed the key elements. Reviewed federal and state regulatory precautions for medical facilities. Reviewed the job description.				
4	Explained and demonstrated procedures to be performed and the use of procedures manuals supporting these procedures.				
5	Demonstrated the use of any specialized equipment (such as time clocks, key entries, etc.). Medical equipment would be demonstrated by clinical staff.				
Student's Total Points					
Points Possible					
Final Score (Student's Total Points/ Possible Points)					

Name ______________________ **Date** __________ **Score** ______

Instructor's/Evaluator's Comments and Suggestions:

____

____

____

____

____

CHECK #1	
Evaluator's Signature:	Date:

CHECK #2	
Evaluator's Signature:	Date:

CHECK #3	
Evaluator's Signature:	Date:

ABHES Competency: VI.A.1.a.7.d Orient and train personnel

CAAHEP Curriculum: IV.P.4 Explain general office policies

Comprehensive Examination

1. Which term describes false and malicious writing about another that constitutes defamation of character?
   a. Slander
   b. Assault
   c. Libel
   d. Invasion of privacy
   e. Battery
2. When reviewing a résumé, the human resources manager does NOT consider the applicant's:
   a. supplemental education
   b. unexplained gaps in employment
   c. training related to the position
   d. age, sex, and race
   e. previous experience
3. The standard of professional conduct for a certified medical assistant should be:
   a. in keeping with the AAMA Code of Ethics
   b. outlined by the provider or employer
   c. based on the Hippocratic oath
   d. in keeping with the AMA Principles of Medical Ethics
   e. determined by the state's medical practice act
4. After an interview, the applicant should:
   a. telephone to say thank you
   b. have his or her references call the interviewer
   c. telephone after three days to check the status of his or her application
   d. promptly send a follow-up letter
   e. send a lavish thank-you gift
5. A medical assistant must NEVER:
   a. perform a venipuncture
   b. perform a laboratory test
   c. imply that he or she is a nurse
   d. dispense a medication after a direct order from the provider
   e. give a medication after a direct order from the provider
6. Which legal principle is violated when a medical assistant practices outside of his or her training?
   a. Public d'uty
   b. Consent
   c. Privacy rights
   d. Confidentiality
   e. Standard of care

7. Which manner of dress is appropriate for an interview?
   a. A medical assistant's uniform
   b. Evening makeup
   c. Spectacular nail polish
   d. Casual clothing
   e. Neat business attire
8. Which statement accurately describes ethics?
   a. Ethics are a personal moral philosophy of right and wrong.
   b. Ethics are a code of minimal acceptable behavior.
   c. Ethics are the state's legal standards established for a profession.
   d. Ethics are the federal legal standards established for a profession.
   e. Ethics are standards for personal behavior as established by organized religions.
9. When stressed, we may exhibit all of the following EXCEPT:
   a. anxiety
   b. objective thinking
   c. depression
   d. anger
   e. irrational behavior
10. All of the following statements about Good Samaritan laws are true EXCEPT:
    a. These laws do not provide legal protection to on-duty emergency care providers.
    b. Providers must act in a reasonable and prudent manner.
    c. The conditions of these laws vary in each state.
    d. No matter what their level of training, providers must do everything for the patient.
    e. Health care providers are ethically, not legally, obligated to assist in emergency situations.
11. What is the purpose of the certification credential for medical assistants?
    a. The certification credential is required for graduation.
    b. The certification credential guarantees a job.
    c. The certification credential meets state registration requirements.
    d. The certification credential indicates a medical assistant's professional and technical competence.
    e. The certification credential meets state licensure requirements.
12. Consent for treatment may usually be given by:
    a. the patient's closest relative
    b. a patient in a mental institution
    c. any minor over 16
    d. the person accompanying the patient
    e. a legally competent patient

13. Who is the most important member of the health care team?
    a. The patient
    b. The provider
    c. The medical assistant
    d. The nurse
    e. The receptionist
14. All of the following cultural influences may affect communication EXCEPT:
    a. education
    b. sexual orientation
    c. ethnic heritage
    d. geographic location
    e. age
15. When the medical office wins in small claims court, the money is collected from the patient by:
    a. the bailiff
    b. the patient's insurance company
    c. the probate court
    d. the medical office
    e. the court-appointed collection agency
16. Which statement is accurate regarding the Americans with Disabilities Act (ADA)?
    a. The ADA applies only to medical practices and health care facilities.
    b. The ADA applies to all businesses.
    c. The ADA applies only to businesses with 15 or more employees.
    d. The ADA applies only to businesses with 50 or more employees.
    e. The ADA applies only to state and federal government agencies.
17. Which governmental agency requires employers to ensure employee safety concerning occupational exposure to potentially harmful substances?
    a. CDC
    b. HCFA
    c. OSHA
    d. USPS
    e. Department of Health and Human Services
18. The certifying board of which organization awards the CMA credential?
    a. AAMA
    b. AMT
    c. ABHES
    d. CAAHEP
    e. RMA

19. The certifying board of which organization awards the RMA credential?
    a. AAMA
    b. ABHES
    c. CAAHEP
    d. CMA
    e. AMT
20. Which of the following might be expected as an Asian expression of pain?
    a. Descriptive words such as "piercing" or "throbbing"
    b. A description of disturbances of the mind
    c. Ranking pain on a scale of 1 to 10
    d. Moaning and crying out
    e. Descriptive terms of body imbalance
21. How often must the CMA (AAMA) credential be renewed?
    a. Annually
    b. Every five years
    c. Biannually
    d. Every three years
    e. With every job change
22. What is the highest level in Maslow's hierarchy of needs?
    a. Safety needs
    b. Love needs
    c. Self-actualization
    d. Belongingness needs
    e. Esteem needs
23. Which of the following information is considered to be public domain?
    a. A person's sexual preference
    b. A person's police record
    c. A person's past drug addiction
    d. A person's HIV-positive status
    e. A person's alcoholism
24. The goal of the National Health Information Network is to create a:
    a. unified EMR for all health care facilities
    b. standard for computer hardware in health care facilities
    c. support network for health care facilities transitioning to EMR
    d. method of communicating EMR software program options
    e. system for exchange of health care information

25. Dr. Bennett's office will be switching to an EMR system. The office manager communicates to staff that they will be using a "remote hosted" system. This means that:
   a. the software will be run from a server in the office, which requires the purchase of only one software license
   b. the software will be installed on each individual computer, and each individual computer will require its own license
   c. the software is owned and maintained by another company, but the office will pay for the right to log in and use the system
   d. a software company will log in to the office computers in order to install and maintain the software
   e. the system will require the use of very complex hardware and additional training for staff
26. An individual who has done something that results in damage to another person or his or her property would be prosecuted under what type of law?
   a. Statute
   b. Case
   c. Breach of contract
   d. Tort
   e. Regulatory
27. Which of the following would NOT be considered an intentional tort?
   a. Defamation of character
   b. Invasion of privacy
   c. Assault
   d. Negligence
   e. Fraud
28. A patient who is undergoing a surgical procedure signs a consent for treatment. The consent would be referred to as a(n):
   a. expressed contract
   b. implied contract
   c. breach of contract
   d. tort contract
   e. consideration contract
29. Licensing for health care professionals, health department regulations, and regulations for mandatory reporting are all examples of:
   a. civil law
   b. administrative law
   c. criminal law
   d. negligent law
   e. contract law

30. A durable power of attorney document indicates:

    a. what type of medical treatment a patient wishes to have during end-of-life care

    b. who the patient would like to make decisions for him if he cannot make decisions himself

    c. what (if any) organs a patient would like to donate

    d. Do Not Resuscitate orders

    e. consent for surgical treatment

31. A medical professional who is convicted of nonfeasance would have:

    a. performed a treatment improperly

    b. performed an illegal act

    c. failed to perform necessary treatment

    d. violated confidentiality

    e. performed a duty outside of her scope of practice

32. Statutes of limitation apply to everything but:

    a. negligence

    b. fraud

    c. malfeasance

    d. dereliction of duty

    e. murder

33. Health care workers are mandatory reporters in all BUT which of the following situations?

    a. Child abuse

    b. Elder abuse

    c. Alcoholism

    d. Communicable diseases

    e. Death

34. Which of the following is true of HIPAA?

    a. Hospitals are prevented from releasing homicide or other crime-related information to law enforcement agencies.

    b. Students performing internships may not have access to computer systems in health care facilities.

    c. The HIPAA prevents health care facilities from sharing information with health care providers who are not their employees even when the information is essential for patient treatment.

    d. Health care facilities should appoint a privacy officer and adopt procedures for handling requests.

    e. HIPAA regulations do not apply to patients seeking care under government assistance programs.

35. The stage of grief in which patients attempt to make promises in order to change their situation would be considered:

    a. denial

    b. bargaining

    c. anger

    d. depression

    e. acceptance

36. End-of-life palliative care is most often provided by:
    a. hospice
    b. acute care hospitals
    c. rehabilitation hospitals
    d. skilled nursing facilities
    e. assisted living facilities
37. The AAMA code of ethics for medical assistants includes statements about each of the following EXCEPT:
    a. honor
    b. confidentiality
    c. continuing education
    d. improving community
    e. supervising provider
38. A medical office that transmits information over a wireless network must ensure that:
    a. the network allows staff to transmit information from home
    b. the network allows the provider to transmit information while doing patient visits at the hospital
    c. each staff member understands the encryption of the network
    d. the network meets HIPAA guidelines
    e. the network can be accessed by the appropriate insurance companies
39. Advanced Beneficiary Notices must be used for patients with what type of insurance?
    a. Medicaid
    b. Workers Compensation
    c. Medicare
    d. Blue Cross/Blue Shield
    e. TRICARE
40. Which of the following helps a medical assistant to manage time well?
    a. Reading email while answering patient calls
    b. Asking patients to jot down their complaints in their charts
    c. Asking patients to email rather than call with questions
    d. Asking front office staff to obtain patients' complaint
    e. Identifying priorities
41. Which of the following is NOT an important quality for a medical assistant?
    a. Ability to manage time efficiently
    b. Ability to delegate
    c. Initiative
    d. Flexibility
    e. Ability to work as a team member

42. Which of the following is an important aspect of verbal communication?
    a. Facial expressions
    b. Appearance
    c. Tone of voice
    d. Body language
    e. Gestures
43. The most important component of the message you communicate is:
    a. Perception of the person receiving the message
    b. Tone of voice
    c. The vocabulary used
    d. Facial expression
    e. Body language
44. Nancy, the medical assistant you work with, always changes the subject when you bring up topics that she does not want to discuss. This behavior would be considered:
    a. assertive
    b. passive
    c. aggressive
    d. professional
    e. passive-aggressive
45. Which of the following is NOT considered a part of negligence?
    a. Duty
    b. Dereliction
    c. Denial
    d. Direct cause
    e. Damages
46. The "base" of a medical word is called the:
    a. prefix
    b. suffix
    c. combining form
    d. root
    e. anatomical
47. The provider you are working with asks you to place a bandage just proximal to the knee. You would place the bandage:
    a. just below the knee
    b. on the front of the knee
    c. on the back of the knee
    d. just above the knee
    e. covering the entire knee area from top to bottom

48. You read a medical report that indicates that a provider made an incision from the superior to the inferior portion of the heart during a surgery. This means that the incision was made in the:
    a. frontal plane
    b. coronal plane
    c. transverse plane
    d. superior plane
    e. horizontal plane
49. The sac that covers the heart is referred to as the:
    a. pericardium
    b. epicardium
    c. endocardium
    d. myocardium
    e. mediastinum
50. The structure that is responsible for the formation of urine is the:
    a. medulla
    b. cortex
    c. nephron
    d. major calyx
    e. minor calyx
51. The congenital disorder that involves one or more vertebrae that do not close is called:
    a. cerebral palsy
    b. muscular dystrophy
    c. Tay-Sachs disease
    d. spina bifida
    e. hydrocele
52. Which of the following is a characteristic of a malignant tumor?
    a. Smooth borders
    b. Irregular shape
    c. Slow growth
    d. Well-differentiated cells
    e. Encapsulation
53. Muscular movements that are out of conscious control (e.g., the heart beating) are called:
    a. voluntary
    b. involuntary
    c. agonist
    d. antagonist
    e. synergistic

54. The type of joint that allows for the greatest range of motion is the:
   a. hinge
   b. suture
   c. pivot
   d. cartilaginous
   e. ball and socket
55. The portion of the brain that is responsible for higher thought processes such as logical thinking is the:
   a. parietal lobe
   b. frontal lobe
   c. occipital lobe
   d. temporal lobe
   e. cerebellum
56. An individual with a blood type of O positive is considered:
   a. a universal recipient
   b. ineligible to donate
   c. able to donate only to people with O positive blood
   d. able to donate only to people with only O negative blood
   e. a universal donor
57. The type of immunity that is developed from being vaccinated is:
   a. naturally acquired active immunity
   b. artificially acquired passive immunity
   c. artificially acquired active immunity
   d. naturally acquired passive immunity
   e. naturally acquired active passive immunity
58. An X-ray that is shot from the back of the person toward the front would be considered:
   a. AP
   b. lateral
   c. oblique
   d. PA
   e. transverse
59. Which of the following is NOT a portion of the large intestine?
   a. Duodenum
   b. Cecum
   c. Transverse colon
   d. Rectum
   e. Ascending colon

60. When performing screening, the medical assistant must:
    a. diagnose patients' symptoms
    b. prioritize patients' needs
    c. allow patients to determine their own needs
    d. schedule patients in the order in which they arrive
    e. evaluate patients' ability to pay
61. A person with a hypersensitivity to a bee sting may go into:
    a. cardiac arrest
    b. neurogenic shock
    c. anaphylactic shock
    d. seizures
    e. respiratory shock
62. All of the following statements about shock are accurate EXCEPT:
    a. There is inadequate circulation to body parts.
    b. The patient's body is kept warm to prevent chilling.
    c. The patient's pulse becomes rapid and weak.
    d. The medical assistant can administer medication as ordered by the provider.
    e. The patient's blood pressure increases.
63. Which of the following is a major disadvantage of NOT seeking care for an illness until it becomes very advanced?
    a. The patient does not have time to deal with death.
    b. Pain management and treatment may not work as well as they could have.
    c. The family can prepare without frightening the patient.
    d. Denial postpones the inevitable.
    e. The patient does not have time to create advance directives.
64. Redirecting a socially unacceptable impulse into one that is socially acceptable is called:
    a. regression
    b. repression
    c. projection
    d. sublimation
    e. denial
65. You are a medical assistant in an ambulatory care facility, and an emergency situation arises. What should you do first?
    a. Notify the provider.
    b. Give first aid.
    c. Assess the patient.
    d. Call 911.
    e. Evaluate the causes.

66. The act of evaluating the urgency of a medical situation and prioritizing treatment is known as:
    a. screening
    b. empathy
    c. trauma
    d. diagnosing
    e. sorting
67. Which condition is detected with the Mantoux test?
    a. HIV
    b. Syphilis
    c. PKU
    d. TB
    e. Infectious mononucleosis
68. Which of the following is used as a contrast medium for a radiographic lower GI examination?
    a. Air
    b. Iodine salts
    c. Water
    d. A barium swallow
    e. A barium enema
69. Which type of pathogen causes mumps, measles, and chicken pox?
    a. Bacteria
    b. Viruses
    c. Spirochetes
    d. Parasites
    e. Rickettsiae
70. Which body system does the acronym PERRLA refer to?
    a. Cardiovascular system
    b. Gastrointestinal system
    c. Nervous system
    d. Respiratory system
    e. Urogenital system
71. Which term means difficulty breathing?
    a. Apnea
    b. Bradypnea
    c. Tachypnea
    d. Eupnea
    e. Dyspnea

72. Which of the following statements is accurate regarding vitamins?
    a. Vitamins A, B, D, and E are fat soluble.
    b. Vitamins are needed in large quantities.
    c. Water-soluble vitamins are stored in fatty tissues.
    d. Vitamins are simple molecules.
    e. Vitamins B and C are water soluble.
73. Which statement is accurate regarding ventricular tachycardia?
    a. Ventricular tachycardia causes severe chest pain.
    b. Ventricular tachycardia is life threatening.
    c. Ventricular tachycardia is often seen in patients using depressants.
    d. Ventricular tachycardia has a cardiac cycle that occurs early.
    e. Ventricular tachycardia occurs in healthy people.
74. Which genetic disorder is characterized by mental retardation?
    a. Sickle cell anemia
    b. Huntington's disease
    c. Down's syndrome
    d. Cystic fibrosis
    e. Pernicious anemia
75. Which type of nutrient contains the most calories per gram?
    a. Carbohydrate
    b. Protein
    c. Mineral
    d. Fat
    e. Vitamin
76. Which term describes a reason why a medication should NOT be administered?
    a. Side effect
    b. Contraindication
    c. Potentiation
    d. Idiosyncratic
    e. Cross-tolerance
77. Robby is coming down with chicken pox but does not have any symptoms yet. He is now at the:
    a. acute stage
    b. convalescent stage
    c. declining stage
    d. incubation stage
    e. prodromal stage

78. Which of the following statements about medical asepsis hand washing is accurate?
    a. Medical assistants should turn the faucet on with a clean, dry paper towel.
    b. Medical assistants should hold their hands upward.
    c. Medical assistants should scrub up to their elbows.
    d. Medical assistants should touch only the inside of the sink with their hands.
    e. Medical assistants should turn off the faucet with a used paper towel.
79. Which of these positions is used for the treatment and examination of the back and buttocks?
    a. Trendelenburg
    b. Dorsal recumbent
    c. Lithotomy
    d. Supine
    e. Prone
80. Which term describes a woman who has never been pregnant?
    a. Multigravida
    b. Nullipara
    c. Nulligravida
    d. Multipara
    e. Primipara
81. Which infection control guidelines are used by all health care professionals for all patients?
    a. Body Substance Isolation guidelines
    b. Standard Precautions
    c. OSHA guidelines
    d. Transmission-Based Precautions
    e. Universal Precautions
82. All of the following are acceptable wrappings for autoclaving EXCEPT:
    a. plastic pouches
    b. muslin
    c. paper bags
    d. aluminum foil
    e. paper wrapping
83. The most common disorder of the urinary system is:
    a. renal calculi
    b. urinary tract infection
    c. glomerulonephritis
    d. cystitis
    e. pyelonephritis

84. Which of the following diseases is sexually transmitted?
    a. Pelvic inflammatory disease
    b. Cervical cancer
    c. Endometriosis
    d. Prostatitis
    e. Ovarian cancer
85. Which term describes an infection of the middle ear?
    a. Otitis externa
    b. Otalgia
    c. Otitis media
    d. Otorrhagia
    e. Otosclerosis
86. Which condition is commonly known as fainting?
    a. Tinnitus
    b. Singultus
    c. Bruit
    d. Syncope
    e. Vertigo
87. Which of the following is a progressive degenerative disease of the liver?
    a. Hepatitis A
    b. Cholecystitis
    c. Hepatomegaly
    d. Hepatitis B
    e. Cirrhosis
88. Which type of injection is made into the fatty layer just below the skin?
    a. Intramuscular
    b. Subcutaneous
    c. Intradermal
    d. Intravenous
    e. Intermuscular
89. An elevation of which blood cell count indicates the presence of inflammation in the body?
    a. Platelet count
    b. Erythrocyte sedimentation rate
    c. Hematocrit
    d. Total hemoglobin
    e. White blood cell differentiation

90. What condition is characterized by an abnormal thickening and hardening of the skin?
   a. Acne
   b. Melanoma
   c. Dermatophytosis
   d. Scleroderma
   e. Psoriasis
91. Who discovered penicillin?
   a. Sir Alexander Fleming
   b. Robert Koch
   c. Louis Pasteur
   d. Joseph Lister
   e. Edward Jenner
92. Homeostasis refers to what?
   a. A sterile environment
   b. A complete procedure
   c. Everyone getting along
   d. Internal equilibrium
   e. Rapid heart rate
93. The classification of drugs with the lowest potential of abuse is:
   a. Schedule IV
   b. Schedule I
   c. Schedule V
   d. Schedule II
   e. Schedule III
94. The provider you are working with asks you to provide a patient with samples of a new medication. By doing so, you are:
   a. prescribing medication
   b. administering medication
   c. compounding medication
   d. mixing medication
   e. dispensing medication
95. Which of the following is information about a medication that is NOT found in the PDR?
   a. Indications for use
   b. The shape of each pill
   c. Dosage and administration route
   d. Precautions
   e. Generic name

96. A drug that increases the effect of another has which type of effect?
    a. Local
    b. Remote
    c. Synergistic
    d. Systemic
    e. Topical
97. A medication that is ordered to be delivered in a sublingual route would be:
    a. placed in the cheek
    b. swallowed
    c. inserted into the rectum
    d. placed under the tongue
    e. placed on top of the tongue
98. A medication that is classified as an expectorant would have what effect?
    a. Dilate bronchi
    b. Prevent coughing
    c. Relax blood vessels
    d. Decrease nausea
    e. Increase the amount of mucus being expelled
99. A medication that increases the amount of urine excreted by the body would be classified as a(n):
    a. diuretic
    b. antiarrhythmic
    c. antiemetic
    d. vasopressor
    e. muscle relaxant
100. All of the following are part of a medication order EXCEPT:
    a. name of drug
    b. who dispenses the medication
    c. form of drug
    d. route of administration
    e. prescribing provider's signature
101. A prescription that indicates a medication should be administered "OD" would go where?
    a. Left eye
    b. Right ear
    c. Left ear
    d. Right eye
    e. In the nose

102. The metric prefix which refers to one-millionth of a unit is:

a. milli

b. kilo

c. meter

d. gram

e. micro

103. Pediatric medication dosages are figured based on the child's:

a. height

b. age

c. weight

d. gender

e. chest circumference

104. A patient weighs 130 pounds. The provider asked you to convert that weight into kilograms. You know that there are 2.2 pounds in 1 kilogram. How many kilograms does this patient weigh?

a. 4.55 kg

b. 59.09 kg

c. 286 kg

d. .07 kg

e. 260 kg

105. Which of the following is NOT 1 of the 6 rights?

a. Dose

b. Provider

c. Route

d. Patient

e. Drug

106. Parenteral medication is administered via:

a. the mouth

b. the rectum

c. the skin

d. inhalation

e. an injection

107. The type of injection that is administered at a 90-degree angle is:

a. subcutaneous

b. intradermal

c. intravenous

d. inhaled

e. intramuscular

108. Hypodermic needles are most appropriate for what?

a. Venipuncture

b. Aspirations

c. Allergy injections

d. Intramuscular and subcutaneous injections

e. Insulin administration

109. Which of the following is NOT an appropriate injection site for an intramuscular injection?

a. Dorsogluteal

b. Biceps

c. Ventrogluteal

d. Deltoid

e. Vastus lateralis

110. Which of the following points is the highest point in a normal ECG graph?

a. P

b. Q

c. R

d. S

e. T

111. The yellow portion of the safety warning label indicates which of the following?

a. Chemical instability

b. Health hazard

c. Fire hazard

d. PPE requirements

e. Biohazard level

112. A chemical that is extremely flammable would be given a safety rating of:

a. 3

b. 2

c. 1

d. 4

e. 0

113. The component of blood that is responsible for clotting is:

a. Erythrocyte

b. Leukocyte

c. Plasma

d. Serum

e. Thrombocyte

114. Which of the following substances is NOT a normal component of urine?

a. Ammonia

b. Blood

c. Creatinine

d. Urea

e. Water

115. The type of urine sample that requires a patient to avoid eating and drinking prior to voiding is:

a. 24-hour

b. first-morning

c. fasting

d. random

e. catheter collection

116. Which of the following is NOT a component of the physical examination of urine?

a. Volume

b. Color

c. Unusual

d. Specific gravity

e. pH

117. Casts found in urine are formed from:

a. carbohydrates

b. lipids

c. calcium

d. proteins

e. potassium

118. Exposing bacterial growth to an antibiotic in order to determine effective treatment of an infection is called:

a. culturing

b. taxonomy

c. sensitivity testing

d. inoculation

e. Gram stain

119. The disease of the eye that is characterized by an elevated intraocular pressure is:

a. cataract

b. glaucoma

c. macular degeneration

d. amblyopia

e. strabismus

120. The mineral that is important for the formation of bone tissue is:

   a. calcium

   b. potassium

   c. zinc

   d. iron

   e. magnesium

121. Which of the following is a type of bacteria?

   a. Streptococci

   b. Helminth

   c. Protozoa

   d. Tinea

   e. Scabies

122. Diseases caused by which type of pathogen are treated by antibiotics?

   a. Protozoa

   b. Fungi

   c. Bacteria

   d. Virus

   e. Parasite

123. Personal protective equipment should always be used in each of the follow situations EXCEPT:

   a. handling processing a urine specimen

   b. taking vital signs

   c. performing venipuncture

   d. assisting with surgical procedures

   e. disinfecting instruments

124. A worker who is exposed to bodily fluids through an accidental needlestick from a contaminated needle should immediately flush the area with:

   a. alcohol

   b. hydrogen peroxide

   c. betadine

   d. bleach

   e. water

125. Which immunization must be available free to all health care employees?

   a. Hepatitis A

   b. Hepatitis C

   c. Hepatitis B

   d. HIV

   e. TB

126. Use of alcohol-based hand rub is acceptable in which of the following situations?

a. Before and after eating

b. Before and after using the restroom

c. After contact with body excretions

d. After decontamination of a work area

e. Following processing of microbiological specimens

127. Which of the following is NOT an OSHA requirement for housekeeping in a medical setting?

a. Routine decontamination of reusable containers

b. Double-bagged soiled linens

c. Biohazard waste collected in impermeable red containers

d. Sharps containers stored in an upright condition

e. Alcohol-based hand rub available at all times

128. When performing CPR on an infant or child, circulation is checked by assessing pulse at which pulse point?

a. Carotid

b. Axial

c. Femoral

d. Brachial

e. Dorsal pedis

129. The method used to clear an airway obstruction in an unconscious adult is:

a. finger sweep

b. back blows

c. chest thrust

d. 2 rescue breaths

e. CPR

130. A burn that has penetrated to the bone would be considered:

a. superficial

b. partial thickness

c. 100%

d. full thickness

e. 75%

131. Which of the following is NOT a step in controlling bleeding from an open wound on the arm?

a. Applying direct pressure

b. Elevating the arm

c. Wrapping the wound tightly

d. Applying pressure to the appropriate artery

e. Disinfecting the area

132. Appropriate first aid for a patient with a case of acute frostbite would include:
   a. immersing the area in warm water
   b. warming the area by creating friction
   c. immediately raising the patient's core body temperature
   d. applying heavy moisturizing cream to the area
   e. immediately debriding necrotic tissues
133. Appropriate treatment for an acute sprain or strain would include all BUT which of the following?
   a. Ice
   b. Rest
   c. Compression
   d. Range of motion
   e. Elevation
134. A medication that is to be taken twice a day would be indicated as:
   a. qd
   b. tid
   c. qid
   d. bid
   e. od
135. Which type of manual identifies the specific methods for performing tasks?
   a. Policy
   b. Training
   c. Procedures
   d. Personnel
   e. Benefits
136. What is the primary purpose of managed care plans?
   a. To allow patients to manage their own care
   b. To control patients' access to providers
   c. To encourage patients to explore alternative medicine treatments
   d. To provide acute care only
   e. To provide comprehensive health care at a reasonable cost
137. How are claims managed when both parents are covered by health insurance?
   a. The father's plan is always primary.
   b. Claims for the family are paid according to the birthday rule.
   c. The mother's plan is always primary.
   d. Double benefits are paid for the children.
   e. The duplication of benefits rule is put into effect.

138. Why are accurate medical records legally important?

a. Because they are needed to provide referrals

b. Because they assist in controlling health care costs

c. Because they aid in billing

d. Because they are written documentation used to prove patient care

e. Because they are essential to quality patient care

139. Which type of check is used most often for writing payroll checks?

a. Voucher check

b. Traveler's check

c. Certified check

d. Cashier's check

e. Money order

140. What is the role of a computer firewall?

a. A computer firewall limits potential damage from viruses.

b. A computer firewall protects the computer in the event of a fire.

c. A computer firewall does not allow outside computers access to your computer.

d. A computer firewall allows outside access to an office computer but not to databases.

e. A computer firewall prevents employees from surfing the Internet for personal reasons.

141. How should a letter that requires a written receipt be mailed?

a. Registered mail

b. Priority mail

c. Third-class mail

d. Certified mail

e. First-class mail

142. Which of the following are used in conjunction with CPT codes?

a. V Codes

b. Preventive care codes

c. Injury codes

d. Modifiers

e. E Codes

143. What must happen when more than one policy pays on a claim?

a. Coinsurance

b. Coordination of benefits

c. Co-pay

d. Deductible

e. Exclusions

144. When alphabetizing and assigning units for filing order, titles are considered:
   a. as part of the last name
   b. as the first indexing unit
   c. as the third indexing unit
   d. as part of the patient's surname
   e. as a separate unit at the end
145. A person who is injured on the job may be covered by:
   a. workers' compensation
   b. CHAMPUS
   c. Medicaid
   d. disability insurance
   e. HCFA
146. Which of the following is an advantage of accepting credit cards in an ambulatory care setting?
   a. Maintaining patient confidentiality is not a problem.
   b. There are no fees to be paid by the practice.
   c. The money is available to the practice within one day.
   d. The money is usually available to the practice within 10 days.
   e. Accepting credit cards eliminates having to file insurance claims.
147. What is the key to having an effective scheduling system?
   a. Accommodating patient preferences
   b. Customizing the system to the type of practice
   c. Tailoring the system to provider preferences
   d. Accommodating the requirements of the insurance carriers
   e. Effectively monitoring the use of time versus the dollars produced
148. Which scheduling system assigns two patients to the same time?
   a. Clustering
   b. Stream
   c. Modified wave
   d. Double booking
   e. Open-hours
149. Which program provides health care coverage for low-income individuals?
   a. CHAMPUS
   b. Workers' compensation
   c. Medicare
   d. CHAMPVA
   e. Medicaid

150. Which of the following is a critical issue regarding the use of a fax machine in a medical office?
   a. The speed at which the machine works
   b. The time required to train personnel
   c. Compromised confidentiality due to access by unauthorized personnel
   d. The clarity of the documents received
   e. The volume of documents the machine can handle

151. Which of the following is used when there is not enough information to find a more specific code?
   a. NEC
   b. NOS
   c. CC
   d. V Codes
   e. E Codes

152. Which of the following tells the computer hardware what to do?
   a. Application software
   b. The motherboard
   c. The modem
   d. System software
   e. Servers

153. Which of the following conditions is most frequently related to the repetitive use of a computer?
   a. Eyestrain
   b. Fatigue
   c. Carpal tunnel syndrome
   d. Lower back pain
   e. Tension headaches

154. When seeking employment, a person who has job experience should use:
   a. a targeted résumé
   b. a functional résumé
   c. a complete résumé
   d. an Information Mapping résumé
   e. a chronological résumé

155. Which type of résumé highlights one's special qualities?
   a. Targeted
   b. Functional
   c. Chronological
   d. Concise
   e. Career oriented

156. Which statement is accurate regarding a cover letter?
   a. The cover letter may be addressed "To whom it may concern."
   b. The purpose of the cover letter is to ask for an interview.
   c. The cover letter includes résumé information.
   d. The cover letter should be bulleted.
   e. The cover letter should include a list of references.

157. Which of the following tasks is NOT assigned to the human resources manager?
   a. Creating office manuals
   b. Hiring and firing personnel
   c. Interpreting legal regulations
   d. Providing employee training
   e. Performing employee evaluations

158. Tiffany wants a well-paying position as a medical assistant. Which statement is accurate regarding her search?
   a. Every CMA (AAMA) is guaranteed a well-paying position.
   b. Using an employment agency is her most effective tool in finding a well-paying position.
   c. Networking is her most effective tool in finding a well-paying position.
   d. Running down all leads is her most effective tool in finding a well-paying position.
   e. Cold calling to offices that are not advertising will produce excellent leads.

159. Which federal law requires employers to verify the right of employees to work in the United States?
   a. Immigration Reform Act
   b. Equal Pay Act
   c. Civil Rights Act
   d. Fair Labor Standards Act
   e. Americans with Disabilities Act

160. Which of these interviewing tips is accurate?
   a. Think carefully before answering questions.
   b. Do not ask questions, as you may appear confused.
   c. Answer questions "off the cuff" so your responses do not seem rehearsed.
   d. Place your personal belongings—coat, purse, and so on—on the interviewer's desk.
   e. Give lengthy answers to all questions, even when you are not sure of the answer.

161. Which of the following statements about completing an employment application form is accurate?
   a. Write "See résumé" rather than repeating information.
   b. Using either a pen or pencil is acceptable.
   c. Try to complete the application without referring to your résumé.
   d. Complete the application quickly to demonstrate how well you work.
   e. Following instructions is very important.

162. Which of the following is the best networking resource for recruiting new personnel?
   a. Newspapers
   b. Family and friends
   c. Current employees
   d. Patients
   e. AAMA's national office
163. All of these interview questions are appropriate EXCEPT:
   a. "What is most important to you about this job?"
   b. "What is your clinical experience?"
   c. "Have you ever been bonded before?"
   d. "Do you have any health-related problems that might affect your job performance?"
   e. "Where did you go to school?"
164. Which of the following is NOT vital résumé information?
   a. Home address
   b. Current telephone number
   c. Education
   d. Date of birth
   e. Work experience
165. Which payroll forms must be submitted to the Social Security Administration each year?
   a. W-4
   b. W-2
   c. W-6
   d. 1099
   e. 941
166. A policy manual should include all of the following EXCEPT:
   a. employment practices
   b. insurance billing techniques
   c. wage and salary scales
   d. evaluation schedules
   e. continuing education policies
167. In order to track inventory in an office, the most appropriate type of software to use would be:
   a. word processing
   b. billing
   c. contact management
   d. spreadsheet
   e. EMR

168. When taking a telephone message, everything BUT the following should be included:
    a. full name of person leaving message
    b. reason for the call
    c. time and date of call
    d. expected action
    e. diagnosis of the patient the message is about
169. An office operating on a wave schedule will:
    a. have groups of patients arriving at relatively the same time throughout the day
    b. schedule two patients for the same appointment time
    c. schedule patients in specific time increments (e.g., every 15 minutes)
    d. allow for walk-in patients at any time
    e. provide "catch up" time for the provider
170. When scheduling an outpatient procedure, each of the following should be completed EXCEPT:
    a. obtaining necessary preauthorizations
    b. making arrangements with the facility
    c. notifying the patient of the arrangements
    d. determining and scheduling preprocedure testing
    e. precertifying the admission
171. A block letter style includes:
    a. centered paragraphs with all other components at the left margin
    b. all components starting at the left margin
    c. centered address and signature lines with paragraphs starting at the left margin
    d. centered address, signature line, and first paragraph
    e. all components centered
172. Source-oriented medical records are organized by the:
    a. cause of a patient's medical diagnosis
    b. location of a patient's medical record
    c. nature of a patient's complaint
    d. treatment methods being used
    e. professionals who have documented in the record
173. Each of the following is objective information EXCEPT:
    a. laboratory data
    b. diagnosis
    c. prescribed treatment
    d. patient's complaint
    e. exam findings

174. Color coding medical records assists with each of the following EXCEPT:
   a. increasing efficiency with filing
   b. increasing the ability to identify filing errors
   c. identifying a patient's diagnosis
   d. identifying patients who are due for a physical during a specific month
   e. removing inactive files
175. Tickler files are helpful in:
   a. sending billing notices
   b. scheduling the provider's time
   c. providing reminders for routine medical appointments
   d. submitting insurance claims
   e. processing payroll
176. Providers' fees are generally set by each of the following EXCEPT:
   a. reasonable
   b. insurance
   c. customary
   d. usual
   e. geographic region
177. Accounts receivable refers to:
   a. money collected by a practice during a day
   b. accounts turned over to a debt collection agency
   c. money owed by the practice
   d. money owed to a practice
   e. petty cash expenditures
178. Manually posting charges usually involves each of the following EXCEPT:
   a. day sheet
   b. ledger card
   c. account summary
   d. encounter form
   e. HCFA 1500
179. The Truth in Lending Act requires:
   a. lower interest rates for medical services
   b. an increased amount of time for repayment of medical loans
   c. use of an independent billing service
   d. accurate information regarding finance charges
   e. routine billing statements

180. Calls made to a patient's home in order to collect money owed to a practice are regulated by:

 a. the Truth in Lending Act

 b. CLIA

 c. the Fair Debt Collection Act

 d. OSHA

 e. AMA

181. Once an account has been submitted to a collection agency, the medical assistant should:

 a. discontinue sending statements to the patient

 b. continue to send routine billing statements to the patient

 c. send copies of billing statements to emergency contacts listed in the patient's chart

 d. file for legal action in small claims court

 e. telephone the patient in order to attempt to collect the debt

182. Best practices with manual bookkeeping involve all of the following EXCEPT:

 a. proficiency with 10-key typing

 b. using consistent methods

 c. writing with red ink

 d. writing numbers clearly

 e. double checking all math

183. In managing practice finances, an adjustment would be used for:

 a. recording payment

 b. recording charges

 c. indicating past due accounts

 d. indicating discounts or write-offs

 e. indicating accounts turned over to collections

184. When preparing a check to a supplier, the medical assistant should:

 a. verify the expense has been approved

 b. endorse with "for deposit only"

 c. reconcile the bank statement

 d. record the payment on the correct ledger card

 e. file a I-9 tax form

185. If an office determines it will accept personal checks as payment, it is important to:

 a. clearly post the policy

 b. implement use of a restrictive endorsement

 c. follow Truth in Lending guidelines

 d. verify policies with the practice's bank

 e. follow Fair Debt collection guidelines

186. Mrs. Jones's insurance requires that she pay for $400 of medical expenses before she is eligible for insurance payment for medical services. The $400 would be referred to as:

a. a co-payment

b. coinsurance

c. a deductible

d. a premium

e. an exclusion

187. Mr. Johnson's insurance company has stated that it will not pay for treatment of his asthma because he was known to have the disease prior to the time when his policy was purchased. His asthma would be considered a(n):

a. exclusion

b. preexisting condition

c. concurrent condition

d. secondary diagnosis

e. subjective condition

188. The type of Medicare coverage that provides benefits for inpatient medical care is:

a. Medicare B

b. Medicare D

c. Medicare E

d. Medicare A

e. Medicare F

189. Most managed care organizations provide a capitated payment for services. This means that:

a. a maximum payment for services is set

b. patients must pay excess charges out of their own pocket

c. they will not pay for services covered by another company

d. the government sets the maximum allowed charge for a service

e. patients' premiums will never change

190. RBRVS payment structures are based on all EXCEPT which of the following?

a. Level of work

b. Malpractice expenses

c. Regional charges

d. Diagnosis of patient

e. Experience of the provider